The
EVERYTHING®
Alzheimer's Book

Dear Reader:

Only a few months before I began writing *The Everything®* *Alzheimer's Book*, my mother died after a five-month illness with acute leukemia. I thought of her constantly while writing this book. She didn't want to burden anybody but was very grateful that three of her four daughters were each able to spend several months of precious time with her. It took her a while, but she came to realize the gift she was giving us by allowing us to care for her as she had cared for us many years before. The time with her remains so precious that it helps take away the sting of her absence.

As I write this letter, the light in my room brightens as she seems to make her presence known. With Alzheimer's, remember that the dear soul you know and love is still there and will be even beyond death.

Carolyn Dean

The EVERYTHING® Series

Editorial

Publishing Director	Gary M. Krebs
Managing Editor	Kate McBride
Copy Chief	Laura MacLaughlin
Acquisitions Editor	Eric M. Hall
Development Editor	Lesley Bolton
Production Editor	Jamie Wielgus

Production

Production Director	Susan Beale
Production Manager	Michelle Roy Kelly
Series Designers	Daria Perreault
	Colleen Cunningham
Cover Design	Paul Beatrice
	Frank Rivera
Layout and Graphics	Colleen Cunningham
	Rachael Eiben
	Michelle Roy Kelly
	John Paulhus
	Daria Perreault
	Erin Ring
Series Cover Artist	Barry Littmann

THE
EVERYTHING®
ALZHEIMER'S
BOOK

Reliable, accessible information
for patients and their families

Carolyn Dean, M.D.

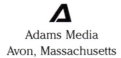

Adams Media
Avon, Massachusetts

To my dear Mum, Alexandernia Grant Wheeler (Rena), who passed
away September 2003, five months after a diagnosis of leukemia.

An Everything® Series Book.
Everything® and everything.com® are registered trademarks of F+W Publications, Inc.

Published by Adams Media, an F+W Publications Company
57 Littlefield Street, Avon, MA 02322 U.S.A.
www.adamsmedia.com

ISBN: 1-59337-050-4
Printed in the United States of America.

J I H G F E D C B A

Library of Congress Cataloging-in-Publication Data
Dean, Carolyn.
The everything Alzheimer's book / Carolyn Dean.
p.   cm.
(An everything series book)
ISBN 1-59337-050-4
1. Alzheimer's disease. I. Title. II. Series: Everything series.
RC523.D425   2004
616.8'31–dc22   2004007859

This book is available at quantity discounts for bulk purchases.
For information, call 1-800-872-5627.

Contents

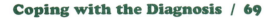

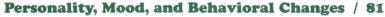

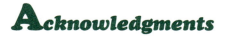

Acknowledgments

I accepted the contract for *The Everything® Alzheimer's Book* knowing it had an incredibly short deadline due to a rigid production schedule set by the machines that run our world.

That's when humans come in and make miracles happen! I want to acknowledge everyone at Adams Media who pitched in to help create this book in record time.

I also want to thank my mother, who inspired me both in dreams and in daylight—showering me with her last gift, unconditional love. Writing about the mental devastation of Alzheimer's, I feel blessed that my Mum was alert, witty, and ever so wise until the end. Striving to keep our parents that way is a goal that we all share.

Top Ten Ways
to Prevent Alzheimer's Disease

1. Learn all you can about the disease and its possible triggers.
2. Exercise your brain.
3. Exercise your body.
4. Lower your intake of saturated fats.
5. Increase your intake of antioxidant fruits and vegetables.
6. Take a good multiple-vitamin supplement containing the B vitamins.
7. Reduce stress in your daily life and take advantage of stress reduction techniques.
8. Drink at least the recommended eight glasses of filtered water a day.
9. Look at life with a positive and optimistic attitude.
10. Get regular physical checkups to prevent or better control problems with blood pressure or hormone levels.

Introduction

▶ WHEN FORMER VICE PRESIDENT DAN QUAYLE made his famous gaffe, "What a waste it is to lose one's mind," he might have been talking about Alzheimer's. In fact, he was talking about education and making an inept stab at the well-known quote, "A mind is a terrible thing to waste." But in the case of Alzheimer's, it is an incredible waste to lose one's mind to the ravages of a progressive disease with no known cause and no known treatment. Alzheimer's disease is a degenerative disorder affecting the brain and causing dementia. It has no one discernible cause, no 100 percent accurate diagnosis, and, as yet, no cure.

Alzheimer's has become so well known that people of all ages blame the disease when they have a memory lapse. Perhaps Alzheimer's disease has always existed in the elderly. Two centuries ago, however, the average life span was only about thirty or forty years of age. In 1900, the average age of Americans was only forty-nine, so very few people grew old enough to develop Alzheimer's, as the typical age of onset occurs after age sixty-five. In the twenty-first century, with almost 20 percent of the population over the age of sixty-five, the numbers of Alzheimer's cases are escalating rapidly. Alzheimer's occurs in one out of every ten households in America, and it is on the rise. The major risk factor for Alzheimer's is growing old, and we are an aging population as the baby boomers are fast approaching retirement age. But we don't have to think that it's inevitable that we will get Alzheimer's.

For those of you who have been diagnosed with Alzheimer's or are caregivers of Alzheimer's patients, there are many treatments and supports that can help slow the progress of the disease and make it more bearable. Alzheimer's is not one of those diseases that you want to ignore; education about the disease is very important. The key to Alzheimer's is being aware of the warning signs and symptoms.

You have picked up this book for a reason. Maybe a loved one has been diagnosed with Alzheimer's or you are wondering about your own failing memory. Within these pages you will find invaluable information about the disease, including other possible conditions that can mimic Alzheimer's. Some of these conditions are much more treatable than Alzheimer's, so it is important to know exactly what is going on in regard to your individual situation.

It is also important to obtain an early diagnosis, which can then lead to early treatment. The current treatments for Alzheimer's will be described in this book. Knowing what's available can allow you to be more interactive with your doctor and proactive in your treatment. Early treatment can mean a much slower progression of the disease and a delay in the onset of more severe symptoms. Another ray of hope is that Alzheimer's research is moving forward at an incredible rate and the chances of a cure in the not-too-distant future are very likely. New drugs and new ways to use vitamins, minerals, and exercise are described in detail, allowing you to discuss these options with your doctor.

The Everything® Alzheimer's Book also contains the latest information on caregiver strategies, both to help the Alzheimer's patient and to keep the caregiver healthy as well. You will also be provided with a resource section to help you further your research and find additional information. You'll be amazed to find out how much support there is for dealing with this very difficult condition. E

Chapter 1

What Is Alzheimer's?

Alzheimer's is a slow-progressing type of dementia caused by a gradual loss of brain cells. Alzheimer's disease disrupts nerve cell communication and interferes with nerve cell metabolism. As a result, damaged nerve cells can't work, can't connect, and eventually die. When nerve cells can't transmit their signals, memory fails, personality changes occur, and daily activities become impossible to perform.

Alzheimer's—One Cause of Dementia

Dementia is a general term that describes a disease that has a set of symptoms related to a deterioration in thinking skills. Common dementia symptoms include gradual memory loss, judgment difficulties, disorientation, difficulty in learning new tasks or performing old ones, and loss of language skills. As these are also symptoms of Alzheimer's, it becomes confusing to try to differentiate between Alzheimer's and dementia, especially since people with dementia also experience personality and behavioral changes like agitation, anxiety, delusions, and hallucinations, which are also symptoms of Alzheimer's. So, in the final analysis, all people with Alzheimer's have dementia, but not all people with dementia have Alzheimer's.

In the case of Alzheimer's, the brain cells are choked off by abnormal deposits called plaques and tangles. Another characteristic of Alzheimer's is shrinkage of the brain. Although almost 100 years have passed since identifying these plaques and tangles, an autopsy is still the only way to make a 100 percent positive diagnosis of Alzheimer's. There are, however, warning signs of memory loss, confusion, and difficulty with language, which can alert us to a brewing problem. The diagnosis of Alzheimer's, with an accuracy of 90 percent, is made by ruling out the different causes of dementia and by administering a highly accurate battery of neuropsychological tests. One thing we do know is that Alzheimer's is not communicable; it can't be transmitted or picked up from someone who has the disease.

The History of Alzheimer's

Many diseases are named after the scientist or doctor who discovered them and tell us nothing about the disease. Alzheimer's is no exception. Its discovery, in 1907, is credited to a German neuropathologist and clinician, Dr. Alois Alzheimer. He was the first person to describe a case of gradual mental decline of a woman he first saw in her early fifties. When she died, he equated her brain autopsy findings with her confusion and memory problems.

When first admitted to Dr. Alzheimer's psychiatric hospital in 1901, Frau Auguste D. had all the signs and symptoms of senile dementia. Her husband described the beginning of her illness as bouts of anger, then memory loss and increasing confusion. Finally, he could not care for her by himself and brought her to the hospital.

Because she was only fifty-one, it meant that her brain had aged ahead of her body and catapulted her thirty years into the future. Dr. Alzheimer had seen nothing like this in the past, and he watched his patient closely over the next six years as she gradually deteriorated and became bedridden. In retrospect, Frau Auguste D. had early-onset Alzheimer's.

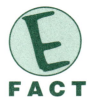

FACT

Early-onset Alzheimer's is a rare form of dementia that strikes people younger than age sixty-five. There is no scientific reason for this cutoff age because early-onset Alzheimer's has the same symptoms as later onset, which is defined as occurring after age sixty-five.

Frau Auguste D.'s Autopsy

When Frau Auguste D. died in 1907, Dr. Alzheimer was still at a loss to diagnosis her condition and asked to perform an autopsy on her brain. What he found was as unusual as her disease. There were abnormal deposits of protein outside and inside the nerve cells in her brain. He called these abnormal deposits surrounding the nerve cells neuritic plaques. Inside the cells, he found twisted and deformed fibers, which he called neurofibrillary tangles. We now know that this woman suffered from early-onset Alzheimer's, but her symptoms mimicked the gradual decline of mental function with age that was, up until that time, thought to be normal.

Plaques and Tangles

Plaques are also called senile plaques, and they are the result of a buildup of a protein that is normally produced around nerve cells. In the case of Alzheimer's, however, this protein, called beta amyloid, keeps on building. Symptoms begin when the excess protein actually prevents electrical signals from being transmitted from one nerve cell to the next.

Tangles have their own story. They occur inside the nerve cell and are a buildup of another protein with the seemingly innocuous name "tau." They build up to the extent that they cause cell death and also impede the passage of information between nerve cells.

It wasn't until the early 1970s that neurologists began focusing their research on the brain. They realized that the plaques and tangles that Dr. Alzheimer had found in 1907 were also found in the normal aging brain but in much less profusion. They began to equate the amount of plaques and tangles with the appearance and severity of Alzheimer's.

Alzheimer's Research

Alzheimer's was recognized in 1907, but Alzheimer's research remained dormant for many decades after Dr. Alzheimer's brilliant discovery. It was not even considered to be a major disease entity until the 1970s. At that time, neurological research expanded, and tremendous amounts of Dr. Alzheimer's plaques and tangles were found in patients that were thought to have dementia or senility.

ESSENTIAL

If you are concerned about memory problems or mood swings, it's important to talk with your doctor; he or she may be able to identify the cause of your concerns, treat the condition, and possibly reverse the symptoms. If your condition isn't reversible—as is the case with Alzheimer's—a diagnosis can give you a head start on managing the disease.

This gave hope to people who had been convinced that aging and senility went hand in hand. By distinguishing Alzheimer's as a disease separate from normal symptoms of aging, researchers could now hope to find a cure.

In the 1970s, researchers named the condition after Dr. Alzheimer since he had been the first person to equate its symptoms with plaques and tangles. Even after Alzheimer's disease was distinguished from senility and dementia by its name, it still wasn't recognized by the government for purposes of research funding. It was, however, being recognized by the families of Alzheimer's sufferers.

Alzheimer's Awareness

In 1979, delegates from five Alzheimer's family support groups across the United States met to form a national Alzheimer's association. A representative from the National Institutes of Health was also present. They called the new organization Alzheimer's Disease and Related Disorders Association, Inc., and later renamed it the Alzheimer's Association.

Getting the Media Involved

Abigail Van Buren of "Dear Abby" heard about the new association that supported families with Alzheimer's or dementia sufferers and wrote about it in her column. An avalanche of 25,000 letters to the national office asked for more information about Alzheimer's. These letters demonstrated a real need for more information, more research, and more funding. The association published a national newsletter and began offering educational seminars about Alzheimer's to help people understand the condition and also to teach caregiving skills.

Getting the Government Involved

Government lobbying led to a 1982 declaration of National Alzheimer's Disease Week, and President Ronald Reagan signed legislation designating Thanksgiving week as National Alzheimer's Disease Awareness Week. In 1983, Congress declared November National Alzheimer's Disease Month for the first time. In that same year, an 800 telephone number handled 100,000 requests from consumers for information on Alzheimer's.

Also in 1983, President Ronald Reagan recommended a task force, the Select Committee on Aging, to oversee and coordinate scientific research on Alzheimer's disease. The Alzheimer's Association then presented its report, "National Program to Conquer Alzheimer's Disease," to the Select Committee on Aging. Its request for major federal investment in medical research for Alzheimer's was met by a Congressional allocation of $22 million.

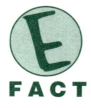

FACT

In 1987, the first government report on Alzheimer's disease, "Losing a Million Minds: Confronting the Tragedy of Alzheimer's Disease and Other Dementias," was published by the U.S. Office of Technology Assessment. This report set off a groundswell of both relief from people dealing with Alzheimer's and fear among the population about this new and dangerous brain disease.

In 1984, the Alzheimer's Association presented a Humanitarian Award to President Ronald Reagan and United States Senator Howard Metzenbaum for their efforts on behalf of Alzheimer's sufferers and families.

The High Cost of Alzheimer's

The tremendous physical and emotional cost of the disease to Alzheimer's sufferers and their families has been known for decades. There is also, however, a financial cost of the disease. Finally, in 1998 and again in 2002, reports were commissioned by the Alzheimer's Association on the costs to U.S. businesses. Both studies were shocking.

"Alzheimer's Disease: The Costs to U.S. Businesses," authored by Ross Koppel, Ph.D., of the Social Research Corporation and the Department of Sociology at the University of Pennsylvania, found that the 2002 Alzheimer's cost to U.S. businesses would be in excess of $61 billion. To put that number into perspective, this amount is equal to the net profits of the top ten *Fortune* 500 companies and exactly double the amount that was calculated in the 1998 report. The costs to businesses to cover medical insurance and disability for workers with Alzheimer's was $24.6 billion. The costs incurred because workers must take on the tremendous responsibilities as family caregivers was $36.5 billion due to absenteeism, productivity losses, and replacement costs.

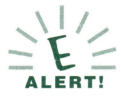

ALERT!

According to a UCLA study published in the *Journal of the American Geriatrics Society* in 2002, caregivers spent an average of eighty-five hours a week caring for patients. Those hours, in part, represent the emotional and physical cost to family and friends of Alzheimer's patients.

This seems like a huge amount of money until you realize that 70 percent of people with Alzheimer's live at home, where almost 75 percent of their care is organized and provided by family and friends. The remaining 25 percent, averaging $12,500 per year, is paid for by families out of their own pocket for private home care. It seems like U.S. business is subsidizing home care for Alzheimer's sufferers, but is it a less expensive option than nursing home care? The average cost for nursing home care is $42,000 per year with a high range of $70,000 per year in some areas of the country.

It's Only Going to Get Worse

In a 1994 report from the *American Journal of Public Health* on the economical and social costs of Alzheimer's, it was the third most expensive disease in the United States after heart disease and cancer. They reported that the average lifetime cost of care for an Alzheimer's patient is $174,000 with a two to twenty year life expectancy after diagnosis. This figure does not include the loss of wages both for the Alzheimer's sufferer or the caregiver.

The costs to Medicare were calculated for the decade beginning in 2000. For Medicare beneficiaries with Alzheimer's, the 2010 costs are expected to increase 54.5 percent, from $31.9 billion in 2000 to $49.3 billion in 2010. Medicaid expenditures for residential dementia care will have an even higher increase of 80 percent, from $18.2 billion to $33 billion in the same time period.

"Alzheimer's Disease: The Costs to U.S. Businesses" was commissioned by the Alzheimer's Association in 2002 and projected the cost of Alzheimer's into the future. The projection was based on a 2002 Alzheimer's incidence of 4 million Alzheimer's sufferers in the United States with a 2002 cost to businesses of $61 billion. The account said that within a decade there could be about 14 million baby boomers with Alzheimer's. An even more dramatic projection was that by 2050 the economy could collapse from the weight of taking care of Alzheimer's patients.

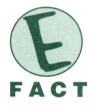

FACT

The National Institute of Aging's Progress Report on Alzheimer's Disease (1998) found that the annual economic toll of the illness in America "in terms of healthcare expenses and lost wages of both patients and their caregivers was estimated at $80 to $100 billion."

Early Treatment Is the Key

As the symptoms of Alzheimer's worsen, the need for more expensive care increases. Therefore, to cut costs, many doctors and researchers warn that we need to diagnose the condition early and institute treatment protocols that can lessen the symptoms.

A UCLA study published in the *Journal of the American Geriatrics Society* in February 2002 found that health care costs for a high-functioning patient were about $20,000 compared with a patient with severe dementia at $35,000.

A Picture of Alzheimer's

The image that comes to mind for many people when they hear or think about Alzheimer's is Ronald Reagan. In fact, Reagan, unknowingly, has made Alzheimer's a household word. When he was diagnosed in 1994, everyone suddenly became aware of this progressive and deadly condition. As with many health conditions that afflict a well-known person, the spotlight on his or her illness helps others to focus on theirs.

For a decade before his diagnosis, Ronald Reagan was known for his self-deprecating jokes about his poor memory. He told these jokes at dinners and even to his doctors. One famous such incident was during a routine physical exam with his doctor in Reagan's second term of office.

Reagan announced to his doctor that "I have three things that I want to tell you today. The first is that I seem to be having a little problem with my memory. I cannot remember the other two."

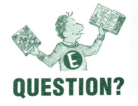

QUESTION?

If we live long enough, won't we all get Alzheimer's?
Ten percent of people currently have Alzheimer's at age sixty-five and 50 percent at age eighty-five. With that progression, the vast majority of centenarians will have Alzheimer's unless we find a cure.

There is no question that after Ronald Reagan's passing there was an incredible surge of media discussion about Alzheimer's that benefitted many sufferers. As with any incurable disease, we need all the attention, funding, and focus on the problem that we can get to find the cause and cure.

Does It Always End This Way?

Sadly, Alzheimer's does eventually lead to the inability to care for oneself, and in the later stages, brain cell death, and death. We tend to see the worst case scenario when we think of Alzheimer's; there are, however, millions of people living a comfortable life with Alzheimer's, given the proper care and support.

There are other conditions that may or may not be associated with Alzheimer's that can affect people and cause a more rapid decline in health. In other words, a heart attack or stroke may be what keeps a person from the end stages of Alzheimer's.

Who Is Affected?

Men and women are equally at risk for Alzheimer's. Women, because they live longer, may make up more of the Alzheimer's population, but they are no more likely to be stricken with Alzheimer's than men. Although Alzheimer's rarely occurs under age fifty, by age sixty, 2 percent of the population has Alzheimer's—that means two out of every 100 people are affected. By age eighty-five, the incidence increases to 50 percent, or five out of ten people.

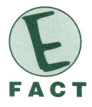

FACT

The World Health Organization in 2000 estimated there are 18 million Alzheimer's cases worldwide. Over 4.5 million Americans have Alzheimer's—that's 25 percent of all the cases in the world. But the United States only makes up 4.6 percent of the world's population.

We would like to believe that Alzheimer's is caused by a gene that we could eliminate. As of 2004, there have been five genes identified that are associated with Alzheimer's. Three of these genes are each a contributing factor in early-onset Alzheimer's disease (before age fifty). They are rarely, however, the cause of Alzheimer's. The fourth gene, called ApoE4, increases the risk of later-onset Alzheimer's. The fifth gene is located on chromosome 10 and is currently under investigation by several groups of researchers.

The Risk Factors

We know that aging is the number one risk factor for Alzheimer's. And except for the ApoE4 lipoprotein gene, Alzheimer's is not specifically a genetic disorder. The lipoprotein gene needs to be triggered or "turned on" by one or more of the following risk factors that are themselves associated with Alzheimer's.

This is the part of diagnosing Alzheimer's that is very frustrating for researchers and doctors. Alzheimer's doesn't seem to have one specific cause that you can immediately point your finger at and say "ah ha." The disease may have several contributing factors.

Head Trauma and Stroke

When you fall and hit your head and go unconscious, even though you can't see through your skull, you are likely bruised and bleeding. We now know that if you are unconscious for over an hour from a head injury, you have twice the risk of developing Alzheimer's. After the bleeding stops and the swelling goes down after head trauma, you can still have scar tissue that may be involved in the future development of Alzheimer's.

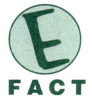

FACT

Researcher Dr. Luise Schmidt from the University of Pennsylvania's Center for Neurodegenerative Disease Research found that brain injury can cause Boxer's Syndrome by activating mechanisms like the ones that cause tau lesions in Alzheimer's. She concluded that, "by extension, it also suggests that a head injury can increase susceptibility to Alzheimer's later in life." Alzheimer's and Boxer's Syndrome have similar physical and memory disorders associated with them.

The same can be said for trauma to the brain from stroke. A stroke usually occurs because a blood clot blocks off a blood vessel, which cuts off all the blood supply to the vessel's designated area. The lack of oxygen, glucose, and nutrients to the blocked off area seems to trigger an increase in amyloid protein, the hallmark of Alzheimer's.

High-Fat Diet

We all know that improperly stored oils and fats will go rancid. Well, that's just what happens in the body when you eat a high-fat diet. Since the brain and nervous system are very high in fat, some researchers take the idea of rancid fat one step further and speculate that rancid fat may be damaging the brain by causing free radicals (unstable molecules that potentially cause cell damage).

Scientists at Case Western Reserve are studying the association between high-fat diets and Alzheimer's. They admit that their work sheds a whole new light on Alzheimer's and diet.

The people with an ApoE4 lipoprotein gene are most at risk from eating a high-fat diet. Eating a diet in which 40 percent of the calories come from fat raises the risk of Alzheimer's in someone who has the ApoE4 gene an incredible twenty-nine times. Younger people aged twenty to thirty-nine with the ApoE4 gene are twenty-three times more likely to develop Alzheimer's in later years than are healthy eaters.

Chronic Stress

Chronic stress produces high levels of adrenaline and cortisol, also called stress hormones. Add stress to a high-fat diet and you create brain atrophy. Researchers at the James A. Haley Veterans Administration Medical Center, at the University of South Florida (USF), and Arizona State University (ASU) found that chronically stressed rats consuming an "American-style" diet of excessive carbohydrates and beef fat developed atrophy in the hippocampus, the part of the brain that is essential for learning and remembering new information.

Test rats at USF were placed in a room where they were safe, but surrounded by cats, every day for a month. At night, the cat-exposed rats were fed high-fat diets in crowded housing conditions. Similarly stressed rats were fed low-fat diets. Following the test period, researchers at ASU analyzed the rats' brains and found the group fed a high-fat diet and living under chronic stress developed hippocampal atrophy, expressed in reduced dendrites length. Dendrites are the connections between brain cells where information is stored.

ESSENTIAL

A study funded by the National Institutes of Health (NIH) and the Alzheimer's Association in 1998 found that some unknown genetic and/or environmental factors are increasing the risk for Alzheimer's among African-Americans and some Hispanics. Even without the ApoE4 gene present, African-Americans had four times the risk of developing Alzheimer's by age ninety than whites. The risk was doubled for Hispanics.

One of the researchers said, "The implication is that the combination of a high-fat diet and stress can interfere with the ability of the brain—in rats or people—to learn new information."

Previous research had shown that rats on a high-fat diet produce an excessive amount of corticosterone in response to stress. Corticosterone, a steroid hormone produced by the adrenal glands, can cause damage to the hippocampus. There was also prior evidence that showed rats fed a high-fat diet did not perform as well in learning tasks as rats fed a low-fat diet. The consequences, however, of both a high-fat diet and stress were unknown. Now we are aware that a high-fat diet and stress are doubly detrimental to the brain.

The Warning Signs

With the level of Alzheimer's awareness in our society, we are very attentive to when we have incidental memory lapses. With Alzheimer's, however, it's a constellation of symptoms including a confusion and disorientation that make us befuddled and apathetic, and so we may just deny it for a time. That's why it's important to be aware of the warning signs of Alzheimer's in yourself, in your parents, and in your friends.

Mind and Memory Problems

Because nerve transmission is the first thing to deteriorate in Alzheimer's, we lose the connection to our thoughts. Everything we do in life is preceded by a thought. Most people don't vocalize their intent to do something, but if we did, it would be something like this: I think I'll get up and have a glass of water in the kitchen; while there, I see the plants need watering, too, and I'll do that; then I notice the garbage can is full, and I must change the bag.

We think of something, and it triggers us to take an action. In Alzheimer's, the thought is initiated, but it often doesn't go far enough along the nerve pathways to trigger an action before it stops dead.

The mind and memory symptoms will appear as if the memory is failing, when you can't remember a name or an event. The inability to find the right word to name a familiar object is another of Alzheimer's problems, which has to do with language. For instance, you may be able to describe what the broom does, but unable to say "broom."

Abstract thinking, which is necessary for balancing your checkbook or when you make analogies or comparisons, becomes almost impossible because of all the electrical connections that have to take place to compare one idea to another. There can even be a disconnection in recognizing your surroundings or what time of day it is. You may go to the mall and then become confused as to where you are. Because you forget what you are doing, you can leave the stove turned on or the kettle boiling dry, and this is often interpreted as poor judgment.

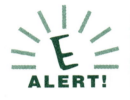

ALERT!

Aphasia describes a brain injury, usually due to stroke, where language is impaired. The sudden appearance of aphasia is a medical emergency. With severe aphasia, you can't speak, understand speech, write, or read. Medically, a stroke, which may produce paralysis and aphasia, can be treated with clot-busting drugs that may be able to reverse some of the symptoms. Milder forms of stroke aphasia may be confused with symptoms of Alzheimer's.

Difficulty Doing Things

The electrical disconnection of Alzheimer's makes it very difficult to accomplish tasks, even if you have done them for a lifetime. You think a thought and really want to do something, like make a cup of tea or pick up the mail, but the electrical connections between thinking the thought and performing the action just won't work. With Alzheimer's, you think of something and you may even begin a task, but then not remember what you are doing midtask and stop in your tracks. As the disease progresses, you may not even have enough memory connections to begin the task. Too many cells are tangled up and blocked by plaque to make the connection. You may pick up the mail because it came through the mail slot and is lying on the floor, but when you look at it you may not know what it is or what to do with it. Or, you may start putting the tea bags in the freezer or your keys in the cat box.

Mood and Behavior Problems

Memory lapses and the misplacement of things are often easy to deny, but when irritability, agitation, and depression begin to descend, you know something is wrong. By the very nature of mood changes and rapid mood swings, however, you often drive away family and friends from getting close enough to find out what's really going on. And it's not just the irritability and depression that are signs of Alzheimer's; it's also the fear. It's a very scary thing to feel you are "losing your mind." That's the very time you really need all the love and support you can gather around you. So, be aware that you might be driving away your support team.

Your family may say you seem different. They may pick up the personality changes that set in because of the memory loss and inability to complete tasks. Understandably, you may be confused and suspicious. You become fearful and either push people away and refuse their help or become dependent and won't let them out of your sight.

The electrical disconnection in the brain also causes apathy to set in. The last thing you want to do is to start a conversation, go out, or get involved in a social activity.

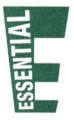

Rather than trying to cover up the fact that you have Alzheimer's, use it to your advantage. When you have the courage to tell people about your disease, you can get their support, and they will better understand your mood swings. Otherwise, people will take your mood swings personally and think you are mad at them, and even worse, they will get mad back.

Chapter 2

The Alzheimer's Brain

Before we dive into the Alzheimer's brain, we need to find out what goes on in the normal brain. Then, we need to find out what is altered with aging. It appears that brain aging markedly speeds up in Alzheimer's and may give us clues as to how to treat and prevent the disease. Not only will this chapter explore the Alzheimer's brain, but it will also take a look at some of the more common theories surrounding the cause of Alzheimer's disease.

The Living Brain

Put your two palms together and then make your hands into fists. If you look down at your thumbs, you can envision the actual size of your brain. Your curled up fingers even look a bit like the incredible convolutions in the brain. Its 100 billion nerve cells weigh about three pounds in total and connect with each other along 100 trillion different pathways. The 100 billion nerve cells in the brain look like bizarre amoeba on hallucinogenic drugs. They have a central body where metabolism takes place, and they have several incredibly long, stretched-out arms, or axons, that conduct electrical signals. At the tips of the axons is where signals jump from one nerve cell to another. That junction is called a synapse. To give you an idea of how many axons there are making connections, there are 100 trillion synapses in the brain.

ESSENTIAL

The brain makes up about 2 percent of the total weight of the body but requires 20 percent of the body's blood supply, utilizes 20 percent of the body's total oxygen supply, and needs 65 percent of its glucose. It's obvious we need to feed our brain properly for it to function.

The brain is also a supercomputer, the likes of which will probably never be duplicated by technology. Just think of all the functions it's involved in: myriad memories, a wide range of moods, sensory perceptions (taste, touch, smell), all muscle movements, breathing, blood circulation, digestion, pressure, pain, swallowing, arousal, abstract thinking, identity, and more. And yes, we take it for granted—that is, until we find we are losing our grasp on it.

The Nerve Cells in the Brain

The main function of nerve cells in the brain is to communicate with one another and pass messages along the chain of command to keep the body functioning. You've already heard that there are 100 billion nerve cells in the brain, and each cell body has several axons or long arms attached. From those axons come multiple smaller arms called dendrites. A nerve cell, like all other cells, has a nucleus in the cell body that controls all the metabolic functions of the cell. The axon, which is the width of a hair, carries messages from one nerve cell to the next. Dendrites also receive messages from axons. The number of nerve cells that connect with their extended axons and dendrite system numbers in the thousands. But the brain isn't just made up of nerve cells. Surrounding each nerve cell are neuroglial cells that provide nutrients, support, and protection.

Nerve cells have specialized functions, such as movement, sensory input, thinking, memory, and learning. But no matter what function they have, it all boils down to communication. The 100 trillion synapses in the brain are constantly sending messages to keep the body functioning.

We can measure the electrical activity in the brain with an electrocardiogram, so it should come as no surprise that the nerve cells send and receive electrical messages. An electrical charge builds up in the nerve cell and then at a certain critical point it travels down to the end of its axon. At the tip of the axon a chemical messenger is released by the electrical stimulation. Chemical messengers are called neurotransmitters. Their job is to travel the short distance from the tip of the axon to bind to receptor sites on dendrites or nerve cell bodies. The junction is called a synapse, and the average nerve cell has about 15,000 synapses.

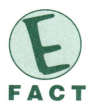

FACT

We hear about neurotransmitters all the time. Prozac works to keep the levels of the neurotransmitter *serotonin* high in the brain. *Adrenalin* is responsible for the fight or flight reaction when you have a sudden fright. *Dopamine* controls movement, emotional response, and ability to experience pleasure and pain. And the major drugs used in Alzheimer's treatment help to prevent destruction of *acetylcholine*, a neurotransmitter that is derived from choline and released at the ends of nerve fibers.

When neurotransmitters attach to receptor sites, it's like opening a door. Then, depending on the chemical nature of the neurotransmitter, the cell may speed up or slow down its activity. The coordination of millions of signals every second results in everything we think and do. The whole process is beyond comprehension. That's why when it begins to fail, we don't have all the answers.

Regeneration and Repair

Cells in the lining of our mouth and intestines live for only a few days; red blood cells live an average of three months. But nerve cells, which arise when we are in our mother's womb, are very long-lived. In fact, they can live 100 years or longer. We used to think that once nerve cells died they weren't replaced, but even that notion is being disputed.

Recent studies show that new nerve cells can arise in a few regions of the brain, even in older brains. As time goes on, we may find out new nerve cells can form in other parts of the brain. This puts a whole new emphasis on how we can best support and stimulate the production of new nerve cells.

Even so, as with anything that is going to be around for a long time, we must make sure to take good care of our nerve cells. The brain and body do their jobs by ensuring an ongoing process of cellular detoxification and repair.

Areas of the Brain

The brain is divided into two hemispheres (remember your two fists held together making up the whole brain). There is the right cerebral hemisphere and the left cerebral hemisphere. Cerebral just means "to do with the brain." The two cerebral hemispheres make up most of the weight of the brain, about 85 percent. The connection between the cerebral hemispheres is called the corpus callosum and is like a major telephone switching station crowded with bundles of nerve connections.

The outer layer of the cerebral hemispheres is called the cerebral cortex and has an average thickness of 2.5 millimeters or $1/8$ of an inch. It is here that incoming sensations are scanned, and from which movement and thinking originates.

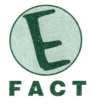
FACT

In Alzheimer's, the cerebral cortex is significantly thinner compared to healthy subjects. Dr. Jason Lerch, the head researcher in one study, found that the worst hit was around the short-term memory area of the hippocampus, where the cortical thickness was 1.2 mm less in Alzheimer's disease patients than in controls.

The cerebellum is located at the base of the brain. It makes up about 10 percent of the weight of the brain. It controls balance and coordination. Frequent stumbling, inability to turn, or inability to balance on one foot are signs that the cerebellum is affected.

Finally comes the brain stem, which sits below the cerebellum at the base of the brain. It forms the important connection between the brain and the spinal cord, relaying messages from one to the other. Its mere 5 percent of the brain is crucial for automatic functions in the body such as breathing, heart rate, blood pressure, and sleep. The brain stem controls these functions that happen automatically to keep us alive. The brain stem is one of the last areas affected by Alzheimer's. The loss of automatic functions in the body such as the heart rate and breathing signal that the end is near.

What Lies Deeper?

The deepest areas of the brain can also be ravaged by Alzheimer's. These areas include:

- The limbic system: controls instinct and emotions, and the sense of smell. That's why when you smell a long-forgotten scent, it can bring up long-forgotten emotions.
- The thalamus: receives information from the limbic system and transmits it to the cerebral cortex.
- The hippocampus: converts short-term memories into long-term memories for storage. Alzheimer's plaques begin in the cortex near the hippocampus and then enter the hippocampus. Memory loss is the first sign of Alzheimer's.

The Brain on Video

Microscopes gave us our first clue into the Alzheimer's brain. Without the ability to see these tiny deposits, which are 5–200 micrometers (a micrometer is a unit of length equal to one millionth of a meter), Dr. Alzheimer would not have been able to associate the symptoms of his patient with her autopsy findings of plaques and tangles.

More intricate technology in the form of PET scans can show blood flow and glucose metabolism deep inside the brain. For example, if an area of the brain is activated with the firing of nerve cells, blood flow and glucose metabolism also increase. The image on the screen of this activity is displayed in colors that show the brain in action. Researchers can even put tracers on neurotransmitters to understand how they differ with age, sex, disease, and drug intervention.

As the Brain Ages

The modern-day electron microscope allows us to view anatomical evidence of changes in the brain that occur with age. These changes mirror a corresponding decline in memory and thinking. With age, our outer skin puckers and wrinkles, and it seems our brain does as well. However, there seems to be an increase in the presence of dementia in these anatomical changes, which results in nerve cell death and brain atrophy.

The tangles and plaques that Dr. Alzheimer found are not unique to the disease; they are found in normal aging. It's the amount of tangles and plaques and the cumulative destruction they result in that signifies Alzheimer's.

Free Radicals, Aging, and Antioxidants

The aging brain is also subject to damage by free radicals. A free radical is an unstable molecule that is formed when molecules within our own body's cells react with oxygen. It is unstable because it has an unpaired electron that steals a stabilizing electron from another molecule, potentially causing cell damage. The body's own metabolism causes free radicals, but there are also external sources that we usually term pollution.

ESSENTIAL E

External free radicals that we have some degree of control over, meaning we can try to avoid them, include: chemicals (pesticides, industrial pollution, auto exhaust, cigarette smoke); heavy metals (dental amalgam, mercury, lead, cadmium); most infections (virus, bacteria, parasites); X-rays; alcohol; allergens; stress; and even excessive exercise. Many researchers advise us to avoid these sources of free radicals as much as possible.

Antioxidants are vitamins and minerals such as magnesium, selenium, Vitamin C, and Vitamin E stored in the body whose job it is to neutralize free radicals. Internal free radicals are automatically turned off by these natural antioxidants. But, if there aren't enough antioxidants available, excess free radicals begin to damage and destroy normal healthy cells. We now know that uncontrolled free radicals, from either inside or outside sources, play a major role in the development of degenerative diseases. They can damage any body structure by affecting proteins, enzymes, fats, and even DNA. Free radicals are implicated in more than sixty different health conditions, including Alzheimer's, heart disease, autoimmune diseases, and cancer. Could some form of free radical be implicated in creating beta amyloid and tangles?

The Impact of Aging

Even if you are healthy, as you age you can have a noticeable decrease in your ability to remember names, learn new information, or retrieve information. Interestingly enough, when asked to perform complex tasks of memory, attention, and learning, healthy seventy- and eighty-year-olds may perform worse, but only if they are under a time constraint. If given enough time, they have the same scores as young adults.

Determining Neurological Symptoms

"What a waste it is to lose one's mind." There are many ways the mind can betray us with diseases and conditions that impinge on parts of the brain that allow us to think, talk, walk, and function as complete beings.

These many diseases make up the differential diagnosis of Alzheimer's. Most of them have similar symptoms to Alzheimer's, and many, like Alzheimer's, are not curable. But the good news is that some are, and you and your family should do everything possible to determine whether your neurological symptoms are in the treatable and curable category.

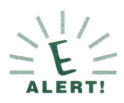

ALERT!

Confusion and memory lapses aren't always due to degenerative disease. Dr. William Philpott wrote a book called *Brain Allergies* in 1987. He described many case studies of people showing signs of confusion and memory lapses when they were exposed to auto exhaust, perfumes, and strong-smelling cleaning products.

Researching Alzheimer's

In scientific research, most investigators focus on one theory and try to prove it right before they admit defeat. Research is also a series of ups and downs, a positive experiment followed by an equally negative one. For instance, when amyloid plaque was discovered by Dr. Alzheimer and rediscovered in the 1970s, researchers sought to explain all the Alzheimer's symptoms on the basis of excess amyloid. They called it a nerve toxin and thought amyloid was produced by a genetic mutation. Subsequent research showed that people with severe dementia didn't necessarily have severe amyloid buildup. In an animal model, amyloid plaque alone failed to produce the neurodegenerative changes seen in Alzheimer's. So, the theory that amyloid alone causes Alzheimer's was not supported by the facts.

ESSENTIAL

Dr. George Bartzokis, a neuroscientist at UCLA, in a January 2004 report says that the cholesterol and fat that coat nerve cells (called myelin) breaks down because of age, genetic factors, and too much cholesterol. Excess cholesterol creates a toxic protein that attacks myelin leading to nerve destruction. That's why a low-cholesterol diet is important in Alzheimer's.

Abnormal protein aggregation, or buildup, seems to be common to most of the neurodegenerative diseases: Parkinson's disease, Creutzfeldt-Jakob disease, motor neuron disease, and Huntington's disease to name a few. Presently, geneticists are trying to find the clue to Alzheimer's abnormal brain protein because early-onset Alzheimer's, which is a rare form of the disease, is linked to a mutation that codes for the beginning stages of amyloid plaque formation.

The following are some of the causes or triggers of Alzheimer's disease that are currently being researched:

- Amyloid plaque
- Tangles from tau
- Genetics
- Inflammation
- Cardiovascular damage
- Oxidative stress

Causes of Alzheimer's

We have known since 1907 that plaques and tangles in the brain may cause Alzheimer's, but what does that really mean since we still don't know what causes the plaques and tangles to appear? In fact, plaques and tangles may be the result of the Alzheimer's process and not the cause. Researchers are hard at work trying to find an Alzheimer's gene and trying to pin down a single cause.

It appears, however, that Alzheimer's may fall in that murky category of diseases that have more than one cause or trigger. Diseases like arthritis or diabetes that come on gradually when a genetic predisposition is triggered by environmental and lifestyle factors never happen in the same way for any two people. Alzheimer's could have the same mix of genetics and environmental triggers.

Doing the Plaque and Tangle

Plaque and tangles do occur in normal brains but not to the extreme extent that they do in Alzheimer's brains. They do not come out of the clear blue. Instead, they are abnormal accumulations of normal structures. Beta amyloid plaques originate from beta amyloid protein, which is part of a larger protein called amyloid precursor protein (APP). The plaques build up outside the nerve cells. In Alzheimer's, plaques develop in the memory, thinking, and decision-making centers of the brain.

The role of APP in the brain is to help nerve cells grow and repair. It sits astride the nerve cell membrane, half in and half out. In Alzheimer's, an unknown variable causes particular enzymes to chop APP into fragments, creating beta amyloid. The beta amyloid fragments clump together outside the nerve cell, and form plaques that won't dissolve.

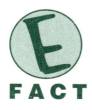

FACT

A study done on mice at Saint Louis University published in *Neuroscience* in October 2003 found that Alzheimer's may occur because the mechanisms that should remove amyloid protein from the brain don't work. Chief researcher, Dr. William A. Banks, says the findings mean a big piece of the Alzheimer's puzzle is solved. Now we just have to find ways to turn on that mechanism.

Neurofibrillary tangles occur inside healthy nerve cells. The inside of nerve cells is held together by a kind of scaffolding that is made up of structures called microtubules that act like guide wires directing nutrients back and forth from the cell body to the tip of the axon. Tau is a special protein produced in the nerve cells that is necessary to make the microtubules stable. In Alzheimer's, for some unknown reason, tau begins to bond with other tau molecules creating the tangles seen under the microscope. Without normal tau molecules, the cell collapses around the abnormal tangles.

Alzheimer's research has centered on finding out what causes plaques and what causes tau tangles and then trying to stop the formation of these structures.

The Genetics of Alzheimer's

It would be easier to diagnose Alzheimer's if it were caused by one gene that we could eliminate or manipulate. It's never that easy, however.

The ApoE4 gene is associated with 60 percent of late-onset Alzheimer's, so it is receiving a lot of attention from researchers. This "Alzheimer's gene" makes a particular lipoprotein, which is involved with transporting cholesterol within the body. It is also directly involved with making plaques in the brain.

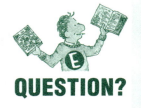

QUESTION?

What is DNA?
DNA occurs in every cell. It is formed by twenty-three pairs of chromosomes. Each chromosome has thousands of individual genes in precise sequences that "read" out directions to make specific proteins. If a gene is altered, even slightly, the protein is damaged; this creates cell failure and either causes disease or increases the risk of disease. Free radicals can cause this type of damage.

If you have the ApoE4 gene from one parent, this increases the risk of Alzheimer's by four times. The ApoE4 gene from both parents increases your risk by sixteen times. Even having two copies of the gene, however, does not guarantee you will get Alzheimer's; you have to have other risk factors as well.

Inflammation and Alzheimer's

Several studies have shown that if you take anti-inflammatory drugs for arthritis, you may have less risk of developing Alzheimer's. Inflammation is an immune system reaction to infection, injury, some diseases, and even obesity.

Extreme inflammation causes fever, swelling, pain, or redness. Chronic inflammation, however, may not cause any external signs—and that may be the case with Alzheimer's. Researchers find collections of inflammatory cells and inflammatory chemicals in and around Alzheimer's plaques. It is well known that once an inflammatory process starts, the chemicals produced by the inflammation trigger an ongoing cascade of reactions. These chemicals break down cell membranes and scatter the contents of the cell, which causes cell death. This process continues to ignite more and more cells to rupture, which results in a widespread area of damage. Many researchers feel this inflammatory process is one of the causes of Alzheimer's disease.

Cardiovascular Risk Factors in Alzheimer's

Surprisingly enough, there seems to be a link between heart disease and Alzheimer's. In 1969, elevated levels of an amino acid called homocysteine were found in the urine of patients with heart disease. Homocysteine is a normal by-product of protein digestion. If it occurs in elevated amounts it can cause cholesterol to change into an "oxidized," or rancid, form, which goes on to damage blood vessels.

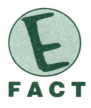

FACT

The association between homocysteine and heart disease was found in people who developed severe heart disease in their teens and twenties along with high levels of homocysteine; these high levels were caused by an enzyme deficiency due to a defective gene. In the general population, 10 to 20 percent of coronary heart disease cases have been linked to elevated homocysteine levels.

For certain individuals who lack specific enzymes for protein digestion, homocysteine can become a real problem. The B vitamins are necessary for proper protein digestion, and if various B vitamins (B_{12}, B_6, and folic acid) are deficient in the diet, homocysteine builds up. Conversely, if these B vitamins are given to people with high levels of homocysteine, the condition disappears and heart disease symptoms are reversed.

A healthy level of homocysteine should be well below 12 micromoles of homocysteine per liter of blood (12 umol/L). If homocysteine levels are greater than 12 umol/L, they are considered high. As it turns out, 20–40 percent of the general population have elevated levels of homocysteine. Individuals with high homocysteine have almost four times the risk of suffering a heart attack compared to people with normal levels. Many doctors and researchers now feel that elevated homocysteine is an even stronger marker than high cholesterol for heart disease and blood clotting disorders.

In the *New England Journal of Medicine* on February 14, 2002, the Boston University Medical Center reported on an eight-year study. In 1,092 patients, an increase in plasma homocysteine level of 5 umol/liter increased the risk of Alzheimer's disease by 40 percent. The highest levels doubled the risk. The relationship between Alzheimer's and elevated homocysteine still needs more investigation, but correlates with data about the brain-protective effects of the B vitamins that we will talk about in the treatment chapter. In essence, if there were enough folic acid, vitamin B_{12}, and vitamin B_6, there might not be an elevation of heart- and brain-damaging homocysteine.

Oxidative Damage from Free Radicals

The free radical aging theory that we talked about in Chapter 1 is being studied as a factor in Alzheimer's. Free radicals are formed normally in the body, but if there is an overabundance, the body can't maintain the proper supply of antioxidants necessary to keep the free radicals under control. With aging, the body's stores of antioxidants become lowered unless they are regularly replenished with an excellent diet or supplements.

Free radicals can build up in all parts of the body, including the brain. When they enter nerve cells they can disrupt function and cause cell death. They can also trigger a cascade of free radical formation. This chain reaction can cause widespread oxidative damage in the brain.

E ALERT!

As we've noted earlier, the brain uses 20 percent of the body's oxygen, 65 percent of its glucose, and 20 percent of its blood circulation. This high level of metabolism makes it extremely susceptible to free radical damage.

The avenues of research regarding Alzheimer's and antioxidants, in the form of comprehensive dietary surveys and laboratory studies, suggest that low-fat, low-calorie diets and certain supplements may be beneficial in Alzheimer's treatment.

Stroke and Alzheimer's

We spoke about stroke as a part of the differential diagnosis of Alzheimer's, but current research, from a long-term study on Alzheimer's and aging, seems to suggest that a stroke can be a significant risk factor for Alzheimer's. It appears that even without an abundance of plaques and tangles, the brain of a stroke patient is susceptible to the ravages of Alzheimer's.

Researchers are intrigued by the Alzheimer's-stroke connection because stroke is very common and a major cause of death in our society. With new research on lifestyle intervention, we can modify the risk factors for stroke, lower the stroke rate, and thereby decrease the incidence of Alzheimer's in this group. Stroke risk factors include hypertension, high cholesterol, and smoking.

Heavy Metal Theories

Aluminum, mercury, zinc, and copper have all been implicated in the cause of Alzheimer's. Different researchers are protective of their particular theory, but perhaps they all have a role in the creation of this complex disease.

ESSENTIAL

Water covers 75 percent of the earth; our bodies are 60–70 percent water. Only 1 percent of the world's water is available to us. Roughly 97 percent of the world's water is seawater, and 2 percent makes up glaciers and polar ice caps. We can die sooner from lack of food than from lack of water. And water that looks safe can contain harmful elements, such as heavy metals, which could cause illness.

In 2000, the *American Journal of Epidemiology* linked drinking water with a concentration of aluminum above 0.1 milligram/liter with an increased risk of Alzheimer's. The study followed 2,700 people for eight years to identify new cases of probable Alzheimer's. In 2001, another study on nerve cells found degeneration of neuritic processes and accumulation of tau protein and beta-amyloid protein appeared after chronic exposure to aluminum chloride for more than three weeks.

A 1997 study fed a group of rats aluminum drinking water. They found brain changes in the hippocampus, and neurofibrillary degeneration, similar to neurofibrillary tangles in Alzheimer's disease. The authors of this study concluded that in spite of very low gastrointestinal absorption (less than 1 percent), aluminum in drinking water might accumulate, in the long term, in vital organs such as the kidney and brain, with distinct cytotoxic and neurotoxic effects.

Mercury Theory

Research at the University of Calgary Faculty of Medicine done in 2001 found that nerve cells exposed to mercury caused the formation of neurofibrillar tangles, one of the two diagnostic markers for Alzheimer's disease. Researchers were able to catch their findings on video and make it available to interested parties.

Previous research by Dr. Boyd Haley at the University of Kentucky has shown that mercury can cause formation of amyloid plaques. Dr. Haley commented on the new research in Alberta. He said, "Seven of the characteristic markers that we look for to distinguish Alzheimer's disease can be produced in normal brain tissues, or cultures of neurons, by the addition of extremely low levels of mercury. In addition, research [in 1998] has shown that Alzheimer's diseased patients have at least three times higher blood levels of mercury than controls" (*NeuroReport*, 12[4]:733–737, 2001).

Dr. William R. Markesbery, director of the Sanders-Brown Center on Aging at the University of Kentucky, in 1990 autopsied the brains of Alzheimer's patients and compared them to patients who died of normal causes. He and his group found that the Alzheimer's patients' brain tissue had almost double the concentration of mercury as that of patients who died of all other causes. One particular area of the brain that transmits memories and sensations to higher brain centers contained almost four times as much mercury as did the normal controls.

A 1995 study by the Alberta University group found that mercury vapor interacts with brain tubulin and disassembles microtubules that maintain neurite structure; this results in the formation of neurofibrillary tangles.

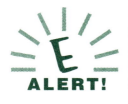

ALERT!

The toxicity of mercury is second only to plutonium. Sources of mercury in our society include "silver" amalgams, which are 50 percent mercury; flu vaccines with a mercury preservative called thimerosal; coal burning power plants; crematoriums, which vaporize people's dental fillings; and deep-water fish such as swordfish, king mackerel, tilefish, and shark.

Zinc and Copper Theory

A December 2003 *USA Today* article reported on another theory of Alzheimer's, that of zinc and copper mixing with beta amyloid protein deposits. It's a decade-old theory of Dr. Ashley Bush, a researcher at Harvard Medical School who published in the journal *Science*. He believes that zinc and copper accumulate in the brain and mix with amyloid plaques, which causes oxidation, and thus destroys brain nerve cells.

In the beginning his views were ignored, but he's the winner of the 2003 American Academy of Neurology prize for Alzheimer's disease research. And he now has a five-year grant from the National Institutes of Health (NIH) to develop a drug that absorbs excess copper and zinc from the brain.

Chapter 3

Alzheimer's: The Differential Diagnosis

Nobody wants to wait for an autopsy to obtain a diagnosis, but that's the state of the art in Alzheimer's. When you first start to have memory loss, you, like Ronald Reagan, may laugh it off for a few years. And with luck, you may just be experiencing normal signs of aging where a few brain cells go down for the count. Family doctors, however, should be alerted to signs of Alzheimer's so that treatment can be started as early as possible.

Early Detection of Symptoms

You know something is wrong because you've put your house keys in the freezer once too often. At first it was a joke, even though you didn't share it with anyone because you knew they would think it was a bit crazy. But then you got confused at the shopping mall parking lot the other day and couldn't find your car for the longest time. That was scary. And, even though you told her there is nothing wrong, your daughter keeps saying that you are more irritable and even paranoid lately. What's going on?

It is a scary feeling when your mind goes blank and you can't remember where you are or what you are doing. Because these feelings come and go in Alzheimer's, you don't really pay attention to them. This slow deterioration of brain cells causes intermittent interruption of signals. The next day can be perfectly normal because the signals all go through, and you can tell yourself that everything is fine. Such is the power of denial.

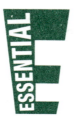

People with Alzheimer's live between eight and twenty years after the first sign of symptoms and between two and twenty years from diagnosis. The question becomes: Why go for early diagnosis if there is no treatment for the disease? The answer: Many drugs, nutrients, and even exercise can delay development of severe symptoms of Alzheimer's.

Chances are that your family doctor will be the first doctor to consider the diagnosis of Alzheimer's. But, he or she may not be the first person to recognize the signs and symptoms. That person is usually a spouse or another family member.

Someone who hasn't seen you for a few months or a year will usually be the first to notice a change in your personality or your level of functioning. Family that sees you every day or every week may not even notice a slow progression of symptoms. And everyone, doctors included, is very quick to dismiss memory problems, saying, "Oh, you're getting on in years, you know." Only someone who saw you do crossword puzzles last year and now sees that you can't remember where you put your glasses begins to raise the alarm.

Fear of finding out that you have Alzheimer's is the main reason why you may delay your first visit to your doctor. But you must remember that knowledge is power. In the case of Alzheimer's, the sooner you know, the sooner you can do something about it.

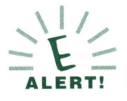

ALERT!

To find Alzheimer's even six months earlier would mean a 65 percent decrease in avoidable months of nursing home care, and a 48 percent drop in unnecessary drug treatment, according to Dr. Daniel Silverman, assistant professor of molecular and medical pharmacology and associate director of imaging for the UCLA Alzheimer's Disease Center.

You will probably see your family doctor and blurt out the question, "Do I have Alzheimer's?" Your doctor may be taken off guard, but if he or she has seen some deterioration in your mental status over the past years, then you have opened the door to finding out why you feel the way you do.

It's a Matter of Exclusion

Even before you finish your sentence, your doctor is running through a list of what other conditions could cause your symptoms. In order to diagnose Alzheimer's, your doctor has to exclude all those other conditions based on your history, physical and neurological tests, lab tests, and scans. Because to definitively diagnose Alzheimer's you have to wait for an autopsy, your doctor must rule out all other possibilities before he or she says you have Alzheimer's. The process of doing this is called *differential diagnosis*. Alzheimer's disease is a type of dementia that may be difficult to distinguish from many other conditions. Some of these other causes of dementia may be more treatable than Alzheimer's:

- Senility and dementia
- Organic brain syndrome
- Cardiovascular disorders

- Trauma-induced brain injury
- Metabolic disorders
- Prescription drugs and drug interactions

Senility and Dementia

Senility and dementia are still considered by many to be a normal stage of aging. They are catchall diagnoses and are freely used to diagnose any memory symptoms in the elderly. With age, we assume that most people will lose some important brain cells and decline in mental function.

The definition of senile is as follows: forgetful, confused, or otherwise mentally less acute in later life; occurring in or believed to be characteristic of later life, especially the period after the age of sixty-five years.

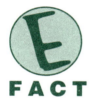

FACT

In 1998, Dr. Morrison-Bogorad of the NIH said, "Our challenge is to educate the family practitioner to make them aware of when they should be concerned about possible dementia." She said forgetfulness is not part of normal aging, and it's important to identify mild cognitive impairment because those people are more likely to develop Alzheimer's within a few years than people without such problems.

The definition of senile dementia is: A form of brain disorder marked by progressive and irreversible mental deterioration, memory loss, and disorientation, known to affect some people after the age of about sixty-five years. What an irony that the age of retirement is also designated as the age when senility sets in.

Organic Brain Syndrome

Organic brain syndrome (OBS) is a general term used to designate diseases that affect mental status. The organic part refers to a physical disease or condition that affects the brain and causes a decrease in mental function. Psychiatric disorders are not included in the organic brain syndrome category. Symptoms vary for different diseases, but in general include confusion, delirium, dementia, and agitation.

OBS is a disease of the elderly. It's as if the brain just gets rusty with age and slows down. But OBS is not inevitable as you grow older. There are many disorders associated with OBS. Many of them can present symptoms similar to Alzheimer's because Alzheimer's disease is also a degenerative neurological disorder; these disorders must be ruled out in the differential diagnosis.

Creutzfeldt-Jakob: Mad Cow Disease

This disease is a rapidly progressing OBS that affects mental function and movement. It is characterized by brain destruction due to a viral-like protein particle called a prion, which can be transmitted from an infected living creature to humans. It's very rare, and occurs in only two per one million people. The average age of onset of this disease is fifty.

E ALERT!

A very rare form of Creutzfeldt-Jakob has occurred in adolescents who have been treated with a human growth hormone that was infected with prions. Because of this condition, all natural human growth hormones were banned and growth hormones are now made synthetically with no possibility of infection.

Creutzfeldt-Jakob distinguishes itself from Alzheimer's because of the rapidly fatal progression of the disease. It begins with personality changes and poor coordination and progresses to severe dementia, muscle tremors, and rigid posture.

Live transplants, such as corneal transplants, from patients who have the disease carry a potential for the disease. A family history of dementia is also a risk factor.

More has become known about Creutzfeldt-Jakob disease because of the British, and now the American, experience with mad cow disease. Creutzfeldt-Jakob disease may be related to other prion diseases including kuru (documented in New Guinea headhunters), scrapie (found in sheep), and bovine spongiform encephalitis (seen in cows).

Huntington's Chorea

This OBS is also rare, and affects five in one million. It's an inherited condition caused by a gene mutation. Huntington's Chorea causes degeneration of the nerve cells in the cerebrum. It resembles Alzheimer's in the personality changes, progressive loss of mental function, and loss of cognitive functions such as speech, calculative skills, and judgment.

It was first described by an American doctor, George Huntington, in 1872. It wasn't until 1993, however, that a team of researchers at the Massachusetts Institute of Technology (MIT) found the gene responsible for this disease on chromosome number four. It is unlike Alzheimer's because symptoms appear from age thirty-five to fifty even though the gene is present from birth.

Huntingon's Chorea causes dementia, but unlike Alzheimer's, it is a hereditary condition. If one parent has the gene, then half of his or her children will have the condition. It also differs from Alzheimer's because it is characterized by frequent abnormal facial and body movements, which include quick jerking movements. Chorea means "dance" and refers to the puppet-like jerking of the body.

Multiple Sclerosis

Multiple sclerosis (MS) is an OBS that involves the brain and the spinal cord. It's a disease that causes scarring or sclerosis of the myelin sheath that covers all the nerve cells in the body. Six out of ten cases affect women, and it is fairly common, occurring in one out of 1,600 people. It is not an "elderly disease" and arises between the ages of twenty and forty. In people under sixty-five, MS is a major cause of disability.

It comes about with repeated episodes of inflammation of nervous tissue in any area of the brain and spinal cord. The inflammation can affect vision, movement, or sensation, and is different in each person. The scarring of various nerves slows or blocks the transmission of nerve impulses in the inflamed area, which results in typical MS symptoms.

We know MS is caused by inflammation, but we don't know what triggers the inflammation in the first place. Researchers theorize that it is triggered by a type of viral infection or some gene abnormality that controls the immune system, or a combination of both.

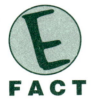

Multiple sclerosis is the most common progressive and disabling neurological condition in young adults, whereas Alzheimer's is the most common in older adults. Scotland has the highest incidence of multiple sclerosis in the world. And the disease is five times more prevalent in colder climates than in tropical ones. The incidence among the Inuit, however, is much lower than in the general population.

Normal Pressure Hydrocephalus (NPH)

This OBS occurs when the normal flow of cerebral spinal fluid (CSF) is blocked. With no way to get out, it builds up and enlarges the ventricles within the brain, and the pressure it puts on adjacent brain tissue causes tissue destruction. As we are finding out, any damage to delicate brain tissue can lead to symptoms of dementia. This condition occurs in one out of 100,000 people and can be reversed or treated if properly diagnosed.

Some risk factors and causes of NPH are head injury, brain surgery, meningitis, and brain hemorrhage. The pressure often diminishes when the swelling subsides over time with these conditions. In addition, a temporary "shunt," or drainage tube, can be put in the brain to release the excess CSF build up.

Pick's Disease

Pick's disease is also called presenile dementia because it occurs in younger adults. In this condition, brain atrophy occurs and on autopsy, abnormal bodies (Pick's bodies) are present in the nerve cells usually in the frontal or temporal lobes of the brain. It is another rare disorder affecting one out of 100,000 people.

Pick's disease is more common in women and may be evident in people as young as twenty but usually begins between forty and sixty years of age. It differs from Alzheimer's because there are no plaques or tangles to be seen, but patients have Alzheimer's-like symptoms. The cause of Pick's disease is unknown but thought to be a genetic disorder.

Parkinson's Disease

This is a much more common disorder than many of the other neurological diseases we have been talking about. It occurs in two out of 1,000 people, but unlike Alzheimer's, it develops early, around the age of fifty. Both men and women are affected equally, and it is becoming one of the most common diseases of the nervous system in the over-fifty population.

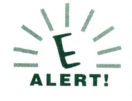

ALERT!

Dr. Grandinetti told the participants of the American Academy of Neurology meeting in Honolulu in April 2003 that eating fruit with pesticides may be a risk factor for Parkinson's disease. In 2000, a Stanford University study linked Parkinson's risk to occupational exposure to chemicals and even home use of pesticides. Researchers believe these poisons may kill specific brain cells.

With this disease, movement is impaired, which makes walking difficult. There is also a general shaking of the head and hands and loss of coordination. Like Alzheimer's, there is progressive damage of nerve cells, but in Parkinson's the damage is confined to nerve cells in an area of the brain that controls movement. Dopamine, a neurotransmitter from these cells, is consequently diminished and produces loss of muscle function. As with Alzheimer's, we really don't know why the cells are destroyed in the first place. Dementia is a symptom of later-stage Parkinson's. Some of the drug treatments for Parkinson's, however, may cause dementia.

Lung Disorders and Alcohol Related Conditions

There are several lung disorders that may cause or aggravate OBS simply because not enough oxygen is getting to the brain. Sleep apnea is an increasingly common condition in which breathing stops for several seconds and oxygen to the brain is reduced. Emphysema may also lower the oxygen supply to the brain. All of these conditions can cause symptoms of confusion and even memory loss that could be misinterpreted as dementia by the casual observer.

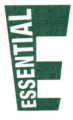

Emphysema is caused by smoking and has the typical early symptoms of labored breathing and shortness of breath while walking, climbing stairs, or doing household chores. Low oxygen levels cause symptoms of anxiety, sleeplessness, confusion, weakness, and appetite loss, which are similar to Alzheimer's symptoms. Quitting smoking and regular exercise are the keys to keeping a good oxygen supply to the brain.

Alcohol-induced dementia is called Wernicke-Korsakoff syndrome. The underlying cause is a vitamin B_1 deficiency caused by malnutrition common in habitual alcohol use. Wernicke-Korsakoff syndrome affects people between forty and eighty years old with a gradual onset. Symptoms are often reversible, however, especially in the early stages, with high doses of vitamin B_1.

Cardiovascular Disorders

The heart and blood vessels are responsible for transporting oxygen-rich and glucose-rich blood to all parts of the body. So, it's obvious that when the heart and blood vessels are impaired or damaged, they can't get enough oxygen or glucose to the brain. Lack of oxygen to the brain for over four minutes can result in death. Shorter periods of no oxygen or prolonged low levels of oxygen can result in nerve cell death in the brain, and in symptoms such as dementia.

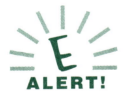

Heart attack and stroke are life-and-death emergencies where every second counts. The warning signs are chest discomfort (pain, pressure, tightness, or fullness); pain or discomfort in one or both arms, the back, neck, jaw, or stomach; shortness of breath; and other signs such as a cold sweat, nausea, or lightheadedness. If you experience any of these symptoms, call 911 immediately.

The following cardiovascular disorders can result in impaired blood flow to the brain.

- **Arrhythmias:** A disturbance of the electrical conduction system of the heart that interrupts the heart rate or rhythm. When the heart beats too fast or too slow and the flow of blood to the brain is impaired for even a few seconds, brain damage can occur.
- **Cardiac infections:** A bacterial or viral infection of the inside lining of the heart, which can impair blood flow to the brain.
- **Multi-Infarct Dementia (MID):** MID affects four out of 10,000 people and accounts for 10–20 percent of all dementias. It happens when atherosclerotic cholesterol plaque in arteries breaks off and blocks off small blood vessels in the brain causing tissue death.
- **Stroke:** Stroke is usually caused by a blood clot or buildup of cholesterol plaque that blocks an artery in the brain. Depending on where it occurs, it can mimic any and all symptoms of dementia. The incidence of stroke is about four out of 1,000 people; it is the third leading cause of death in the United States. Risk for stroke includes high blood pressure, heart disease, smoking, high cholesterol, and diabetes.
- **Transient Ischemic Attack (TIA):** TIAs are also called mini-strokes, and are defined as blood flow disruption and decreased brain function for less than twenty-four hours at a time.

Trauma-Induced Brain Injury

Motor vehicle accidents, sports trauma, bike accidents, and serious falls can all result in head injuries that cause swelling and bleeding; this puts pressure on delicate brain tissue, and sometimes results in symptoms of dementia. Of course, you should remember if you have had a head injury, and suspect any mental impairment could be due to that. Sometimes, however, the symptoms come long after a traumatic event.

Even a minor trauma, when combined with taking blood thinners or aspirin or alcohol intake will thin the blood and could turn a minor bleed into a major one. The symptoms may come on so gradually that the trauma and the symptoms are not connected. The result could be dementia-like symptoms due to chronic subdural hematoma, intracerebral hemorrhage, subarachnoid hemorrhage, or a concussion.

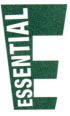

If you feel that your doctor is not digging deep enough into your case to find other possible causes for your symptoms or conditions that can make your Alzheimer's worse, it is your right to change doctors and find someone you can trust to be 100 percent supportive of your needs.

Metabolic Disorders

Disorders of metabolism can produce chemicals in the body that are toxic to the brain. This form of dementia occurs in about one in 10,000 people. This type of dementia may be reversible and deserves a close investigation by your doctor. Outright liver and kidney failure can cause dementia but are usually not reversible.

Endocrine Disorders

Metabolic causes of dementia may include endocrine disorders such as:

- Addison's disease: failure of the adrenal glands.
- Cushing's disease: overproduction of adrenal hormone.
- Diabetic nephropathy: diabetic kidney disease.
- Diabetic ketoacidosis: overproduction of ketones.
- Insulinoma causing hypoglycemia: low blood sugar.
- Hypoglycemia: low blood sugar.
- Hypoparathyroidism: imbalance of calcium in the body.
- Hyperparathyroidism: imbalance of calcium in the body.
- Hypothyroidism: low thyroid hormone.
- Thyrotoxicosis: overproduction of thyroid hormone.
- Pheochromocytoma: overproduction of adrenalin.

Electrolyte Imbalance and Nutritional Deficiency

Metabolic disorders causing dementia can manifest as disorders of electrolytes creating acid/base disorders, low sodium, high calcium, low potassium, and low magnesium. Nutritional disorders such as vitamin B_1 deficiency, vitamin B_{12} deficiency, niacin deficiency, and protein-calorie malnutrition can produce dementia. Studies show that the majority of nursing home patients are malnourished and deficient in most vitamins.

Prescription Drugs and Drug Interactions

Prescription medication may cause toxic OBS. There is, of course, a scientific basis with each prescription drug tested in extensive clinical trials. Most drug research subjects, however, are healthy, white males. A drug may pass all the tests required for it to become an FDA-approved medication, but it's not until the drug gets into the general population that it is used by all ages.

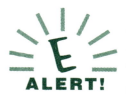

ALERT!

The over-sixty-five population consumes more than a third of all the drugs prescribed in the United States. Dr. Robert Epstein, of Medco Health Solutions, Inc., conducted a 2003 study on drug trends. He found that seniors go to multiple physicians, get multiple prescriptions, and use multiple pharmacies. The average senior receives twenty-five prescriptions annually.

In the elderly, however, drug metabolism is usually slower, which means it takes longer for a certain amount of medication to clear the body. The bowels move slower; the digestion is slower; the liver doesn't work at top speed. Therefore, if high drug doses are given to an elderly person, there is the potential of a toxic drug reaction. Seniors often also take multiple prescriptions; this creates a complexity of drug interactions that may cause toxic OBS. Nearly one quarter of our elderly are admitted to hospitals or nursing homes because of medication side effects. Ⓔ

Chapter 4

Your Physical Examination and Staging of Alzheimer's

Perhaps you go for an annual health exam, and you always pass with flying colors. Usually these exams include the standard: taking your blood pressure, listening to your heart and lungs, tapping your knees, and then you are out the door. Maybe every few years you get some blood tests for hemoglobin or cholesterol, but they are often within normal range. A physical exam is pretty basic, unless your doctor is looking for something specific. That's why you almost have to prod your doctor into checking you for Alzheimer's.

Medical History and Physical Exam

With the list of dementias in the forefront of his or her mind, your doctor will take a medical history and find out when you first started having memory problems, confusion, and personality changes. You will be asked about any past head trauma, surgery, medication, and exposure to toxic chemicals. Then your doctor will ask for a detailed family history, which includes any family member who has or had neurological disease.

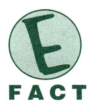

FACT

An *Annals of Internal Medicine* report in the May 7, 2002, issue examined the "Public expectations and attitudes for annual physical examinations and testing." Recent guidelines for adult disease prevention do not recommend a comprehensive annual physical examination. They found, however, that the U.S. public would be upset if measures were taken to withdraw the annual physical or not have it covered by insurance.

Your doctor performs your physical examination. If he or she does suspect some neurological disease, you will also be referred to a specialist. In the meantime, your doctor will do the following examination.

- **General Appearance:** Look for apathetic appearance and flat stare to rule out Parkinson's disease.
- **General Appearance:** Nutritional status—check for dehydration, muscle wasting, bruising, brittle hair and nails, and dry skin.
- **Eyes:** Perform an eye examination to rule out brain tumors, which cause pressure that can be seen at the back of your eye.
- **Head:** Test your cranial nerves to rule out brain tumors.
- **Neck:** Feel your thyroid to help diagnose hypothyroidism or hyperthyroidism.
- **Heart:** Check your heart sounds, pulse, and blood pressure to help rule out arrhythmias, valve problems, and hypertension.
- **Lungs:** Listen to your lungs to help rule out lung disease.
- **Reflexes:** Test your reflexes to help rule out other neurological diseases.
- **Abdomen:** Feel your liver to rule out liver disease.

The Neurologist

If your family doctor suspects you may have a neurological disease, he or she will probably send you to see a neurologist to help decide on your diagnosis. Your family doctor most likely already performed a mental status evaluation, but your neurologist will perform a more detailed exam. Neurologists have standard tests for memory, reasoning, vision-motor coordination, and language skills. In fact, scientists are finding that memory and recall tests may give the most accurate diagnosis of Alzheimer's. Researchers are working hard to improve a series of standardized tests that can be given to people at risk in order to detect early Alzheimer's or to predict whether you are at a higher risk of developing Alzheimer's in the future. These tests are also used to monitor the progression of Alzheimer's.

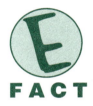

FACT

The Mini-Mental State Exam consists of thirty questions. Your doctor asks the set list of questions and your answers help determine your mental status. The questions cover various aspects of mental capability, including orientation, your ability to register the questions, attention, recall, and language skills. This test is widely used to diagnose and assess the progress of Alzheimer's disease.

The first examination will become the baseline test. The current tests in use include the Mini-Mental State Examination (MMSE) or Physical Self-Maintenance Scale (PSMS). They assess cognition (thinking) and function. To begin, you may be asked what day, month, and year it is, followed by more and more difficult questions. You'll be asked to name common items from pictures and maybe to use building blocks to reconstruct drawings of block structures. It does sound a bit like preschool, but these simple tests give important information about how the brain is functioning.

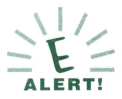

ALERT!

According to a report in the January 2004 issue of *Neuropsychology*, smart people beat the normal Alzheimer's tests. As a result, they need to have tougher testing if they are to be correctly diagnosed for early signs of Alzheimer's disease.

Other neurological tests for sensation, balance, and temperature are carried out. Then decisions have to be made about scans and laboratory tests. Usually a brain scan is done to detect other causes of dementia such as stroke. Laboratory tests can help exclude metabolic diseases, organ diseases, and endocrine diseases.

Alzheimer's Testing

Alzheimer's testing is focused in several areas. There is no one definitive test for the condition, so it becomes a process of excluding other possible conditions, doing intensive memory and language tests, and performing more and more sophisticated brain scanning technology. Testing for Alzheimer's includes memory and language tests, tests for existing brain damage and its association with Alzheimer's, tests for blood chemistry changes and the association with Alzheimer's, and neuroimaging.

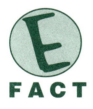

FACT

On April 24, 2001, BBC News reported on the "ten-minute test for Alzheimer's," also called the CANTAB Paired Associates Learning Test. The test's authors, who have published results of its early trials in the journals *Dementia* and *Geriatric Cognitive Disorders*, say that the test can distinguish Alzheimer's sufferers from patients with depression and those without any neuropsychiatric disorder with 98 percent accuracy.

A Picture Is Worth a Thousand Words

We could learn a tremendous amount about Alzheimer's if we could catch it on one of the many types of scans available in medicine. Sections of the brain are stained and viewed under a microscope, and it is only then that the tangles and plaques can be visualized. In the last ten years, however, several imaging systems have been developed that may show some promise in the diagnosis of Alzheimer's.

According to 2002 research, Magnetic resonance imaging (MRI) scans of the brain may detect Alzheimer's disease decades before the first clinical signs of dementia occur. When you have an MRI, you are injected with a dye called gadolinium; this isn't the iodine dye used in CT-scans or x-rays. There is no x-ray radiation; a magnet produces the images.

According to a UCLA study, positron emission tomography (PET) scans can detect Alzheimer's disease at its earliest stage. When you have a PET scan, you are injected with radioactive glucose (sugar) and exposed to radiation similar to a chest x-ray.

Single photon emission computed tomography (SPECT) scans depend on a radioactive material injected into the bloodstream. A nuclear medicine camera then picks up the radioactivity in the brain. This scan is in the research stages and may help diagnose Alzheimer's, neurodegenerative diseases, strokes, and seizures. It may also be useful in following Alzheimer's drug treatments.

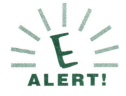
ALERT!

In November 2002, Charlton Heston was diagnosed with Alzheimer's using a PET scan and made a statement to the press that he believes in the early diagnosis of Alzheimer's using PET. In December 2000, however, Medicare refused to allocate funding for $2,000 PET scans to screen for Alzheimer's.

With increased emphasis on the need to diagnose Alzheimer's while people are still alive, brain-scan researchers are rushing to find an answer. Some doctors, however, feel that this type of scan-based screening is premature because we don't have a definitive Alzheimer's prevention program or even a treatment program that stops the disease.

I'd Still Rather Not Know

Please don't give up. Every day research comes to light with new information about Alzheimer's disease. There are, however, other practical benefits to an early diagnosis. Sometimes it's just good to know that there is something physical going on, and even a bad diagnosis is still a diagnosis. Also, the sooner you and your family know that you have Alzheimer's, the more time you have to plan for the future. It's just wise to make financial decisions, think about living arrangements and power of attorney, and create your support system early on.

Possible or Probable Alzheimer's

When you get your final diagnosis from your doctor it will be couched in one of two terms, Possible, or Probable Alzheimer's. Probable Alzheimer's means your doctor has tried to rule out all other dementia disorders and has concluded that your symptoms are probably due to Alzheimer's. The less precise diagnosis of Possible Alzheimer's implies that even though Alzheimer's is likely the main cause of your dementia, there may be one or more other conditions that are causing similar symptoms and possibly making your Alzheimer's symptoms appear worse. Your doctor may or may not know what these other conditions are.

Documenting the Progression of Alzheimer's

Even if we don't know what causes Alzheimer's, we have been able to discover what happens in the brain when Alzheimer's attacks, and to correlate it with progressive physical and mental changes. In a late diagnosis, the time until death can be as short as three years, especially in patients over age eighty, or as long as ten years or more in younger patients.

ESSENTIAL

MRI hooked up to video can follow the progression of Alzheimer's and the effects of treatments. A study in the February 2003 issue of the *Journal of Neuroscience* used sequential brain MRI scans every three months for two years in twelve patients and showed how the damage usually begins in the left hemisphere and eventually encompasses the whole brain, something usually not seen until autopsy.

Over the last number of years there has been a concerted effort to document the progression of symptoms in Alzheimer's disease in stages in order to determine medical treatment options, and to assess home care and long-term care needs.

Progression of Alzheimer's symptoms seems to follow the buildup of plaques and tangles and nerve cell degeneration in the brain. We know that plaque first builds up near, and then in, the hippocampus, the memory center. Plaque may, however, appear a full ten to twenty years before any actual symptoms begin. As plaque builds and spreads, memory is affected first, and then slowly but inexorably, all aspects of behavior, thinking, and judgment are affected. The final stages involve the areas of movement and coordination, causing immobility.

The Seven Stages of Alzheimer's

Doctors commonly assign Alzheimer's symptoms to one of the following three stages: mild, moderate, or severe. These will be compared with the more precise Seven Stages of Alzheimer's.

- Stage 1: No cognitive impairment.
- Stage 2: Very mild cognitive decline; forgetfulness.
- Stage 3: Mild cognitive decline; early confusional state.
- Stage 4: Moderate cognitive decline (mild stage); late confusional state.
- Stage 5: Moderately severe cognitive decline (moderate stage); early dementia.
- Stage 6: Severe cognitive decline (moderately severe stage); middle dementia.
- Stage 7: Very severe cognitive decline (severe stage); late dementia.

No two people experience the same degree of symptoms or even fall clearly into one stage or another at any one time. The purpose of staging in Alzheimer's is not to force people into one category or another; it's to help give the patient, the doctor, and the caregivers a clear picture of how the disease is progressing. These symptoms can be listed in a health diary and checked off periodically to keep track of the disease's progress.

Stage 1: No Cognitive Impairment

This designation implies that we are all at Stage 1 Alzheimer's, with no noticeable symptoms. Sixty percent of the general population has the ApoE4 gene that creates a susceptibility to Alzheimer's. Many of us are at risk for stroke or have high levels of homocysteine, which also increases our risk for Alzheimer's. This is the stage where lifestyle intervention, in the form of a good diet, exercise, and certain nutrients, could mean the difference between health and Alzheimer's. This is the stage in the brain where plaques and tangles could start to build up, but take ten to twenty years to be recognized as impaired memory.

Stage 2: Very Mild Cognitive Decline

This is the memory lapse stage. Names, keys, and glasses disappear in the twinkling of an eye. But you are the only one that seems to be concerned about it. It's a stage that is equated with aging, being stressed, or having too much on your plate, and for many people this is exactly what is happening. You are juggling too much in your hectic life, and you're on overload.

ESSENTIAL

It is essential that you feel comfortable with your family doctor and that you are referred to a neurologist with whom you also feel comfortable. You need to know that as your memory fades, someone will be there to help take care of you. Determining this at the onset of your condition can relieve a lot of stress.

Even if you mention memory lapse to your doctor, he or she usually doesn't think it's important, and no one else seems to notice. It's not even denial at this stage; it's just part of life. If you do go on to develop full-blown Alzheimer's, this stage is equated with the increasing buildup of plaques and tangles in the brain.

Stage 3: Mild Cognitive Decline

This stage corresponds with Mild Alzheimer's. Your family and friends remark on your memory problems. Physically, you are just fine. What's happening in your brain is beginning to affect memory, language, and reasoning, but has not reached your movement centers.

In a society that equates illness with physical distress, this disease gives no early physical clues. Yet, you are finding it more and more difficult to keep your world in control. You may just liken your symptoms to normal aging at this time. A diagnosis of Possible Alzheimer's, however, could be made at this time based on detailed mental status testing. The symptoms are all mild, but if you put them all together, they form an undeniable pattern. Symptoms that stand out include: problems remembering names or finding the right word, inability to remember reading material, losing important things, inability to plan or organize, taking a long time with tasks, inability to perform effectively at work, and a growing sense of anxiety.

Stage 4: Moderate Cognitive Decline

Mild Alzheimer's encompasses Stages 3 and 4. In Stage 4, even a cursory medical examination would detect neurological deficits. Personality changes become obvious at this stage, with the most common being shy and withdrawn behavior, especially in groups of people.

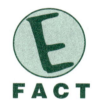

Engaging someone with Moderate Alzheimer's in mentally stimulating social activities is very important. Games, exercise, dance, creative activities, reminiscing, and telling stories can all help to keep the brain active and the body healthy. Try to overcome your resistance, or that of your loved one, to these activities because of embarrassment about memory lapses.

Symptoms that stand out at this stage are a decreased knowledge or awareness of current events, difficulty counting backward from 100 by sevens, difficulty making a shopping list and shopping, making mistakes in paying bills and managing finances, forgetting aspects of personal history, getting lost in familiar places, making bad decisions through bad judgment, loss of spontaneity, and mood changes.

Stage 5: Moderately Severe Cognitive Decline

This is the Moderate Alzheimer's stage. This stage shows evidence of major memory gaps and obvious problems with thinking, language, and tasks. In the brain, plaques and tangles have spread from the hippocampus memory center and are increasing in the areas of the cerebral cortex that control thought, language, reasoning, and sensory processing. As the cells are damaged and killed, they create areas of atrophy that can be diagnosed with a brain scan.

In Stage 5 Alzheimer's, the problems are such that some daily caregiving and support are essential. The Alzheimer's patient may forget addresses and telephone numbers but will know children's or spouse's names. There will be additional symptoms such as confusion as to time and place; confusion that is worse at sundown; agitation, restlessness, anxiety, and crying; inability to cope with new situations or stress; inability to count backward by twos from forty; problems with reading and writing; a very short attention span; inability to think logically; inability to dress appropriately for weather or events; and inability to eat or use the bathroom unassisted.

Stage 6: Severe Cognitive Decline

On the Mild, Moderate, to Severe Alzheimer's scale, Stage 6 is Moderately Severe. At this stage, symptoms are obviously worsening in memory and personality. The amount of care needed is increased to cover all activities of daily living. Behavior problems, such as wandering and agitation, are common. More intensive supervision and care are necessary to prevent wandering or dangerous activities such as leaving the stove turned on or leaving doors and windows open.

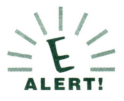

ALERT!

Please don't try to care for your loved one alone. Ask for help. There's your family as well as dozens of national, state, and community services available to help. Not only will you become ill yourself and no longer be able to give care at all, but you'll double the burden of another family member or the community to care for you both!

This is the stage when local services should be called in to help the family. Alzheimer's sufferers in Stage 6 may be unaware of their surroundings or recent experiences; have great difficulty remembering personal history; may still remember their own name; may forget a spouse's name but seem to know familiar faces; must be assisted getting dressed; experience sleep disturbances; must be assisted in the bathroom with wiping, flushing, and washing hands; begin experiencing urinary or fecal incontinence; express major personality changes and behavioral symptoms such as suspiciousness, delusions, hallucinations, and compulsive, repetitive behaviors; forget where they are and wander away and get lost; have little to no impulse control and may undress at inappropriate times or places or use vulgar language; or have trouble getting out of a chair.

Stage 7: Very Severe Cognitive Decline

This is the Severe stage of Alzheimer's; this final stage includes loss of all contact with the outside world, inability to respond or speak coherently, and inability to move. In the brain, plaques and tangles are widespread, leaving devastation and atrophy. Symptoms are those of total incapacity, and patients need assistance in eating and going to the bathroom; in addition, they have incontinence; are unable to walk, sit, smile, or hold their head up; their only vocalizations are groaning, moaning, or grunting; muscles become rigid; swallowing is impaired; they experience weight loss and seizures; have skin infections; and sleep for long periods.

How Alzheimer's Patients Succumb

Due to lack of activity and prolonged confinement to bed, most Alzheimer's patients die from other diseases. One frequent cause of death is pneumonia, either after a cold or flu, or due to aspiration of food into the lungs because of impaired swallowing.

No, it's not a pretty sight; it's not anything we or our loved ones should go through. That is why it's important to have all the facts about Alzheimer's, find all the sufferers, and do all the research necessary to find a cure to stop this tragedy. Ⓔ

Chapter 5

My Doctor Says I Have Alzheimer's

After several visits to the doctor and extensive testing, your doctor informs you that you have Alzheimer's. While the diagnosis may be the same, no two people ever cope with the news in the exact same way. Let's follow two people, Mary and John, as they are told they have Alzheimer's. Eavesdropping on individual cases might make it easier to understand the condition and even come to grips with it yourself.

Mary's Story

Mary has been experiencing memory lapses for years. She calls herself seventy-years young, but forgetting her grandson's name was the last straw. She finally got up the nerve to go to her doctor. He and her new neurologist say she has Possible Alzheimer's. She's in shock for days. She can't get the phrase, "What a waste it is to lose one's mind" out of her mind. Where does she go from here?

Of course the first thing she wants to do is run. After all, it's a disease that has no cure. But, with the way medical research is progressing, it's not going to be long before they find a cure. And she knows there is nowhere she can go to hide from her brain. Denial over the last few years has probably cost her some valuable time that she could have used to begin Alzheimer's treatments. So, it's time to face the music.

Here's where Mary starts. She begins to read all she can find about Alzheimer's. Her doctors gave her some information about Alzheimer's and local support groups. She takes a deep breath and starts to learn about the disease and about what she can do to make the best out of a bad situation.

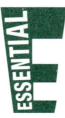

There are a variety of Alzheimer's support systems readily available. You can call an 800 number (✆ 800-272-3900) at the Alzheimer's Association that is answered twenty-four hours a day. The Alzheimer's Association has thousands of chapters and outreach programs all over the country.

Her family already knows her diagnosis. Her daughter was there at the neurologist's appointment when he told her the preliminary results. So, now may be the time to sit with her family and discuss what's on their minds. At first this may be difficult. There is a lot of emotion involved with Alzheimer's because it is such a devastating disease. But she will have to wade through that and hopefully come out on the other side with a plan of action.

Getting a Second Opinion

The second thing to do is get a second opinion. Mary's neurologist said she had Possible Alzheimer's. That could mean that there are other causes of her symptoms or other physical conditions that could be making mild Alzheimer's worse. She really wants to make sure she is checked for all those possibilities, and she is going to do this either with her original doctors, if they are open to more investigations, or with a new set of doctors.

In Mary's case, let's go over the list of differential diagnosis for Alzheimer's in Chapter 3 and make sure they are all investigated. Under organic brain syndrome, it's highly unlikely that Mary could have Creutzfeldt-Jakob or hereditary Huntington's Chorea. They are both very rare and appear below age fifty. Multiple Sclerosis and Pick's disease also appear at a much younger age. In addition, she has not suffered from head injury, brain surgery, meningitis, or brain hemorrhage.

Cardiovascular Complications

Cardiovascular disorders are a more likely cause or contribution to Mary's mild symptoms of dementia. After all, she smoked for twenty years, and only gave it up because her kids wouldn't tolerate it.

Mary was diagnosed with mitral valve prolapse in her twenties, which occasionally sets off arrhythmias. She developed high blood pressure about ten years ago when her husband died, and is on two pills: One is a diuretic, and one is an antihypertensive. She has never had a brain infection, multiple brain infarcts, or a stroke. But transient ischemic attacks (TIAs) might explain the sudden episodes she gets every few months. They seem to pass, and she has just equated them to being overly tired. But they cause symptoms of numbness, tingling, and changes in sensation; speech difficulty (garbled speech, slurred speech); weakness or a heavy feeling of extremities; vision changes (decreased vision and double vision); dizziness; lack of coordination; staggering; and confusion.

Whether due to denial or just her forgetfulness, Mary neglected to tell her neurologist about these symptoms. She asked for an appointment with a cardiologist to do a thorough heart and blood vessel workup.

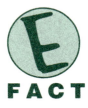

FACT

A study in the journal *Archives of Neurology*, December 2003, found that people who had a history of stroke have a 1.6 greater chance of developing Alzheimer's. In a cumulative fashion, if a stroke patient also had hypertension, the risk for Alzheimer's was 2.28; if they also had diabetes, the risk was 4.59; or if they also had heart disease, the risk was 1.95.

Mary's cardiologist found that she had almost complete blockage of her right carotid artery in her neck. The two carotid arteries are responsible for bringing most of the blood to the brain. After discussing the risks and benefits, Mary decided to have a procedure called an endarterectomy. A skin incision was made over the artery in the neck. The artery was clamped off; an incision was made in the artery; and all of the blockage was removed. She was only in the hospital for three days and recovered very quickly.

Trauma-Induced Brain Injury

Brain hemorrhages she would remember, but the only thing that ever happened to Mary in terms of head trauma was getting knocked out when she was skating once; she fell and hit her head on the ice. She did have a concussion because she couldn't remember falling, and her mother had to watch her all day after that to make sure nothing developed.

Dementia Due to Metabolic Causes

Metabolic causes occur more often than organic brain syndromes. Various types of organ decline and failure affects about one in 10,000 people. Mary doesn't have liver or kidney failure because they are end-stage diseases, and none of her blood tests have ever shown liver or kidney damage.

As she goes over the list of metabolic causes, thyroid and hypo-glycemia stand out most for Mary. She has always seemed to have a low body temperature, slow metabolism, constipation, and dry hair. She recently read that all those symptoms can relate to low thyroid. In terms of hypoglycemia, she sometimes can't go for more than two hours without feeling headachy and hungry.

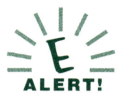

ALERT!

The brain becomes extremely vulnerable to excitotoxins such as MSG and aspartame (NutraSweet) during episodes of low blood sugar or hypoglycemia. Low blood sugar often occurs in malnourished people and when people skip meals. Magnesium and balanced meals help prevent low blood sugar and protect the brain from excitotoxins.

Blood testing for thyroid did show a low level of thyroid hormone. It was low enough for Mary to be placed on a thyroid hormone supplement. Her family doctor also gave her a diet sheet for hypoglycemia that told her to avoid sugar, alcohol, and coffee, and to eat small frequent meals to avoid low blood sugar episodes.

Electrolyte Imbalance

A few years ago, Mary's bone density testing showed the beginning signs of osteoporosis, and she began taking calcium. But she found out with her recent blood tests that her calcium levels were high, probably because she was taking it every day; she also found that her magnesium was low, because too much calcium pushes out magnesium, though it is as important as calcium for the bones. Magnesium is also very important for normal heart muscle action. Mary's potassium levels were also low, probably because she has been taking diuretics for years without taking potassium. Her doctor told her to take extra magnesium to balance out the calcium and add more oranges, bananas, and green vegetables to increase her potassium.

Nutritional Imbalance

Mary didn't really know about the status of her vitamins and decided to ask her doctor about them. When she did, she found out that he was very excited about a recent study from Johns Hopkins University, which showed that people who took extra vitamin A and vitamin C, above the amounts in their diet, had a lower incidence of Alzheimer's.

He said clinical trials giving these vitamins to Alzheimer's patients would determine if this was indeed true. But he felt that the safety of these supplements and the finding from this study and several others gave him enough data to tell her to take vitamin A and vitamin C. When he tested for homocysteine, he found it elevated and told Mary to take folic acid, B_6, and B_{12} to reduce those levels.

Respiratory Disorders

The main lung disorders that can worsen Alzheimer's are sleep apnea and emphysema. Mary had no symptoms of apnea, but she did have a history of smoking. When she was evaluated by her cardiologist, her chest x-ray showed very mild emphysema from her years of smoking. Mary was told, however, that she could overcome those symptoms by getting more oxygen into her lungs with regular exercise.

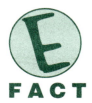

FACT

In 2001, a study published in the Proceedings of the National Academy of Sciences found that the following physical activities led to a lowered risk of Alzheimer's: sports, working out in a gym, biking, gardening, ice skating, walking, and jogging.

Miscellaneous Conditions

The rest of the differential diagnosis includes drug and alcohol associated conditions, Parkinson's disease, and prescription drugs. Mary has never been involved with taking street drugs, so that was not a factor in causing brain damage. But she realized that the stress of her memory loss had caused her to begin drinking more wine in the past year. She may even have three glasses a day. When she found out that alcohol can reduce some important B vitamins and may not be the best way to relax, she decided to stop it.

What Mary Learned

The simple exercise of going through the list of conditions that can mimic or worsen Alzheimer's was a gold mine for Mary. She took care of the side effects from her medications and calcium supplements that caused low levels of potassium and magnesium. She began taking B vitamin, and she ate a more balanced diet and decreased her alcohol intake.

The list led her to a cardiologist who decided she needed an operation to protect her from a stroke and prevent further TIAs. Stroke is one of the most common causes of Alzheimer's, and by unblocking her carotid artery, Mary eliminated a dangerous risk factor. The TIAs also stopped, along with their periodic damage to the brain. The quick recovery happens because the TIA was only causing temporary blockage of oxygen to a specific area; or a TIA can be an actual tiny piece of debris breaking off the carotid artery blockage and causing a clot in part of the brain. With a tiny clot, the nerve cells reconfigure and work around the damaged area. Over time, however, the damage from TIAs can grow.

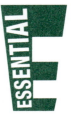

At an Alzheimer's Association conference in Stockholm, Sweden, in July of 2002, lifestyle research was presented to 4,000 scientists. It confirmed that a healthy diet, exercise, and weight management can protect against Alzheimer's. Because the disease may develop twenty or thirty years before any symptoms, doctors say that keeping healthy all your life can lead to healthy aging.

With increased blood carrying oxygen, glucose, and more supplementary nutrients to the brain, Mary actually felt that her mental status improved. When she had a three-month checkup, she was thrilled to learn that she was in much better shape than before the diagnosis of Alzheimer's. Her doctor was also very excited to see that she could improve and felt she was a wonderful example of what medicine could do with an early enough diagnosis and a person who was determined to not give up.

John's Story

Mary had the best possible outcome from having her memory impairment symptoms fully investigated. She may be able to prevent her symptoms from worsening for the rest of her life. John isn't quite so lucky. His symptoms started about ten years before he finally was forced to go to a doctor. He has just turned sixty-five and did not want to think he had already hit retirement age.

In addition, John's normal aggressive, hardworking personality kept people at arm's length anyway. Even his wife and children didn't really know he had been having problems with memory blackouts until the police picked him up going the wrong way on a freeway off ramp. He was lucky he wasn't killed. The police found John argumentative and almost incoherent. Their first thought was that he had been drinking. A breathalyzer test proved them wrong. When John appeared before the judge, he was told to undergo medical tests to determine why he was incapacitated.

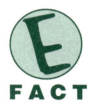

FACT

For every male with Alzheimer's, there are two females with the disease. But that doesn't mean that fewer men get the disease. It's because there are more older women than older men. Women live an average of five years more than men, and the incidence of dementia increases with age, which accounts for the greater number of women with the disease.

John's Medical Exam

The neurologist who examined John was trying to place a label on John's symptoms of memory blackout and belligerence. When the doctor asked about specific symptoms, John finally admitted that he had been having problems remembering names and finding the right words in conversation; he also admitted that he had trouble retaining new information, losing important things, organizing, and taking a long time with simple tasks; he also had a growing sense of anxiety. He said the only reason why his work didn't suffer was because his secretary did most of his routine work and covered for him quite a bit. In fact, John had all the symptoms of Stage 3 Alzheimer's.

He also has a family history of Alzheimer's. His father and his uncle both died of the disease when they were in their eighties. Actually, John knows quite a lot about Alzheimer's because he has seen it up close. He also knew that his symptoms were probably Alzheimer's, but with a combination of denial and willpower, he tried to ignore it for as long as possible.

The Detective Game

In John's differential diagnosis, most of the organic brain syndromes were ruled out quickly except for normal pressure hydrocephalus (NPH). John had had a number of falls in recent years and suffered a few head injuries. He attributed the falls to a "trick knee," but they were probably due to the progressive structural damage occurring in his brain.

A thorough eye examination, which looked at the back of his eye, would reveal any pressure buildup in the brain as a sort of building on the back of the eye. John's eyes were normal. Then a CT scan of the brain was done to look for a buildup of fluid on the brain that would make the cavities in the brain bigger. All the spaces in the brain were of normal size, so NPH was ruled out.

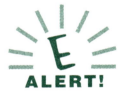
ALERT!

Repeated head injury carries a risk for Alzheimer's. For example, if a boxer also carries the ApoE4 gene, he or she can be advised by their doctor to curtail their career. Having an ApoE4 gene, however, does not as yet prevent a boxer from entering the ring.

The CT scan also looked for areas of subdural hematoma, which is a buildup of blood, like a big bruise, under the skull. There was no hematoma from his head trauma during his falls. A brain tumor, which puts pressure on the memory center, was high on the differential diagnosis list, but that was ruled out on the CT scan as well.

What about Heart Disease?

Heart disease was a factor in John's overall health. He suffered a mild heart attack at age sixty but cut out smoking, changed his diet, and began to exercise after this wake-up call. John was rigorous about his health program, and there were no signs of high blood pressure, arrhythmias, TIAs, or stroke.

John's blood tests, however, came back showing high levels of homocysteine, slightly elevated cholesterol, and low levels of B_{12}. We've already spoken about homocysteine as a marker for heart disease and possibly also a risk factor for Alzheimer's. This amino acid builds up when there is a deficiency of certain B vitamins to break it down. It clogs up the arteries and possibly also the brain. Taking folic acid, vitamin B_6, and vitamin B_{12}, however, easily controls high levels of homocysteine. John's low levels of B_{12} were another indication that he was at risk for high homocysteine.

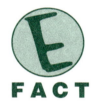

FACT

In the July 1994 *Neurology*, the Consortium to Establish a Registry for Alzheimer's Disease (CERAD) was established. It began by developing a standardized Family History Assessment of Alzheimer's to identify the presence of Alzheimer's, Parkinson's disease, and Down syndrome in family members. It was of note that the risk for Alzheimer's among female relatives was significantly greater than that among male relatives.

The Final Diagnosis

None of the metabolic syndromes fit into John's picture, and neither did electrolyte imbalance, lung disease, or the final neurological condition, Parkinson's disease. He did have a vitamin B_{12} deficiency that was picked up through blood testing. Remarkably, he had a very clean bill of health. His mental status examination, however, confirmed what the neurologist suspected from his symptoms. He had Probable Alzheimer's disease. Even so, the neurologist was quite surprised that John was functioning so well. The usual time from onset of symptoms to succumbing from

Alzheimer's is eight years. John had already had symptoms for ten years. There are people who survive for twenty years or more, and it seemed that John was in that category.

John seemed to take his diagnosis in stride. Actually, he had become quite overwhelmed trying to keep his secret, and he was somewhat relieved that it was out in the open. By his very nature, however, he wanted to know if there was more testing that could be done to further define his particular case, testing that would lead to some definitive treatment.

Additional Testing

Because of John's family history, his doctor recommended specific genetic testing for ApoE4. The gene was only discovered in 1992, and the test is by no means standard. At first, researchers thought it would make an excellent screening tool for the general population, but without an Alzheimer's treatment to offer people with the gene, it became a less viable option. In people who show signs of mild dementia, have family histories of Alzheimer's, and histories of heart disease, however, doing an ApoE4 test is a very good idea.

John did have two copies of the ApoE4 gene, one from each of his parents. That put his risk for Alzheimer's at sixteen times above the normal population. It also helped explain why he was at risk for heart disease and why he had an earlier heart attack.

ApoE lipoprotein (ApoE) transports cholesterol, and when the ApoE4 variant is present, cholesterol becomes elevated and the risk for Alzheimer's is increased. The gene alone is not responsible for causing Alzheimer's. Other factors like infection, head trauma, a high-fat diet, and oxidative stress on the brain have to be present.

John's Risk Factors

John did have a history of head trauma, and before his heart attack, he did have high cholesterol and ate a high-fat diet with lots of meat, butter, milk, cheese, and fried foods. After his heart attack, he drastically cut back on his fat intake, reduced his calories, and lowered his cholesterol. John took a "statin" cholesterol drug for a few years, but after a while his doctor said he didn't need it because his diet was taking care of the problem.

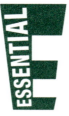

Someone who has the ApoE4 gene should not eat a high-fat diet. Find a nutritionist or dietician who can put you on a palatable low-fat diet. Watch out for low-fat, processed foods; they usually contain high amounts of sugar, which raises triglycerides.

What John and maybe his doctor didn't know was that statin drugs can lower inflammation in the brain that is associated with Alzheimer's by about 30 percent. And a high-fat diet is thought to increase the level of free radicals and oxidative stress in the brain, which may cause or worsen Alzheimer's. A low-fat and low-calorie diet is the recommended way to treat someone who has an ApoE4 gene.

PETs and MRIs

John's doctor told him about MRI, PET, and SPECT scans. John and his doctor decided to have a PET scan and an MRI done for two reasons. His doctor wanted baseline tests to help follow the progression of the disease and hopefully see the positive benefits of any drug treatment John took. John also wanted to have the tests to see if there were areas of the brain that were more affected than others. He wanted advance warning of where his next level of disability might hit so he could be prepared for it.

Chapter 6

Coping with the Diagnosis

People diagnosed with Alzheimer's have to cope. It's a matter of making the best of a bad situation and marking time until a definitive treatment plan is proven to halt the disease. But it's not as if you'll be lying back and waiting for the end to come. Coping isn't a passive activity when it comes to Alzheimer's. There are a million things for you to do to plan for your best possible future.

Bringing Out the Best

It's been said many times that we rise to our highest potential when faced with adversity. When faced with the diagnosis of Alzheimer's, we are certainly put to the test. As with Mary and John, you begin by finding out all you can about the disease and doing what you can to maintain your health. Then you must come to grips with the fact that within a decade, your mind is not going to be able to make decisions. You have to make ten times the decisions now to make up for not being able to do so in the future. You have to plan your future and plan your death.

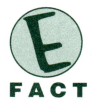

FACT

Dr. Robert Griffith, on the Web site Health and Age (✐ *www.healthandage.com*), writes about Chip Gerber, a fifty-four-year-old diagnosed with early-onset Alzheimer's disease in 1997. His eighty-year-old mother also has Alzheimer's. In July 2000, Chip started an online diary for anyone to read. This has encouraged many people to write their own diary.

If you stand up in front of a roomful of people and ask them if they are going to die, nobody will put up their hand, even though, intellectually, we all know we are going to die one day. It's never happened any other way. But we just can't admit it. When you have Alzheimer's, you just have to admit it much earlier than most. Maybe that, in itself, is a small bonus, the tiny bit of silver lining in this dark cloud. You can spend your years with a new appreciation of life and gather a support team around you that loves you and will give you comfort, dignity, and respect.

Bringing Out the Worst

There is no right or wrong way to respond to your diagnosis of Alzheimer's. Everyone has a different experience. There is also no set way of coping with Alzheimer's. If you are already stressed to the max, are financially burdened, have no health insurance, and your symptoms are getting worse day by day, you might not even feel like coping is an option for you.

You might feel like this diagnosis is the straw that breaks the camel's back, and you just can't cope with it. It may feel like you are being punished and bring up the "why me" question. The following stages of grieving may begin to play out in your head. They are presented in a linear order, but you can go in and out of several of the stages at one time before you reach acceptance. Dr. Elisabeth Kübler-Ross, in her brilliant work *On Death and Dying*, was the first to define the stages of grieving as:

- Denial
- Anger
- Bargaining
- Depression
- Acceptance

Denial

You've probably become quite good at denial for the past few years about the true nature of your symptoms. There is something to be said for denying minor aches and pains and getting on with life. In fact, the opposite of hypochondria may be denial. But, if you have really made all efforts to make sure the diagnosis is accurate, now is the time to accept it. Now is the time to put your energy and attention on living the best life you can.

Anger

Anger is a normal reaction. You are mad at God, at your doctors, at your family, and you may show it. It is good to express your true feelings at this stage and not bottle them up. By holding back strong emotions, you can actually cause more stress and physical symptoms. But, there's a time for anger and a time to put it aside. Work with a counselor to express your feelings of anger and come to terms with them.

Bargaining

Bargaining is an internal process that usually occurs when you are alone and praying for a miracle. For some, bargaining with God takes the form of promising you'll be a better person, devote yourself to service, become a priest, a nun, or a Mother Teresa if only this punishment will be lifted.

Depression

A level of depression is probably with you when you first suspect you have Alzheimer's. And you have a right to be depressed. If you have a history of depression, this type of bad news will further burden you. With good support and counseling, however, you can strive to keep yourself from feeling weighed down and find some joy in life.

Acceptance

Acceptance is the final stage in the process of grieving, and most people do get to it. Sometimes it comes in a flash of understanding, after a period of prayer and meditation. You learn that the reason, or the lesson, or the need for you to have this terrible condition does not matter, and you say, "So be it!"

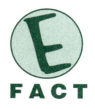

FACT

Gerry Trickle, writing in 2002 for the Web site PageWise, Inc. (✎ *http://fl.essortment.com/stagesgrief_rbdm.htm*), talks about the following stages of grief: shock and a feeling of unreality; emotional release with crying and insomnia; panic and a feeling of mental instability; guilt over what happened; hostility and anger; an inability to resume business-as-usual activities; reconciliation of grief; and finally hope.

Some people even get to see the gift in the tragedy. Families can become reunited, and resources that you never realized were in yourself or others, surface. Acceptance is the state that will help you stay the healthiest and make your caregiver's work that much easier.

Creating a Checklist

The checklist that you must make is one that can branch out into many different areas. It covers your whole life. Following it through can serve as a distraction from harsh reality, and it can also make your future as comfortable as possible.

❏ Talk with your family about your future needs regarding long-term home care and future nursing care.

❏ If you work, talk with your employer or employees.

❏ Join a local Alzheimer's support group.

❏ Discuss your health insurance with your insurance agent.

❏ Discuss your finances with a financial advisor or banking counselor.

❏ Talk to a lawyer about who you want to have your power of attorney and to be executor of your estate.

❏ Alzheimer's-proof your house.

❏ Talk to an Alzheimer's counselor about when you should stop driving.

Take Care of Your Health

During the times when you are depressed and say, "What's the use?" you are probably not in the best frame of mind to take care of yourself. The negative self-talk floods your mind with, "Why not have as much junk food, fried food, sugar, and alcohol as I want? That's not going to kill me, Alzheimer's is!"

ALERT!

The Americans with Disabilities Act (ADA) offers limited protection to individuals diagnosed with Alzheimer's disease. It requires companies with fifteen or more employees to make "reasonable" accommodations for job applicants and employees with physical or mental disabilities. Protection against job discrimination can be discussed with the Equal Employment Opportunity Commission at ☎800-669-4000.

We do know, however, that taking care of your health is the best thing to do for Alzheimer's. Just look at staying as healthy as possible as your new job, your new role in life, until the best treatment for Alzheimer's is found.

Get Physical

Take care of your physical health. See your doctor regularly to keep up on the latest Alzheimer's treatments. Every week there is a new report or study coming out that may help you. Over the past decade, hundreds of millions of dollars have been poured into Alzheimer's research. Some of these studies take years to complete, and now we are seeing the results.

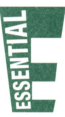

The Alzheimer's Society in the United Kingdom says the fewer drugs you have to take, the better, both for dementia and general health. Check with your doctor to eliminate unnecessary drugs. Sometimes people continue with repeat prescriptions longer than is needed. Also, drugs that manage behavior should be reviewed very regularly, and taken in the lowest possible effective dose.

The best advice is to eat a healthy, low-fat, low-calorie diet and exercise daily. Take supplements and medications as directed. Keep alcohol intake to a minimum, and get eight hours of sleep a night.

Strengthen Your Mental Health

Take care of your mental health. Exercise your brain as much as you do your body. Turn off the television. Join a book club; add new words to your vocabulary; and work on crossword puzzles. Start writing a diary; use big words; express yourself. A diary is also a way to write down what you need and keep lists of what you have to do as a memory jogger. Take your diary to family meetings and read from it when you forget something. Stretch your brain.

And while you're at it, do your best to keep a positive mental attitude. You have a right to be down but try to realize that negative thoughts just attract more negative thoughts. Being positive, especially around friends and family, will make it easier for them to do the same.

Support Your Emotional Health

Take care of your emotional health. Denial, anger, fear, isolation, depression, loss of confidence, and frustration are normal emotions in your situation. Find a counselor, social worker, or psychotherapist to discuss your emotions with and to put them into perspective.

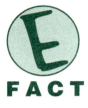

FACT

The Religious Orders study, published in the December 9, 2003, issue of *Neurology*, followed almost 800 nuns and priests. In this study, researchers found that people who most often experience negative emotions such as depression and anxiety were twice as likely to develop Alzheimer's disease as those who were least prone to these negative emotions.

Just as you work on a positive mental attitude, keep your emotions on a positive note as well. Negative emotions attract more negative emotions and can greatly influence the people around you. It actually takes less energy to smile than it does to frown.

Take Care of Your Spiritual Health

We don't have all the answers and now is the time to ask for help from a higher source. Prayer and meditation can help in these difficult times. Talk to a minister, priest, or rabbi. And if you need proof that prayer can help, there are hundreds of actual scientific studies that prove prayer has healing and helping powers. The way to tap into this universal power is to open your heart and ask for guidance.

Just Ask

The resources you will need to take care of yourself can include your family, doctors, social workers, counselors, and a support group. Creating contacts with all these support systems is important when you are first diagnosed. Don't wait until you can't fully communicate what you want from these people before asking for their assistance.

One of the hardest things for Alzheimer's patients to do is to ask for help. Actually, it's the hardest thing for any of us to do. But we all know that life is a "give and take." You have to look at this time of your life as a time when you need to take and others have to give. You will also find that caregivers don't look upon their role as a "have to" at all. Giving from the heart is a reward in itself because it opens up the heart to receive in so many other ways.

E ALERT!

In order to find the most effective tests for predicting driving performance, researchers reviewed twenty-seven studies on dementia and driving that had been published between 1988 and 2003 in the January 2003 issue of *Neuropsychology*. Better than observations from family members were specific skills tests and simulated on-road and non-road tests that evaluated mental status and visuospatial skills.

Talk with Your Family

Your family probably already knows you have Alzheimer's. They know because they have been watching the signs for a while now, or they were right there with you when you got your diagnosis. But what they don't know is what you are going through. Nobody can know exactly what you are experiencing.

That's where your strength and courage come in. You can actually find yourself in the role of comforting them! And what a gift that is. When you can tell a little joke or create a little laughter in the midst of this devastating news, your family will think you're a saint. Laughter breaks the ice. The best is when you can mix tears of sadness and tears of laughter together; it's a wonderful combination that makes it easier for everyone to cope.

In the midst of the laughing, crying, and sharing, try to make sure that your family understands that it's not just an aging process that you are going through. They need to know that Alzheimer's is a brain disease that will impair your memory, thinking, and behavior. And there will be a time when you aren't able to take care of yourself. They also need to know that you require real honest interaction. You don't want anyone to put on a superficial Pollyanna front when they are with you. You want to keep it real and keep it honest.

You've probably been through many of life's challenges with your family and friends. Let them know that this disease will change your life and their lives, but together you can meet the challenge.

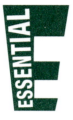

ESSENTIAL

Laughter is good medicine. Since Norman Cousins wrote *The Anatomy of an Illness* and revealed the power of laughter, science has proven it can do more than tickle our funny bone. Laughter can relieve depression, lower blood pressure, alleviate stress, increase endorphins (pleasure hormones), increase oxygen in the blood, and make you feel healthier and more alive.

Talk about Your Present Needs

This is a conversation apart from talking about your diagnosis and your feelings. You need to be very clear with your family about what you can and can't do. You can tell them about your plans for improving your physical, mental, emotional, and spiritual health and ask for their support. Then you need to discuss who is able to help you with:

- Meetings with your employer, insurance agent, financial advisor, and lawyer
- Doctor's appointments
- Alzheimer's-proofing your home for security
- Finding an Alzheimer's support group

Talk about Your Future Needs

The most important thing to get clear about your future is where you will be spending it. About 70 percent of Alzheimer's sufferers are taken care of at home. So, that's the place you'll likely be for most of your illness. With the increased government and public awareness of Alzheimer's, it is becoming easier to get assistance from the community and Alzheimer's groups. Alzheimer's support groups, caregiver training, access to the latest research, and a determination to find the "cure" are driving the Alzheimer's movement.

Discussing a time when you will be completely dependent on others is very difficult. The tables are turning. We are taken care of as infants; then we take care of our children or nieces and nephews; then we are taken care of as we decline. It happens as regularly as day flows into night. But, like death, we don't expect it to happen to us. It takes some getting used to.

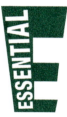

A 2001 American Association of Retired Persons (AARP) study discovered 75 percent of adult children are very concerned about the future care of their parents whether they are healthy or ill. At least one third, however, never discuss these thoughts with their parents. Proper long-range planning would help parents and adult children cope when a crisis hits.

Talk with Your Spouse

This, of course, is a special conversation, an ongoing conversation. You and your spouse may already know about the worst aspects of Alzheimer's through the media, and you know it's going to be rough. But it's not like that in the early stages, and it's not rough all the time. You need to talk to one another about your concerns. A support group for your spouse may be very helpful.

Talking with a counselor can help answer questions about the stages of Alzheimer's and what resources you need to cope with the emotional side of losing someone who is still there beside you. Your counselor may also initiate a frank discussion about changes in intimacy and sexual relations and how you each can meet your needs.

But it's important not to live in the future. Live in the present: Take a trip; go on outings; enjoy life to the fullest. If you have no physical handicaps, there is nothing preventing you from doing all those things you always wanted to do.

Along with the rest of the family, decide on caregiving duties. You and your spouse need to make sure there is enough support, and if not, plans should be made for hiring help with housekeeping, additional caregivers, or working with Medicare for coverage.

Talking with Children and Teens

Children and teens, whether you are their parent or grandparent, are going to have a whole different take on what's happening than adults. They can't be expected to know what the disease is all about, and may think you're going "crazy."

For teens, showing them a picture of the cross section of a brain and telling them that a disease is damaging your brain may help them understand. Younger children mainly want reassurances. They can feel something is shifting in the family dynamic. Hugging and holding them is the best thing. Reassure young children that they cannot "catch" the disease from you.

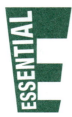

A January 2001 Associated Press article titled "Teens pierce cloudy world of Alzheimer's patients" reports on a weekly visit from four teens and a counselor, as part of a study, to determine whether this type of attention can improve quality of life for Alzheimer's patients. As one patient put it, "This is a big treat when you all come because we wake up again."

Explain to preadolescent kids that you have a disease where you are going to forget things, even their names, and that you still love them very much. You must decide whether the school nurse and teachers should know about your illness. There are also Alzheimer's support groups especially for children and teens. Stay involved in important future events in your children's or grandchildren's lives. Write letters or make audio- or videotapes with your advice, thoughts, and feelings about their first date, their graduation, their marriage, and even your death.

Talk with Others

Once you have discussed Alzheimer's with your family, you will need to inform others. While this may make you feel uncomfortable or embarrassed, preparations need to be made and people need to be informed.

Talk with Your Boss, Coworkers, or Employees

Many Alzheimer's workers are reducing their workload, taking early retirement, and eventually going on long-term disability. But because Alzheimer's is becoming more common, many employers are working on their own coping strategies. Speaking directly about your limitations is important in order to create the best possible working relationship.

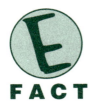

FACT

Alzheimer's in the workplace was investigated by Stacey Burling in the *Philadelphia Inquirer* of November 30, 2003. She found that doctors know little about how employers handle Alzheimer's. Jason Brandt, who runs an Alzheimer's research program at Johns Hopkins University School of Medicine, wants to research this area starting with Congress and the Supreme Court, where members are not forced to retire at age sixty-five.

You may need less of a workload and someone to assist you so that you can do what you do best, and not have to rely on short-term memory if that is your biggest challenge. It's going to be difficult to speak about your limitations, but it's better than doing a bad job and trying to cover it up.

Discuss Insurance, Finances, and Legal Matters

These three aspects of your future are crucial to take care of as soon as possible. You need to know how much your current health insurance will cover, and whether you need to apply for Medicare or Medicaid. Your finances have to be organized so that someone else can take them over for you when it becomes necessary. If you own a home, you have to decide whether or not to transfer it over to a family member. And you have to decide on power of attorney and the executor of your estate. These are all thorny matters in the best of times. Sitting with professionals who do this every day is the key to doing it right.

Join a Local Alzheimer's Support Group

Most communities have Alzheimer's support groups either connected to a local hospital or run by a volunteer agency such as the Alzheimer's Association. Your doctor may have already given you some contact names and numbers.

These are groups that will welcome you with open arms from a place of great caring and sharing. They are there so you don't have to reinvent the wheel when it comes to what needs to be done for your care and support for your family. Ⓔ

Chapter 7

Personality, Mood, and Behavioral Changes

Personality and mood changes in Alzheimer's are more than brain damage. The feeling that your memory is slipping sets off alarm bells in the protective mechanisms of your body. Those alarm bells cause you to worry and get stressed out about the strangeness of what is happening. That stress can actually cause release of stress hormones that can then cause inflammation, even in the brain, and make your symptoms seem worse.

Everyone Is Different

There are no two people alike on this planet of eight billion people. Twins aren't even totally alike. In general, Alzheimer's symptoms, and their ceaseless progression, seem to happen the same in all sufferers. But, your plaques and tangles, and reasons for getting Alzheimer's differ, and the way you react to your condition is going to be different from everyone else.

Various Alzheimer's groups and foundations such as the Alzheimer's Association, Alzheimer's Disease Education and Referral Center, and the American Health Assistance Foundation try to bring these symptoms to life in their various online and printed publications. Taking cues from their decades of tireless work, we've come up with detailed guidelines for you and your caregivers.

ESSENTIAL

Alzheimer's rating scales and Alzheimer's stages will try to make the disease a black-and-white condition on paper, but we all have to remember that everyone's different. The only thing that should be universal is the way Alzheimer's people are cared for—with comfort, dignity, and respect.

As described earlier, what is happening deep inside the structure of the brain is a buildup of plaques and tangles. These deposits create enough damage to nerve cells to interrupt their communication and lead to the brain defects we call behavioral problems.

Personality, mood, and behavioral changes, like all other symptoms in Alzheimer's, begin so slowly and imperceptibly that you don't know they are happening; then they seem to intensify.

The list of behaviors that are present in Alzheimer's are long and varied, but forgetfulness seems to be the first, while hallucinations and delusions come in the final stages:

- Forgetfulness
- Frustration
- Irritability

- Anxiety
- Depression
- Confusion and mood swings
- Agitation
- Compulsive and ritualistic behavior
- Restlessness
- Delusions
- Psychosis
- Hallucinations

Forgetfulness and Frustration

Forgetfulness and frustration typically manifest in Stage 2. Memory loss is the first symptom that you get with Alzheimer's. Memory is an internal faculty, but the outward signs of distorted memory are seen through unusual behavior. For example, because you forget a meeting or a family gathering, or even someone's birthday, that behavior is interpreted as "strange." People will say, "It's just not like Jane to forget Sam's party, I wonder what's going on."

As the list of forgotten events and the comments from your friends and family grow, so does your frustration. At first, you think it's just a matter of being more diligent and making constant notes for yourself as reminders. You try to laugh it off, but when it doesn't seem to go away you become concerned.

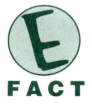

FACT

In 2003, the *Journal of Gerontology: Psychological Sciences* reported a study that examined the relationship between leisure activities and the loss of mental function in 107 pairs of twins; in each pair, one twin had some degree of cognitive impairment. They found that reading, going to movies, visiting museums, and socializing with friends during early and middle adulthood helped lower the risk of developing Alzheimer's disease.

Frustration is not necessarily a behavior; it's more a reaction to what's going on, and it completely describes how you are feeling in the early stages of Alzheimer's. You're used to being in charge, handling any situation, and getting things done. But, as you see your memory slipping, this chips away at your confidence.

There are some basic things you can do to help relieve some of your frustration. You're already making notes to yourself, but here are some more tips.

- Exercise your brain cells. It's been said that we only use 10 percent of our brain. So, dust off the cobwebs in your mind and start doing crossword puzzles, join a reading club, and read more "intellectual" books.
- Turn on your computer's memory alert function to remind you of things to do.
- Use bright-colored reminder Post-Its.
- Take another look at those books you already have on how to improve your memory.
- Eat fish; we've always known it's "brain food," now science has proven it's so.
- Cut down on alcohol, sugar, aspartame sweetener, and MSG. They all interfere with brain function. Alcohol makes you dull; sugar makes you foggy; aspartame and MSG are brain "excitotoxins" and can lead to brain cell death.

Irritability and Mood Swings

Irritability and mood swings typically manifest themselves in Stages 3 and 4. Frustration leads directly to symptoms of irritability. You grind your teeth; you grimace; you scream in frustration, and then you get irritable. You get irritable at things and people. You get irritable at people mostly because they complain that you've changed and ask you why you are so upset at seemingly insignificant things. The other side of irritability is that it serves to push people away who might be asking too many questions about what is going on with you. Mostly you are frustrated and mad that you are feeling confused and disoriented and don't know why.

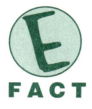

FACT

ABC News reported on August 18, 2003, that researchers had discovered the reason for teen mood swings. Dr. Jay Giedd, following teens from age thirteen using MRI scans, thinks it's because the self-control and judgment area of the brain, the prefrontal cortex, matures in the twenties. Researchers previously thought that the brain had reached 90 percent of its full size by age six.

Mood swings are another aspect of Alzheimer's that is hard to ignore. From tears to tantrums in a split second is not unusual. And you don't seem to have any control over these dramatic emotions.

If you already know your diagnosis is Alzheimer's, your irritability and mood swings express the fear and frustration of having this disease. In order to deal with your emotional symptoms, it may be very helpful to seek out a psychologist or psychotherapist. Support and counseling can help you learn ways to cope with your diagnosis. A counselor can meet with you and your family to help you express your needs and offer support in putting your needs first. Counselors also can help sort out the difficult decisions of future living arrangements.

Confusion and Depression

Confusion and depression typically manifest in Stage 5. Confusion is not really a behavior, but it's how you feel when you can't find something or get lost in a familiar place. One recommendation is to always keep a card with you that says, "I have Alzheimer's, sometimes I get confused, please be patient, here is my address and a number to call for help."

This may sound a lot like a note that you gave your kids when they were young, and it may feel like you are just too dependent on others. But the reality is that bouts of confusion do occur even though you may still be quite independent, and carrying a note is the best way to handle such emergencies.

E ALERT!

It's often difficult to sort out depression from dementia. In the *Psychiatric Times*, February 1998, Dr. Susie Blackmun said that depression, certain types of dementia, and normal aging can all cause the same types of behaviors. Only by using a series of neuropsychological tests for normal aging, dementia, and depression can we differentiate between the three.

Depression is also a common part of the Alzheimer's picture. Who wouldn't be in low spirits to know that their memory is failing? The period of not knowing can be very difficult. In finding the diagnosis, while it relieves the anxiety of not knowing, the reality of having a diagnosis of Alzheimer's is in no way comforting. You are entitled to feel depressed, but there are ways to cope, people that will support you, and steps you can take to treat depression. Ways of dealing with depression include:

- Talking with a therapist, social worker, or psychotherapist to help put your symptoms into perspective.
- Getting some exercise every day to help your whole body, including your mind, feel more energized.
- Eating well, getting your sleep, and taking a good multiple vitamin and mineral to make sure you are getting appropriate nutrients.
- Sharing your concerns with your family and planning together for the future.
- Seeing your doctor about taking low levels of appropriate medication for your depression.

Agitation

The dictionary definition of agitation is nervous anxiety. It's not just nervousness and not just anxiety, and it's more than the sum of the two together because it also includes depression and irritability. Agitation is a feeling of not being quite right in your own skin. As the frustration and irritability build, a complex set of behaviors results in agitation. It may present itself as constant pacing, screaming, asking the same question constantly, repeating the same words over and over, or aggressive behavior; it typically manifests in Stages 5 and 6. Complicating matters even further is the possibility that agitation may be due to coexisting medical conditions and medications that are used in the treatment of Alzheimer's. Physical symptoms of tiredness, lack of sleep, and fatigue can all lead to an increased level of agitation.

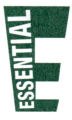

French gerontologist Dr. Elisabeth Kruczek reported in the May 1993 issue of *Lancet* that "contact with pets can spontaneously induce extended periods of calm, on occasions even permitting a reduction in amount of sedative therapy required." Dr. Kruczek remarked on "a particularly agitated patient, who would spend the whole day pacing to and fro, would stop to caress a cat for a whole hour."

Changes in the surrounding environment can also lead to agitation or an increase in symptoms of agitation. Such changes could be moving to a new home or to a nursing home, a change in caregivers, or anything that seems to threaten security and stability. The obvious recommendations to prevent or treat agitation include trying to keep the living environment as stable and structured as possible.

Agitation can be scary for caregivers as well as for the afflicted individual. Depending on the level of anxiety, agitation can "paralyze" a person and make it difficult for them to go about their daily routine. This makes the role of caregivers even more necessary, yet at the same time, they can become more exhausted by giving constant reassurance to someone who is agitated.

When to Bring in the Doctor

At the onset of noticeable agitation or if the level of agitation increases drastically, a medical assessment is warranted. Especially if the level of communication is low, someone who is agitated might not know that they have an underlying infection, for example, that could be triggering internal alarms such as fever, pain, dehydration, and general discomfort.

People with Alzheimer's who need glasses and hearing aids often pull them out and discard them when in an agitated state. This can only lead to more agitation, however, if they are unable to properly hear or see. During the possible years of confinement with Alzheimer's, it is also important to recognize that hearing or vision may become impaired and should be corrected.

Do a Medication and Nutrition Check

Specific medications may cause agitation; it may happen more often, however, in the case of multiple prescriptions. A pharmacist can often, with or without the use of a computer program, analyze a list of medications and their possible interactions.

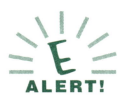
ALERT!

Sarah Green-Burger wrote a June 2000 report called "Malnutrition and Dehydration in Nursing Homes" for the National Citizens' Coalition for Nursing Home Reform. She found that from 35 to 85 percent of U.S. nursing home residents are malnourished, and 30 to 50 percent of residents are substandard in bodyweight. The Nursing Home Reform Act of 1987 was enacted to prevent both malnutrition and dehydration.

Simple dehydration can cause the brain to react in strange ways. Fogginess, dizziness, and lack of concentration are all symptoms of dehydration. And in the Alzheimer's brain, we don't even know the possible effects. The same goes with nutrition; it's crucial to get the right protein, carbohydrates, and fats from the plate into the mouth. Keep a diet log; if you don't, several meals can go by with different caregivers, and your patient hasn't eaten more than a few bites.

Treatment for Agitation

Agitation is treated first with behavioral modification and second with the addition of prescription drugs. In order to apply behavioral modification, you first have to find out what is aggravating the behavior. We must concede that a certain amount of agitation is part of the Alzheimer's picture. But if there is excessive agitation of recent onset, then we must identify the cause and then either eliminate the cause or circumnavigate it.

As mentioned above, there are many potential causes in the living environment that may increase agitation; changes can be as seemingly insignificant as a new tablecloth. We have no way of knowing what a person may focus on to give them a sense of continuity and stability. The major changes, however, can be arrived at through a commonsense evaluation of the person's environment.

It could be a new room, a new house, moving to a nursing home, loss of a caregiver or change in caregiver, a recent trip outside the home, a recent hospitalization for an acute illness, visitors or overnight guests, or simply being dressed or bathed by a caregiver. Any of these day-to-day routines can present a mental or emotional overload to an Alzheimer's person.

This Is Not a Debate

In a situation where you are the caregiver dealing with someone who is agitated, it's not a matter of trying to convince them that what you are doing is the right thing. They don't care; they don't even know what you are talking about. They just know they don't like it, and it's making them very anxious and agitated. In a way, it is very much like dealing with a small child. You distract; you reframe; you redirect the conversation or the activity, and hopefully the agitation will calm down. A commonsense approach to keeping the level of anxiety and agitation down is to "Keep it simple."

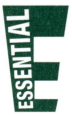

Decluttering may seem like another huge task, so make it a family affair. If it's your parents' home with decades of accumulation, make a plan first. This is the time to organize the family album. Sort out what needs to go and what stays, and when it comes to moving furniture and appliances, don't be afraid to hire some help.

You need to cut down on clutter in the home and remove unnecessary stimulation from radio and TV. Use neutral colors in the bedroom;

create a daily routine; build in a rest period after each activity; have a few stuffed toys as a "security blanket"; use good lighting especially late in the afternoon and evening to reduce agitation (full spectrum lighting that mimics the rays of daylight might be most beneficial); play soothing music, and offer healthy meals, limiting the stimulants coffee and sugar.

How to Avoid and Handle Agitation

Usually a heightened level of agitation can't be sustained for a long period of time. It just takes too much energy. So agitation tends to occur episodically. It's important for caregivers to learn how to handle these episodes. Remember, the guiding principle of a caregiver is to offer comfort, dignity, and respect. Your mother, father, or client is agitated for some reason; you may or may not know the reason, but it's important to bring the situation under control.

First of all, let's consider ways to avoid agitation. Eliminate the frustration factor. Organize eating, dressing, and bathing after a rest period and be ready to curtail or modify at the first signs of frustration. Become a master of distraction. Their attention span is very short, and distractions do work. If buttering toast causes frustration, offer a cup of tea. Keep explanations simple. Gently guide activities. Use loving and kind words and gestures. Keep the exit doors locked to prevent wandering. Try to avoid the use of restraints, which causes more agitation.

How to Divert an Episode of Agitation

It's not always possible to prevent agitation. The following guidelines can help you learn how to guide them right out of the picture. First, you physically and verbally back away. If arms are flailing or objects are being thrown, don't endanger yourself; don't confront; step back until the moment passes. Be calm and reassuring; when you speak, offer reassurances, apologies, and safety.

Use what you know about your Alzheimer's patient to offer them something they usually see as positive. Of course you must always be aware that there could be an injury, a need to use the bathroom, a need for more light, a hunger, a thirst, or just fatigue. Assess whether a change of scenery or shutting off all stimulation would be appropriate.

It's Time for Medications

If you've stabilized the home environment and are using behavioral modification, but the level of agitation is escalating, your next step is to turn to medication. Especially when medications become part of the treatment program, an accurate way of monitoring improvement and side effects must be employed. Sometimes, if side effects occur, you can't really tell if they are due to the drug or part of the complex of Alzheimer's symptoms.

E ALERT!

The caregiver must be in charge of medications. You can never assume an Alzheimer's patient will take his or her own medications. In order to make sure it is taken you might have to put the medication in your patient's food. Be aware that if paranoia is an issue, they might think they are being poisoned.

Make a list of current symptoms before starting any medications. There are various types of charts that are available from your doctor for following Alzheimer's symptoms. Pharmaceutical companies use these charts in clinical trials to determine the effect of their drugs, and caregivers use them to chart progress or decline. Doctors like to see these charts on a regular basis so they too can monitor progress.

The rules in implementing medication are universal, but even more important in Alzheimer's patients. Only start one medication at a time; begin with the lowest dose possible; chart any change in symptoms; and chart any side effects.

Compulsive Behavior and Restlessness

Humans, in an attempt to influence their fate, will often develop a set of ritual behaviors. It's a minor variant of obsessive-compulsive behavior. Athletes often express ritualistic behavior: They wear the same socks or carry some "lucky" talisman. Some people count or repeat phrases like, "oh my, oh my," over and over. Some Alzheimer's sufferers also shout out profane words in what appears to be a compulsive way. It's a form of trying to get control of a seemingly uncontrollable situation. Other compulsive behaviors include dry-washing the hands or rubbing parts of the body.

Restlessness is a form of burning off energy that builds up due to frustration and agitation. It can take the form of constant pacing back and forth or checking to see if the stove is off or the doors are locked.

These behaviors are in the later stages of Alzheimer's, and they are very difficult for caregivers to deal with. If you attempt to stop a compulsive or ritualistic behavior, you can cause a considerable amount of distress and agitation in the Alzheimer's sufferer. The most appropriate response is to try to offer a distracting activity, but if that doesn't work, just allow the behavior until they have no more energy for it.

Severe Mood Swings, Aggressiveness, and Combativeness

Alzheimer's treatment programs call this set of behaviors the "challenging" ones. That's putting a positive spin on behavior that to the outside observer seems to be intent on driving you, the caregiver, crazy. If you have had children, you can relate to the terrible twos; now you have to adopt that same mindset for the "terrible eighties." Of course, you may not have handled it well back then, but now with guidance and specific instructions, you will do just fine.

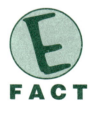

FACT

A November 2003 issue of the *New England Journal of Medicine* reported that family members who care for relatives with dementia experience even more stress in the year before the patient dies. According to the study, more than six million adults in the United States presently provide long-term, unpaid care to elderly members of their family, of which two million have dementia.

The tension and frustration you feel as a caregiver is absolutely normal. Don't feel guilty about these feelings. The main thing to remember is not to take it personally. The behavior you are witnessing has nothing to do with you and everything to do with the person you are caring for.

Repetition of words, although not an aggressive activity, can be very annoying. One way of dealing with this behavior is to say your own repetitive mantra, "this is the disease talking, this is the disease talking." It helps you remember that all these symptoms are, indeed, the result of Alzheimer's.

Assessing the Cause

As with the other behaviors mentioned, it's time to assess what is causing the mood swings, aggressiveness, and combativeness. The reasons could be so varied that you need a checklist. After a while, the checklist may become automatic and you can, almost intuitively, know what's causing the outrageous behavior.

The reason could be that a new person becomes involved with the patient's care. There could be excessive activity and overstimulation on a particular day. They could have pain or symptoms of an acute illness, or be experiencing side effects of medications. They could suddenly be unable to do tasks or activities that they were once able to do and become agitated, or are no longer able to communicate their desires or needs.

Responding to Challenging Behaviors

How to respond to the challenging behaviors is much like responding to agitation and irritability, but there is a heightened level of intensity and even a feeling of danger that as a caregiver you can't help but feel. After all, we have grown up associating aggressive behavior and combativeness with danger. But this behavior is occurring in someone who may be your mother or father or a client, and who has no intentions of harming you.

ALERT!

Creating a safe space for you and your Alzheimer's patient is very important. As with a small child, you must keep all sharp objects (scissors, knives, letter openers) and golf clubs, baseball clubs, or anything that can be thrown, hidden away out of sight. With no other way to express themselves, Alzheimer's patients often hit and throw.

First, become very calm and centered, take deep breaths, and relax. Sometimes your calmness actually rubs off, just as an angry tone or impatience will also be felt. Be very patient and realize you are doing exactly what you should be doing by being very quiet. In our very busy and stressed-out lives, we think we always have to be doing something, and there is no question that there is a lot to do when you are a caregiver for someone with Alzheimer's. But at this moment, you want to stop time and just be.

Don't Argue

This is the worst time to argue or try to make your mother, father, or client do something they don't want to do. That is often the reason they start to fight you. If they ask or motion to do something else, be flexible and go with their wishes.

As in dealing with agitation, after the dust settles, do a retrospective assessment and try to find the possible cause of the escalation in behavior. Afterward, chart the behavior and make notes about corresponding events and try to understand the pattern of behavior leading up to the event. Above all, seek support and guidance from the doctor or local support groups on coping skills.

Paranoia, Delusions, and Hallucinations

Paranoia, delusions, and hallucinations are the hallmark symptoms of the final stages of Alzheimer's. Individuals experience symptoms of paranoia during which they really believe someone is breaking into the house, or someone is trying to poison them. Paranoia is an extreme and unreasonable suspicion of other people and their motives. Reassurance is the best way to deal with paranoia.

Delusion is a persistent false idea. Delusions can range from patients believing they are being held hostage to being a member of a royal family. In order to deal with delusions, you don't want to enter into the delusion, but you nod and listen and never contradict what the Alzheimer's patient says.

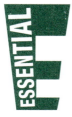

Hallucinations should be checked out by the doctor who will evaluate medications and physical symptoms. Other physical disorders such as kidney or bladder infections, dehydration, intense pain, or alcohol or drug abuse must be ruled out. In rare cases, hallucinations are caused by schizophrenia that coincides with the Alzheimer's condition.

Hallucinations are due to false perceptions; patients may imagine that there are people or things in the room that are not really there. The patient may also experience an auditory hallucination, during which he or she hears voices or singing. Sensory hallucinations of touch, taste, and smell can occur when the patient feels something touching or crawling on them, tastes something in their food that isn't there, or smells something. Often the taste and smell hallucinations turn into paranoia about being poisoned or gassed. These are very frightening occurrences.

Dealing with Hallucinations

Constant reassurance is the best way of dealing with paranoia; hallucinations, however, can be much more difficult to contain. Nodding and agreeing is the best approach. You don't want to start telling them that yes, you see their hallucination, because you can't. But you don't want to deny what they are seeing, either. That will only cause more agitation.

If hallucinations become constant, it's time to check with the doctor. They may be a result of medication side effects or some acute physical problem not related to Alzheimer's. Even simple dehydration can cause brain irritation that can worsen Alzheimer's symptoms.

Get an Eye and Ear Checkup

Now is the time to make sure your patient's eyes and ears are functioning optimally. Poor eyesight can make shadows appear real, and poor hearing can turn normal sounds into mumbles.

All the advice for agitation and challenging behaviors applies here as well. Be calm; be centered; be reassuring; and be supportive. Be ready to talk about your patient's experience if he or she wants to. Distraction works for hallucinations as well as other symptoms of Alzheimer's.

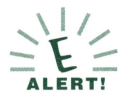

ALERT!

It is important for caregivers to have back-up support, time off, respite, and a chance to recharge during these intense periods. You need time with other people who don't have Alzheimer's so that you don't get pulled entirely into an unreal world. Remember, by taking care of yourself, you are also taking care of your Alzheimer's patient.

When you see the telltale signs of eyes focusing on nothing, an ear cocked when there is no sound, or hands flicking off imaginary bugs, just put a reassuring hand on the patient's shoulder, and they may snap out of their hallucination when they look at you. Increasing the lighting can help remove shadows or reflections. Putting on some gentle music or moving to another room can also banish hallucinations. One common recommendation is to remove or cover mirrors, because at this stage, your patient may see a stranger looking back at them. Ⓔ

Chapter 8

Medical Treatment for Alzheimer's

Worldwide funding for Alzheimer's is currently split between researching the cause and the treatment. As we understand what causes damage to the brain and consequent symptoms, we learn how to prevent and delay the process. The current focus of treatment is on the alleviation of symptoms and on early diagnosis. Many of the newer drugs available can help people improve their mental symptoms for months to years, increasing the chances of finding a cure in time to help them.

Medical Treatment Strategies

There are three aspects of Alzheimer's disease that can be treated with medications: cognitive symptoms (memory, thinking, and perception), behavioral symptoms (agitation, anxiety, and irritability), and insomnia.

It is important, however, to begin with only one medication at a time, use the lowest dose possible to achieve the most benefit, and chart any and all changes in symptoms. You should also be aware that sedative medications, which are used to treat insomnia or sleep problems, may cause grogginess, confusion, incontinence, instability, falls, or increased agitation. These drugs must be used with caution, and caregivers need to be aware of these possible side effects.

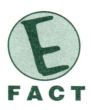

FACT

Alzheimer's Disease International keeps records of the worldwide incidence of Alzheimer's disease. Based on current statistics and the increasing proportion of people that are over sixty-five, they estimate that by 2025, the number of people in the world with dementia will rise to a frightening 34 million.

The U.S. Food and Drug Administration (FDA) has approved two classes of drugs to treat cognitive symptoms of Alzheimer's disease: cholinesterase inhibitors and NMDA(N-methyl-D-aspartate) receptor antagonists, also called glutamate blockers. To date, five drugs are FDA approved for use in treating Alzheimer's cognitive symptoms. (Many more are in the research pipeline.) The following four are from the class of drugs called cholinesterase inhibitors:

- Cognex (THA)
- Aricept
- Exelon
- Reminyl

Cholinesterase Inhibitors

Cholinesterase inhibitors act to prevent breakdown of a very important neurotransmitter called acetylcholine. Acetylcholine is found in the brain and spinal cord and in nerve/muscle junctions. It is made from acetyl CoA and choline. After acetylcholine is produced, it normally transmits a message and is then broken down, by a special enzyme called cholinesterase, back to its original constituents—acetyl CoA and choline.

Cholinesterase inhibitor drugs prevent the breakdown of acetylcholine, thus allowing it to build up, and make more acetylcholine available in the brain to carry messages between the brain cells. A lower-than-normal level of acetylcholine in the brain is one of the characteristics of Alzheimer's. This decrease is caused by destruction of brain cells that normally make and release acetylcholine.

E ALERT!

The poison curare is able to paralyze muscles because it blocks the transmission of acetylcholine. Some nerve gases act by preventing acetylcholine from breaking down, causing constant stimulation of the receptor cells; this leads to intense spasms of the muscles, including the heart. In myasthenia gravis, the body produces anti-bodies against its own acetylcholine receptors in the neuromuscular junctions and causes muscle weakness and paralysis.

Research shows that cholinesterase inhibitors that act on the brain increase cerebral blood flow when measured by SPECT scans. The increased blood flow is in brain regions affected by Alzheimer's disease. They only work, however, in the mild to moderate stages of Alzheimer's disease because functioning nerve cells are necessary to make acetylcholine in the first place. These cells are gradually lost, and in the late stages of Alzheimer's, there are not enough to make any acetylcholine or pass any messages.

Cognex—The First Alzheimer's Drug

Cognex deserves a special place in the Alzheimer's Hall of Fame. It was the first Alzheimer's drug approved by the FDA (1993). It has a long and unpronounceable scientific name, Tetrahydroaminoacridine; the short form is THA, and the drug name is Cognex. It's a "crossover" drug. It's a cholinesterase inhibitor, but it also has beneficial effects on behavior.

In most patients who took Cognex, doctors found moderate improvement in cognitive symptoms with no change in the progression of the disease. It also has a dramatic effect on the behavior of an Alzheimer's sufferer. Most notable is a decrease in symptoms such as apathy, irritability, and agitation.

Along with effects come side effects. The downside of Cognex is a high rate of liver enzyme elevation; 50 percent of all people who take Cognex have a rise in liver enzymes after a month or six weeks on the drug. For this reason it is rarely prescribed.

Drug interactions can occur with other medicines that increase acetylcholine activity. These include medicines for myasthenia gravis (e.g., neostigmine, edrophonium chloride, distigmine bromide, and pyridostigmine bromide); other Alzheimer's medicines (e.g., galantamine and donepezil); and medicines for urinary retention (e.g., carbachol and bethanechol chloride pilocarpine).

Aricept

Aricept, approved in 1996, was designed to be a substitute for Cognex and its toxic liver effects. Its generic name is donepezil. In the U.K., it became the first Alzheimer's drug to be approved, in 1997. It is specifically intended for people with mild to moderate Alzheimer's disease, but it won't help everybody, and it is not a cure. It does one of four things: It can do nothing; it may cause symptoms to improve; it may halt the progression of symptoms; or it could cause side effects.

In one study, compared to the effects of a placebo, 50 percent of the placebo group got worse, which is the normal course of events. But only about 33 percent of those on Aricept got worse. Those people on Aricept were twice as likely to show some improvement in thinking, understanding, problem solving, and overall symptoms. In those patients that improved, if they stopped Aricept after two years, it took another six months for Alzheimer's symptoms to become worse.

Aricept comes in two strengths, 5 milligrams and 10 mg, to be taken once a day in the evening. It is a good idea to start on the lower dose to lessen any side effects. There is no need for blood testing because there is no liver enzyme elevation with Aricept. It does, however, have side effects of diarrhea, nausea, vomiting, muscle cramps, insomnia, loss of appetite, and fatigue; they mostly occur at the beginning of treatment and usually subside. Aricept could possibly worsen the symptoms of stomach ulcers, asthma, and some heart diseases.

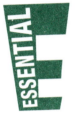

If you have side effects from your cholinesterase drug and your doctor decides that you should stop it, you can do that without experiencing rebound effects or worsening your condition. After about four to six weeks, however, any benefits that you may have had will wear off.

Aricept is usually safe when taken with common drugs such as theophyllin, warfarin, cimetidine, and digoxin. Aricept may interact with some antidepressants, anesthetics, antihistamines, and some painkillers. Your doctor or pharmacist should be aware of all your medications.

Reminyl

Reminyl was approved for the treatment of mild to moderate Alzheimer's in 2000. Its generic name is galantamine. It has much the same indications and moderately successful effects as Aricept, as it is also a cholinesterase inhibitor. Large placebo-controlled, double-blind studies on about 3,000 patients over six months have been done on Reminyl. In one study, on an Alzheimer's scoring system, there was no change in score; in another study, one-third of patients improved their score by four points. The usual annual increase in symptoms is between five and eleven points. 15 percent of people taking the placebo, however, also improved by the same amount in exactly the same way.

Reminyl treats cognitive symptoms, but it is also beneficial for behavioral symptoms such as anxiety, hallucinations, and wandering. In one five-month study, patients' behavioral symptoms as well as activities of daily living did not worsen, whereas those on placebo worsened significantly.

Reminyl comes in 4 mg, 8 mg, and 12 mg tablets. The initial dosage is 4 milligrams twice per day. After one month, the dose may be increased.

The most common side effects are nausea and vomiting, which usually go away with time. Other less common side effects may include abdominal pain, confusion, diarrhea, decreased appetite, dizziness, falling, headache, indigestion, nasal congestion, tiredness, sleep disturbance, urinary tract infection, and weight loss. Rarely, trembling, a slow heartbeat, or fainting may occur.

E ALERT!

Anticholinesterase inhibitors have the opposite effect of anticholinergic medicines, which work by decreasing the activity of acetylcholine. Therefore, they may oppose the effect of the following classes of medicines, making them less effective: anticholinergic medicines for Parkinson's disease, asthma drugs, antispasmodics for gut disorders, and medicines for urinary incontinence.

Drug interactions with Reminyl come mainly from Parkinson's drugs, drugs that treat diarrhea and asthma, as well as heart drugs (digoxin, quinidine, or beta-blockers). A lower dose of Reminyl may be necessary if you are taking antidepressants such as paroxetine, fluoxetine, or fluvoxamine; an antifungal drug, such as ketoconazole; or an HIV drug, such as ritonavir. Reminyl should not be taken if you have severe liver and/or kidney disease. Your doctor will watch you closely if you have acute abdominal pain, asthma, epilepsy, heart disease, liver or kidney problems, ulcers, urinary retention, an allergy to the pill's lactose or yellow dye coating, or have had recent surgery.

Exelon

Exelon is the brand name for rivastigmine, a cholinesterase inhibitor approved by the FDA in 2000 for mild to moderately severe Alzheimer's disease. By the time it reached the market, about 5,200 people had been treated. Exelon increases the level of acetylcholine in the brain to improve thinking, learning, memory, and the symptoms of dementia and daily functioning in Alzheimer's disease.

1.5 milligrams of Exelon is taken twice daily in capsule form with meals. The maximum dose is 6 milligrams twice daily. The main side effects may include nausea, vomiting, abdominal pain, and loss of appetite, which lessen as your system gets used to the drug. Other less common side effects include agitation, chest pain, confusion, depression, dizziness, fainting, hallucinations, headache, indigestion, rash, seizures, sleep disturbance, sweating, tremors, ulcers, and weight loss.

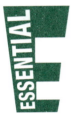

At least half of the people who take cholinesterase inhibitors do not respond to them. But when they do work, they can make a significant difference in quality of life and activities of daily living. That's why a trial period, in which you take one or more of these drugs, is usually recommended by your neurologist.

Exelon should be used with caution in those with asthma, chronic obstructive pulmonary disease, epilepsy, heart rhythm problems, decreased kidney function, Parkinson's disease, peptic ulcer, and sick sinus syndrome.

The Fifth Drug

Namenda, with the brand name of Memantine, was approved by the FDA in 2003, but it has been used in Germany since 1989. It is used to treat cognitive symptoms, but it acts by a different mechanism than the cholinesterase inhibitors. The Alzheimer's brain is flooded by excess neurotransmitters called glutamate, which leak out of damaged cells. Namenda prevents this excess glutamate from interfering with learning and memory. Namenda's side effects are mostly mild. They are nausea, restlessness, stomachache, and headache.

An important aspect of Alzheimer's research is that MSG is a potent glutamate precursor. Its real name is monosodium glutamate. MSG is called an excitotoxin. Excess levels, when taken into the body through processed food or Chinese food, can cause overstimulation of brain cells to the point of collapse. Neurologists who know about the dangers of MSG recommend their Alzheimer's patients avoid it. The same can be said for another excitotoxin called aspartame. It's the artificial sweetener in all processed diet foods and drinks. It too can cause brain cell death and should be avoided.

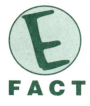

Namenda is the only FDA-approved Alzheimer's drug that appears to work on the late stages of Alzheimer's. Your doctor will only be able to determine if this drug is going to work for you on an individual basis. Your caregiver's careful record keeping of your progress will help decide whether you will remain on the drug or be taken off.

Because Namenda works by a different mechanism than the cholinesterase inhibitors, researchers hoped that the drugs could work together to achieve better control of Alzheimer's symptoms. In June of 2003, however, the Fisher Center for Alzheimer's Research at Rockefeller University announced the bad news.

There is no additional improvement in the action of the three widely used cholinesterase inhibitors when Namenda is added. Alzheimer's patients in the study who took a cholinesterase inhibitor and Namenda together exhibited no improvements on memory tests. And even those taking a cholinesterase drug and placebo did not decline as much as would have been expected. Scientists are at a loss to explain why this occurred. Most geriatricians, however, know that the more medications that elderly people are on, the greater their symptoms of dementia.

Are There Any Other Drugs for Cognition?

There are several drugs with some evidence of benefit for Alzheimer's patients: a Parkinson's drug called selegiline, prednisone, nonsteroidal anti-inflammatory drugs (NSAIDs), and estrogen. Prednisone was not considered for Alzheimer's treatment because of its long list of side effects that include diabetes, osteoporosis, and adrenal gland suppression. The Parkinson's drug selegiline (also known by the brand names Carbex and Eldepryl), at a dosage of 5 milligrams twice a day, may slow the progression of Alzheimer's, but further research is needed. It may have some antioxidant properties but has several side effects. It lowers blood pressure and can cause nausea, dizziness, or vivid dreams.

Not NSAIDs

Several studies, which were not specifically looking for an association between NSAIDs and Alzheimer's, pointed out that people who used these drugs did seem to have a lower incidence of Alzheimer's. People using NSAIDs such as aspirin, ibuprofen, and naproxen had as much as a 30 percent reduced risk of Alzheimer's. Since the drugs still carried the risk of stomach ulcer formation and internal bleeding, specific studies were initiated to determine whether the drugs really do lessen the risk of Alzheimer's.

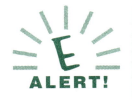

Studies are necessary to show whether a drug will be beneficial for Alzheimer's because their negative side effects may outweigh their benefits. In two studies by Dr. Marie Griffin and her colleagues, NSAIDs have been associated with about 20 to 30 percent of all hospital admissions and deaths due to stomach ulcers in patients aged sixty-five and older.

Researchers enrolled 351 mild to moderate Alzheimer's patients in a NSAID study and reported their results in the *Journal of the American Medical Association* in 2003. Two drugs used for arthritis, rofecoxib and Vioxx, and an over-the-counter (OTC) analgesic, naproxen, were tested for one year. The results showed no reduction of mental deterioration in people given the drugs when compared to another group given a placebo.

Besides the expected nausea, ulcers, and internal bleeding, those who took the drugs had a higher incidence of dizziness, fatigue, dry mouth, and high blood pressure than people who took a placebo. The conclusion was that Alzheimer's patients should not use NSAIDs in the hopes that it will treat their disease.

What about Estrogen?

Estrogen apparently affects the memory center of the brain, the hippocampus, which is also one of the first areas to be impacted by

Alzheimer's. Decades of research, mostly in animals, show positive effects of estrogen on memory. In large studies of women on estrogen, there seems to be a decreased risk of Alzheimer's and an associated increase in cognitive function. Research shows that it enhances the growth of nerve fibers from specific memory nerve cells. Estrogen, like most hormones, has some antioxidant and anti-inflammatory effects. The combination of all these beneficial effects created frenzied activity around the use of estrogen in Alzheimer's treatment. Estrogen was even found to decrease amyloid production by cells and to lower amyloid levels in the brains of living animals.

Finally, the National Institute on Aging sponsored a clinical trial to prove whether estrogen actually altered the course of Alzheimer's. The results were disappointing. In a population of older women with moderate to severe Alzheimer's, it did not improve cognitive or functional outcomes or slow the progression of the disease. Another study of women with mild to moderate Alzheimer's disease, which treated the patients for sixteen weeks with estrogen, showed no significant differences between the treatment and placebo groups.

ESSENTIAL

Indirect marketing of Premarin, an estrogen made from pregnant mare's urine, began in 1966 with a book by Dr. Robert A. Wilson called *Feminine Forever*, sponsored by Wyeth Pharmaceuticals. In order to remain "young, attractive, and sexually active," women were told to take the hormone. With no evidence to back up these claims, women who were in the menopausal age group were immediately placed on hormone replacement therapy.

Several more studies were done, all with the same negative results. Even worse, in May 2003, statistics developed at a five-year follow-up of the large and rigorous Women's Health Initiative called WHIMS (Women's Health Initiative Memory Study) revealed that healthy women aged sixty-five and older who took Prempro, a popular combination of synthetic estrogen and progestin, had twice the rate of dementia, including Alzheimer's, as women who did not take the medication. The study certainly didn't prove that this drug causes Alzheimer's, but it proved that it isn't an effective treatment.

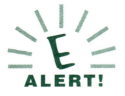

ALERT!

Based on recent definitive studies, on February 11, 2004, the U.S. FDA announced that hormone replacement therapy (HRT) products containing either estrogen or a combination of estrogen and progestin must show a warning label to the effect that combined estrogen/progestin treatment increases the risk of developing dementia.

Medications for Agitation

There really isn't a specific "agitation" medication. Since agitation in Alzheimer's is a combination of anxiety, depression, and irritability, there are a variety of medications that might prove useful. Antidepressant medications that can help the depression and irritability include Celexa, Paxil, Prozac, and Zoloft. Shorter acting drugs that are used for the treatment of anxiety, restlessness, verbal aggression, and resistant behavior include anxiolytics such as Ativan and Serax.

If the anti-anxiety and antidepressant drugs don't work or if the patient is within the worsening stages of agitation, stronger medications called antipsychotics are used. For these patients, agitation is accompanied by delusions, hallucinations, aggressive behavior, hostility, and a total lack of cooperation. The names of these medications are Zyprexa and Risperdal.

Additional drugs that treat agitation include anticonvulsants such as Tegretol; these drugs also treat mood swings. Depakote has been used to partially treat hostility and aggression.

Sleeping Medications

Sleeping medications are called sedatives. They slow down a person's functioning on all levels, not just the nervous system. They may cause drowsiness, but they also cause a lot of other side effects. They can cause incontinence, imbalance, falling, and increased agitation.

At first you might think the side effects of these drugs are symptoms of worsening Alzheimer's. Stopping the medication, however, will cause a reversal of symptoms. If these drugs are used, they must be used very cautiously with awareness of their potential side effects.

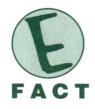

FACT

According to sleep experts, nine out of ten people experience insomnia at some point in their lives, and one in three adults has a problem with insomnia every year. With age, sleep becomes fragmented. Some reasons include lower levels of melatonin, the hormone that helps control sleep; increased sensitivity to noise; more illness, depression, and anxiety; and neurological conditions such as Alzheimer's disease and Parkinson's disease.

Clinical Trials

It is possible that you or your loved one may be asked to participate in a clinical trial. It seems like every month, drug companies are announcing a new Alzheimer's drug that they feel will be *the* answer. All these drugs must eventually be tested on Alzheimer's patients, and you may be one of them. You and your family may even want to be proactive about entering a clinical trial so you can be in on the latest developments from pharmaceutical companies.

The Alzheimer's Association and many other Alzheimer's organizations and hospitals have specific information about clinical trials. You will want to know what they are, how they work, who gets to participate, and the risks and benefits; you will also need help with making a decision about entering a trial.

What Is a Clinical Trial?

Briefly, a clinical trial is a necessary part of drug research to find out if a new drug is safe and effective in a human population. By the time a drug gets to the human trial stage, it has been proven safe in animals. A clinical trial protocol defines who can participate in a study and all the tests, procedures, medications, and dosages that are prescribed, as well as the duration of the study. Drug companies usually pay for clinical trials, and the trials are run by researchers and doctors in hospitals or universities.

The best part of a clinical trial is that frequent appointments are made for patients to see the research staff in order to monitor symptoms, both good and bad. The worst part is that you may or may not get the real drug. If the trial is a placebo-control, you may get the placebo (the inactive pill).

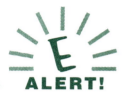

ALERT!

Jerry Phillips, from the Office of Post Marketing Drug Risk Assessment at the FDA, confirms that, "in the broader area of adverse drug reaction data, the 250,000 reports received annually probably represent only 5 percent of the actual reactions that occur." Dr. Jay Cohen comments that there are, in reality, five million medication reactions each year. These are found after the drug is licensed by post marketing surveillance.

The Institutional Review Board

An Institutional Review Board (IRB), usually in a hospital or university, is set up to oversee and monitor every clinical trial in the United States. The IRB members are independent physicians, statisticians, and community advocates who ensure that a clinical trial is ethical and the participants' rights are protected. The IRB ensures that the risks of a particular study are as low as possible and that the benefits outweigh the risks.

Informed Consent

Most of us are familiar with signing an informed consent paper for surgery. It's the same with a clinical trial. Researchers are obliged to inform you of all the important aspects of the research trial, including the type of drug or treatment, the side effects, the expected benefits, whether similar treatments are available, and your right to leave the trial at any time. After you and your family are clear on all aspects of the trial, you will be asked to sign an informed consent.

Regular Checkups with Your Doctor

It's important to have regular checkups with your doctor to monitor your condition and your response to any medications you may be on. Your doctor will have done what's called a baseline assessment, using specific tests, during your initial visits for Alzheimer's. This assessment is kept on record, and at all other visits, the tests are repeated and compared to the first. It's important to have this baseline to know how you felt and what symptoms you had when you were first diagnosed and also to help evaluate medications.

The most common medical test is the Mini-Mental State Examination (MMSE) given by a doctor. Another test is a questionnaire called the Physical Self-Maintenance Scale (PSMS), which can be filled out by a caregiver. Both of them together help establish baseline memory, thinking, language, and functional ability. Behavioral symptoms, such as agitation, psychosis, anxiety, and depression, are also on record as part of the baseline assessment.

Ongoing Evaluation

Your doctor will usually see you every three to six months after your initial diagnosis, and every three months if you have started any medication. When you are stabilized on the medication, the visits are usually every six months.

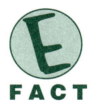

FACT

In 2000, *The American Journal of Psychiatry* published a study of ninety Alzheimer's patients' sense of smell compared to those without Alzheimer's. Since the olfactory tissues, which are responsible for our sense of smell, are damaged along with other parts of the brain, it makes sense that a smell test might work to predict Alzheimer's. Some clinics use a smell test as part of their Alzheimer's workup, while others wait for more research.

Your doctor will perform the MMSE, PSMS, and a behavioral assessment at each visit to follow any change in your symptoms. If you begin experiencing more severe symptoms like depression, agitation, hallucinations, or delirium, you may be started on a different medication and see your doctor more often. If you develop other conditions or symptoms, not necessarily associated with Alzheimer's, regular visits with your doctor will help monitor these as well.

Treatment Evaluation

When your doctor evaluates your response to medication, it is mainly to see if there is stabilization of your condition. Sometimes dramatic improvements do take place but not as often as we would wish. If a sharp decline is noted after initiating a new medicine, your doctor may ask you and your caregiver to stop the medication or slowly wean off it.

Your doctor will also make sure you and your caregiver understand that there is, as yet, no cure for Alzheimer's; the current medications are limited and cannot stop or reverse the natural progression of the disease. They do allow a longer period of independence and may help delay the need for a nursing home or other institutionalized care.

Caregiving at Your Appointments

Your caregiver, for many reasons, should accompany you to every doctor's appointment. You may need assistance getting to the appointment and undressing and dressing for your physical exam. Your caregiver can also help recount your symptoms since your last visit, any major life changes (such as a move or a hospitalization), and what medications you are taking. Your caregiver will bring your medications to the appointment.

Assessment Tools

You or your family and caregivers may want to know what assessment tools are used in Alzheimer's. There are four categories.

1. Cognitive Assessments, which measure thinking, learning, and memory.

    *   Alzheimer's Disease Assessment Scale, cognitive subsection (ADAS-cog)
    *   Blessed Information-Memory-Concentration Test (BIMC)
    *   Clinical Dementia Rating Scale (CDR)
    *   Mini-Mental State Examination (MMSE)

2. Functional Assessments, which measure activities of daily living and ability to function on a daily basis.

- Functional Assessment Questionnaire (FAQ)
- Instrumental Activities of Daily Living (IADL)
- Physical Self-Maintenance Scale (PSMS)
- Progressive Deterioration Scale (PDS)

3. Global Assessments, which assess both cognitive symptoms and functional symptoms.

- Clinical Global Impression of Change (CGIC)
- Clinical Interview-Based Impression (CIBI)
- Global Deterioration Scale (GDS)

4. Caregiver-Based Assessments.

- Behavioral Pathology in Alzheimer's Disease Rating Scale (BEHAVE-AD)
- Neuropsychiatric Inventory (NPI)

The Expanded Role of the Caregiver

In the medical setting, the role of the caregiver in Alzheimer's is much greater than for any other chronic disease. Because the patient is often not able to communicate their needs and concerns to their doctor, it is up to the caregiver to assume this role of communicator. The doctor must establish a good relationship with the caregiver, and often the whole family, to be able to provide effective treatment and care. Any treatment plan introduced by the doctor will be implemented and monitored by the patient's caregivers.

Having a strong and confident caregiver is important for the health of the Alzheimer's patient. In fact, if a caregiver is unduly burdened, that means the treatment approach is not working and needs to be reassessed. (E)

Chapter 9

Treating Alzheimer's Symptoms with Diet and Nutrients

All activity in the body occurs through a process called metabolism in which cells break down chemicals and nutrients to generate energy and form new molecules like proteins. Efficient metabolism requires blood loaded with oxygen, glucose, and nutrients. Enzymes are the molecules that make metabolism happen, and nutrients are vitamins and minerals that act as essential co-enzymes. When a nutrient is deficient in the body, certain metabolic functions are impeded and symptoms of disease can arise.

Water

The human body is mostly made up of water—anywhere from 90 percent when we are babies to 70 percent when we are older. Part of the wrinkling and shriveling with old age is actually dehydration. If everyone were to drink six to eight large glasses of water a day, we would all be in much better shape.

You just need to look at the proliferation of bottled water companies and water filtration devices to know that water comes in many forms—some good and some bad. Marketers for bottled water and water purifiers do tend to exaggerate the problems of tap water, but there are daily reports about our contaminated water supply.

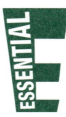

Although no agency has made a recommendation about drinking water and Alzheimer's, it seems to make sense to use a water purifier or a reputable bottled water supplier. Environmentalists who have a growing concern about the chemicals in our environment and their effects on our health call this type of preventive action the Precautionary Principle.

In the *Proceedings of the National Academy of Science*, a cholesterol study showed that a group of rabbits with elevated levels of cholesterol, that had absorbed too much copper from tap water, had an acceleration of Alzheimer's symptoms. A previous study had used distilled water with no copper, and the animals did not develop Alzheimer's. It was an accidental finding, but gave enough evidence to look for a relationship between copper intake in people with high cholesterol and Alzheimer's.

Most researchers and doctors think the aluminum-Alzheimer's connection has been refuted. Several reports published since 2000, however, find that there may be a connection. The aluminum-Alzheimer's connection is discussed in Chapter 2. Another concern is fluoridated tap water. A 1996 study in France showed that fluoride enhanced aluminum absorption in a group of rats.

The Food Factor

A high-fat diet has been implicated as a risk factor for Alzheimer's in those who have the ApoE4 gene. A high-fat diet with 40 percent of calories from fat raises the risk by twenty-nine times. The risk also applies to young adults aged twenty to thirty-nine who eat a high-fat diet; if they have the ApoE4 gene, they are twenty-three times more likely to develop Alzheimer's in later years than healthy eaters.

Whether or not you have the ApoE4 gene, it's still a good idea to cut back on fat. A high-fat diet is a factor in increasing the risk of heart disease, stroke, diabetes, and some cancers. A low-fat diet would have less animal protein, very little fried food, and increased amounts of whole grains and vegetables.

It's well known, however, that over half our brain matter consists of fats or lipids that create all the cell membranes in the body. If you eat bad fats, you make low-quality nerve cell membranes; if you eat good fats, you make higher-quality nerve cell membranes and influence positively the action of nerve cells.

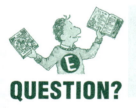

QUESTION?

What is the difference between good fats and bad fats?
Good fats are polyunsaturated, such as flaxseed oil, olive oil, sunflower seed oil, and safflower seed oil. Bad fats are saturated, such as lard, shortening, and fats used in deep-frying.

The more you eat, the more B vitamins you need to metabolize your food. After years of eating a high-calorie diet with consequent weight gain and high levels of cholesterol and homocysteine, the B vitamins may become deficient in the body. We know that when certain B vitamins (B_{12}, B_6, and folic acid) are deficient in the diet, homocysteine builds up. And conversely, if these B vitamins are given to people with high levels of homocysteine, the condition disappears and heart disease symptoms are reversed. (Data from the abundance of homocysteine studies have also found a correlation with Alzheimer's.)

Nutraceuticals and Alzheimer's

The role of diet and nutraceuticals in Alzheimer's is a very hot topic, sparking a lot of debate among Alzheimer's researchers. Nutraceuticals is the umbrella term for nutritional supplements. They used to be called vitamins and minerals, but with each passing year, new categories of nutrients are being found—carotinoids, bioflavinoids, and essential fatty acids, to name a few.

The following causes of Alzheimer's are being researched specifically regarding nutraceutical intervention:

- Homocysteine damage to the brain—with B vitamin treatment.
- Free radical damage to the brain—with vitamin E and vitamin C.
- Nervous system nutrients as essential co-factors—with B vitamins, omega-3 fatty acids, and magnesium.

Homocysteine Damage to the Brain

In 1998, researchers who published in *Archives of Neurology* examined the association of homocysteine and Alzheimer's in a group of elderly people. They confirmed that blood levels of homocysteine were significantly higher, and serum folate and vitamin B_{12} levels were lower in patients with Alzheimer's than in controls. The patients were followed for three years, and x-ray evidence of disease progression was greatest in those with initial high levels of homocysteine. The researchers felt that their study proved that high homocysteine is not just a consequence of having Alzheimer's, but may play a much more important role in the disease; the researchers called for further investigation.

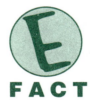

FACT

The National Institute of Aging is sponsoring a homocysteine trial called VITAL (VITamins to slow ALzheimer's disease). It was designed to determine whether reduction of homocysteine levels with high-dose folate (folic acid), B_6, and B_{12} supplementation would slow the rate of cognitive decline in persons with Alzheimer's disease. It recruited 400 patients and began on January 2003, and will be completed by February 2006.

Researchers at the National Institute of Aging found that mice fed a diet deficient in folic acid had elevated levels of homocysteine in their blood and brain. The researchers suspected that the elevated homocysteine concentration damaged the DNA of nerve cells in the brain. When the mice were then fed a diet with a normal amount of folic acid, they were able to repair the damage, but those with continued inadequate folic acid in their diet were not.

Free Radicals and Antioxidants

Vitamins C and E are natural antioxidants that may play a role in preventing and treating Alzheimer's by cleaning up roving free radicals before they inflict damage on the brain. In 2002, one large study from the Netherlands found that eating a diet high in these vitamins was associated with a lower risk of Alzheimer's.

Vitamin E is a natural substance found in oils from soybeans, sunflower seeds, corn, cotton seed, whole-grains, fish-liver oils, and nuts. Vitamin E has various functions in the body and acts as a natural antioxidant.

A 1997 study comparing the effects of vitamin E and selegiline (used in Parkinson's disease) found that vitamin E slowed the progression of symptoms in moderately severe Alzheimer's. The Alzheimer's Association quotes this study as a basis for recommending the vitamin. Vitamin E has few side effects. It can cause mild blood thinning and should be used with caution in patients on blood thinning medication.

E
ALERT!

The best form of vitamin E contains mixed tocopherols and mixed tocotrienols. Synthetic vitamin E is less effective than natural vitamin E. The synthetic vitamin E is labeled dl-alpha tocopherol compared to the natural d-alpha tocopherols.

A review of vitamin E and its ability to act as a beneficial antioxidant for Alzheimer's was published in 2000. Researchers found that only the 1997 vitamin E study fit the inclusion criteria for their review. Their conclusions were that there is still insufficient evidence of the efficacy of vitamin E in the treatment of people with Alzheimer's disease. This review may be misinterpreted to mean that vitamin E doesn't work. What it does mean is that more funding needs to be given to this type of research.

In the June 26, 2002, issue of the *Journal of the American Medical Association*, two studies highlighted the association between dietary vitamin E and decreased risk of Alzheimer's disease. The first study found that the risk of developing Alzheimer's was 70 percent less among people who consumed the most vitamin E foods such as almonds, vegetable oils, seeds, wheat germ, spinach and other dark green, leafy vegetables, compared with those consuming the least amount of vitamin E. The second study found that high dietary intake of vitamin E and vitamin C together may lower the risk of Alzheimer's.

Vitamin C has the ability to cross the blood-brain barrier. Researchers in Italy have theorized that this ability may be used as a means to attach certain drugs to vitamin C to help those drugs penetrate into the brain and reach damaged nerve cells. This research is still in the laboratory stage.

One Vitamin Is Good, Two May Be Better

Science isolates variables by studying only one thing at a time. Otherwise it's impossible to know the exact cause of a disease or which treatment is working. By studying each nutrient individually, scientists think they will find out whether that nutrient is beneficial for treating or preventing Alzheimer's. That's not the way the body works, however.

The body is an ongoing symphony of hundreds, even thousands, of variables working in harmony. Taking one variable out of the concert can sometimes just give you dissonance, but sometimes it's all we can do to reach some general conclusions.

Study on Vitamins E and C

A study on vitamin E and vitamin C is a case in point where two vitamins proved to be better than one. In January 2004, *Archives of Neurology* published findings from a Johns Hopkins study in Utah on 4,470 older residents of Cache County. The study investigated the use of the antioxidant vitamins C and E to protect against Alzheimer's. From 1996 until 2000, 304 new cases of Alzheimer's were diagnosed.

The researchers found that the 17 percent of elderly people who took individual supplements of both vitamins C and E had a 78 percent reduction in the risk of Alzheimer's when the study began, and a 64 percent reduction over the duration of the study. Further refinement of the results showed that the individuals who took only one of the two vitamins and the 20 percent of individuals who took them both in small amounts in the form of a multivitamin did not have a reduced risk of Alzheimer's.

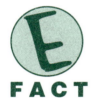

FACT

The profile of people taking vitamins E and C showed individuals who were significantly more likely to be female, younger, better educated, and of better general health when compared to nonsupplement users. A study now needs to be done to follow this group of women to see if any of them develop Alzheimer's.

The authors of the study were very excited by the results and said that regular use of vitamin E in nutritional supplement doses, especially in combination with vitamin C, may reduce the risk of developing Alzheimer's disease. This makes sense because vitamins C and E are powerful anti-inflammatory nutrients that inhibit interleukin (inflammatory) factors produced in the brain.

One Alzheimer's drug, Namenda, prevents excess glutamate from interfering with learning and memory. In a 2000 German study, both natural and synthetic vitamin E were shown to be more effective than estrogen in protecting neurons against oxidative death caused by beta-amyloid, hydrogen peroxide, and the excitatory amino acid, glutamate.

Essential Nutrients for the Nervous System

The B vitamins have long been associated with nervous system health. When they are deficient, many different symptoms can occur such as fatigue, anxiety, numbness and tingling, and depression. Although researchers may study them separately, the B vitamins stick together in the body. Vitamin K, the omega-3 fatty acids, and magnesium are also essential for nervous system health.

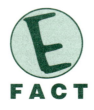

FACT

The idea of using brain nutrients is so new that they are often referred to as "nootropics." Nootropics comes from the Greek words *noos*, meaning "mind," and *tropein*, meaning "toward." It identifies nutrients that readily cross the blood-brain barrier and increase blood flow, neurotransmitter function, and support eye and ear health.

A study published in *Brain Research Bulletin* in 2003 reported that vitamin B_6 was able to act as an antidote to aluminum toxicity in nerve cells in the hippocampus of a rat. The researchers felt that aluminum toxicity mimicked the main characteristic of Alzheimer's disease with a loss of synaptic transmission. They said that vitamin B_6 may be considered a potent antidote to aluminum toxicity and neurodegenerative disorders such as Alzheimer's disease.

Vitamin B_6 helps regulate mood and mental function. Research shows that people with Alzheimer's disease have low levels of vitamin B_6. Studies are underway to determine the effects of long-term supplementation with vitamin B_6 in preventing the progression and development of Alzheimer's.

B_{12} and Folate

A three-year study at the Karolinska Institute in Stockholm, Sweden, was published in the journal *Neurology* in 2001. Researchers followed 370 people who were seventy-five or older and had no signs of dementia. During the study period, the researchers measured the participants' blood levels of vitamin B_{12} and folate, and compared them to normal ranges. The results showed that patients with below-normal levels of both vitamin B_{12} and folic acid had twice the risk of developing Alzheimer's disease than those with normal levels.

The researchers postulated that vitamin B_{12} or folate deficiencies affect Alzheimer's disease by influencing neurotransmitters or the levels of the neurotoxic amino acid, homocysteine, in the body. Both vitamin B_{12} and folate deficiency can increase homocysteine levels. Researchers also admit that low B_{12} and folate levels have been found in the elderly for over thirty years.

Vitamin B_{12} deficiency is associated with a decline in mental function as well as an increased risk of Alzheimer's. In a 1994 study, the presence of hereditary Alzheimer's disease was found to be associated with lower serum vitamin B_{12} values compared with unaffected family members. The conclusion was that additional research must be done to determine if supplementation is effective in people with existing Alzheimer's or whether it is primarily a preventive nutrient.

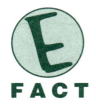

FACT

Vitamin B_{12} is naturally found in animal foods including fish, milk and milk products, eggs, meat, and poultry. Folate, also called folic acid or Vitamin B_9, is found in all leafy greens such as spinach and turnip greens, dry beans and peas, fortified cereals and grain products, and some fruits.

Magnesium and Alzheimer's

A world-renowned magnesium researcher, Dr. Jean Durlach, published "Magnesium Depletion and Pathogenesis of Alzheimer's Disease" in the journal, *Magnesium Research*. Durlach's research showed that magnesium depletion, particularly in the hippocampus, seems to be an important factor in the development of Alzheimer's disease. He also reported that low magnesium is associated with high levels of aluminum incorporation into brain nerve cells.

A 2002 study published in *Brain Research Bulletin* found that a magnesium compound, magnesium D-aspartate, prevented aluminum deposits in rat brain cortexes. Researchers concluded that magnesium protected rat brain cortexes from aluminum accumulation and suggested that this treatment may be useful in preventing aluminum toxicity in the brain.

Natural Anticholinesterase Treatment

In 1995, a Chinese herbal extract called huperzine A, an alkaloid found in the Chinese herb *Huperzia serrata*, underwent preliminary studies to block cholinesterase. It proved to be even more potent than Cognex, the first anticholinesterase drug, and with little to no side effects.

In a multicenter, prospective, double-blind, parallel, placebo-controlled study involving 103 Alzheimer's patients, 58 percent of patients taking huperzine A had an improvement in memory, cognitive, and behavioral functions without any side effects.

Fish Equals Brain Food

We all grew up hearing that fish feeds the brain. What we know now is that it's the omega-3 fatty acids in certain cold-water fish that have the real potential to help the brain. They are so powerful, in fact, they may even reduce the risk of Alzheimer's. A 2003 study organized by the Rush-Presbyterian-St. Luke's Medical Center in Chicago asked a group of people over the age of sixty-five about their diets. Researchers found that those who ate fish at least once a week had a 60 percent less chance of developing Alzheimer's than those who rarely ate fish.

ESSENTIAL

The best fish sources of omega-3 fatty acids are sardines, salmon (especially wild), cod, mackerel, herring, and tuna. Nonfish food sources include fresh ground flaxseeds and flax oil, soybeans, spinach, mustard greens, wheat germ oil, and English walnuts.

Each nerve cell in the brain is surrounded by a protective cell membrane. Receptors for many brain neurotransmitters are found on the membrane. This membrane is composed mostly of different types of fats, which include phosphatidylcholine (PC), also called lecithin; phosphatidylserine (PS); and phosphatidylethanolamine (PE). The cell membrane also contains cholesterol.

The function of the nerve cells and the neurotransmitters is highly dependent on the quality of fats that make up the cell membrane and therefore highly dependent on the type of fats and oils in the diet. The makeup of a cell membrane is always in a state of transition; it is constantly influenced by diet, stress, and the immune system.

Brain Fats

In 1991, researchers from the Karolinska Institute determined that the amount of healthy and beneficial polyunsaturated fatty acids present in the brain declines with age in Alzheimer's patients. Polyunsaturated fatty acids, such as DHA and arachidonic acid, which are normally found in the brain, were replaced by monounsaturated and saturated fatty acids. This change was not nearly as prominent in the brains of patients who did not have Alzheimer's.

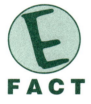

FACT

The brain lipid phosphatydilserine has been studied for decades with double-blind trials conducted in Italy, Belgium, Germany, and the United States. Results of these studies show that phosphatydilserine is helpful in improving memory, learning, concentration, and word choice as well as mood and the ability to deal with stress. Phosphatydilserine is very well tolerated, has few side effects, and is compatible with many prescription medications.

The researchers speculate that brain cells in Alzheimer's patients are unable to make the proper fatty acids for their membranes from saturated and monounsaturated fatty acids in the diet. The researchers concluded, "The substantial decrease in polyunsaturated fatty acids may have serious consequences for cellular function. This could hamper the production of important active metabolites, such as prostaglandins and leukotrienes, which, in turn, could cause the changes observed in Alzheimer's disease."

In a University of Kentucky study, a similar decrease in arachidonic acid and DHA was also noticed. The researchers speculated that oxidative damage to fatty acids reduces the amount of long-chain polyunsaturated fatty acids in the brain.

Omega-3 Fatty Acids and Depression

Many studies have shown that omega-3 fatty acids help balance cholesterol and triglyceride levels and promote heart and vascular health to prevent heart disease and stroke. In terms of brain function, however, a recent study shows that omega-3 fatty acids may play a role in elevating mood in depression. Initial studies showed that people diagnosed with depression appear to have lower levels of omega-3 fatty acids compared to individuals who are not.

ALERT!

Check with a doctor knowledgeable in nutrition before taking omega-3s with other health supplements. Omega-3s, as well as biloba, garlic, and saw palmetto, are all mild blood thinners and should be avoided if you are on blood thinning medication. Omega-3s may lower blood pressure, so if you are already on antihypertensive drugs, you must tell your doctor before you start taking them.

In a recent study published in the journal *European Neuropsychopharmacology*, a small group of thirty-two patients with depression were given either a placebo or a supplement containing 440 milligrams of eicosapentanoic acid and 220 milligrams of docasahexanoic acid (omega-3 fatty acid components) in addition to their regularly prescribed antidepressant medications. The patients who were given the supplement exhibited significantly greater benefits than those who were given the placebo.

Another way that omega-3s may work in the brain is due to their ability to suppress inflammation. In fact, they also work to decrease the pain associated with rheumatoid arthritis.

Herbs and Alzheimer's

We have often heard that the drugs of modern times originally came from plants. For example, aspirin comes from the white willow bark. Over the centuries, people would use the bark of the white willow tree to relieve pain and inflammation.

In the last century, we have been able to analyze white willow bark and, through lab experiments, come up with the most active ingredient, called salicylic acid, which causes the analgesic and anti-inflammatory effects. With this information, we will be able to analyze the chemical structure of salicylic acid and make it synthetically out of petroleum.

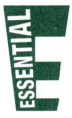

Aspirin can have serious side effects, which are usually related to the amount you take. Take the lowest effective dose to minimize side effects. It can cause ringing in the ears, rash, kidney impairment, lightheadedness, ulcerations and abdominal burning, pain, cramping, nausea, gastritis, and gastrointestinal bleeding and liver toxicity. Black tarry stools, weakness, and dizziness upon standing may be the only signs of internal bleeding.

It's a modern miracle, but along with the miracle come side effects. Some herbalists feel that by using the whole plant, the other constituents of the herb counteract some of the side effects. It's another interesting debate.

Although used for inflammation, white willow bark is not used for the inflammation in Alzheimer's. Researchers at the University of California have studied one special herb, called curcumin, that is used in making curry dishes. They found that in both low and high doses, curcumin was able to reduce the inflammatory immune factors secreted by microglia cells.

Ginkgo Biloba

Ginkgo biloba is said to be the oldest surviving species of tree on earth—possibly 200 million years old. Its leaves have been used for thousands of years in herbal teas for lung problems, increasing circulation, improving digestion, and to boost memory.

Presently, ginkgo biloba extract is one of the most commonly used herbs in Europe and, to a lesser extent, in the United States. In Europe, it has been officially approved by the German Commission E, which has rigorously studied over 200 herbs for both safety and function. In Germany, ginkgo may be used for memory loss, ringing in the ears, vertigo, and circulation disorders. A wealth of studies shows that ginkgo biloba has proven to have beneficial effects on dementia, poor memory, and poor concentration, as well as on certain cardiovascular and circulation problems.

There are more than forty chemical constituents of ginkgo, but the main ones linked to health benefits are flavonoids. Flavonoids are antioxidants that act to eliminate free radicals in the body.

Ginkgo Studies

A popular ginkgo extract was tested in a placebo-controlled clinical trial in the United States in 1997 and reported in the *Journal of the American Medical Association.* The study participants who had Alzheimer's disease or multi-infarct dementia were given 40 milligrams three times per day. Another group received placebo pills.

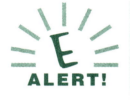
ALERT!

The chemicals in ginkgo biloba that are related to blood thinning are called terpenoids. They may make up from 7 to 13 percent of the total content of a bottle of ginkgo found on the shelf. Therefore, if you are taking blood-thinning medication such as warfarin or heparin, you should avoid taking ginkgo.

When researchers measured both groups on a cognitive assessment scale, 27 percent of the group that took ginkgo improved by at least four points compared to 14 percent of those taking placebo. Clinically, a four-point improvement equates to a six-month delay in disease progression. The ginkgo group had twice as many patients with cognitive improvement and half as many whose social functioning worsened. There were no side effects reported from its use.

Dipsacus Asper

In a 2003 study published in *Life Science,* an herbal medicine used in China was studied for its effects on beta amyloid protein. Animals were exposed to a solution of aluminum in their drinking water for ninety days. Two groups were formed: One was given Dipsacus and one was given vitamin E. The treatment phase lasted five months. Compared to a group of animals not given treatment, both groups of animals taking Dipsacus and vitamin E showed no impairment in their performance of measured tasks; in addition, the hippocampus did not show a buildup of white blood cells indicating an immune reaction from the aluminum as did the controls. It was also noted that the beneficial effects of Dipsacus asper extract, but not vitamin E, increased with time.

Chapter 10

Exercise Is the Key

When astronauts first went into space, they rapidly lost muscle bulk and even began losing bone density. They also got very bored. Billions of dollars spent in space research had missed the essential factors of exercising the brain and the body. We're missing that information as well because most people don't exercise and don't do mentally challenging work or play. And as you can see, if we are going to make any headway in slowing down this epidemic of Alzheimer's, we all have to develop the exercise habit.

Exercise Your Brain

Memory is made and reinforced by the strength of connections between nerve cells and the formation of memory-storage protein molecules inside nerve cells. When a memory of a new idea is formed, like a name or an address, thousands of nerve cells are involved. If you don't use that bit of memory shortly after, it will soon fade away. But if you use it and reactivate the memory many times, you reinforce the stored chemical protein molecules that make up that memory. Reading these words creates thousands of electrochemical reactions in your brain. Often the brain is referred to as a computer, but the malleability and interactivity of the brain is far beyond any computer that is presently in use or on the horizon.

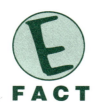

FACT

Computer developers continually try to match the brain's function and capacity. In June 2000, IBM produced a supercomputer called ASCI White, which is able to perform 12.3 trillion operations per second. IBM says it's ten years away from matching the brain. Presently, ASCI White covers 9,920 square feet of floor space, equal to two NBA basketball courts, and weighs 106 tons.

We must exercise the brain as if it were a muscle. We have all heard the stories of the dangers of retiring and not having a plan of how to fill your time. The stories are true, and the science is there to prove it. Most work, even the commute, the interaction with others, and the daily challenges, are stimulating. When you retire, if you don't build in challenges for your brain and body, then you can suffer physical decline and even mental decline.

Studies also find that the more intellectually stimulating the job, the less likely Alzheimer's will strike. But up until the past few years, there has been little human research on the effect of leisure activities and the risk of Alzheimer's disease.

Experiments in Exercising the Brain

A 1993 experiment with two groups of mice shows the importance of exercising the brain. The first group was placed in a barren cage with no mental stimulation. They just ate, slept, or wandered around their cage. The second group was trained in running complex mazes.

After a few weeks, an electron microscope was used to compare the nerve cells of the trained mice to those of the untrained group. There was a noticeable difference between the two groups. The maze mice had developed wider and longer nerve dendrites and more synapses than the couch potato mice.

Use It or Lose It

In the next phase of the study, the maze group was put in solitary confinement without stimulation. At the end of several more weeks, their brains were examined. They no longer had enhanced dendrites and synapses; they had all shrunken away, and their brains were as if they had never been trained. "Use it or lose it" was the conclusion of this study. In another study, it took only four days for dendrites and synapses to flare out and grow when toys were put in cages along with laboratory animals.

Mentally Active Nuns

A 2002 study from the *Journal of the American Medical Association* made big headlines when it was published. The subjects of the study were not mice, but 800 nuns, priests, and brothers from ongoing health research called the Religious Order Study. The topic of the study was a simple one: Can the mind improve with mental stimulation? But the results were nothing less than shocking. Researchers reported that by stimulating the mind with common tasks such as reading, listening to the radio, or playing simple memory games like cards and checkers every day, you may be able to ward off the ravages of Alzheimer's.

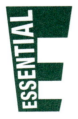

Nuns, priests, and brothers may not be the ideal people to test for Alzheimer's because their lifestyle habits do not necessarily reflect the general population. They tend to be nonsmokers, nondrinkers, and probably eat a balanced diet. These factors must be taken into consideration when looking at their beneficial mental activities.

The participants in the group were 800 Catholic nuns, priests, and brothers over the age of sixty-five. Points were assigned to seven different activities including visiting museums; playing board games; reading newspapers, magazines, and books; listening to the radio; and watching television. Value was also given to the amount of time spent on each activity on a scale of one to five.

When compared to people who participated very little, those who had the greatest number of mentally challenging activities lowered their risk for Alzheimer's by 47 percent. People who participated a moderate amount had a 28 percent lower risk.

Keeping Active Mentally and Physically

A study published in the *Proceedings of the National Academy of Sciences* (PNAS) in 2001 investigated the benefits of keeping active both mentally and physically during leisure time to prevent Alzheimer's. A group of adults between twenty and sixty years of age was compared to more active peers. Researchers took into account all variables and still found that the risk of developing Alzheimer's in inactive people was four times that of active people.

ALERT!

It was found in the *PNAS* study that the main activity of Alzheimer's patients, which they participated in more frequently than the healthy controls, was watching television. One could speculate that watching television is a much more passive activity than reading a book or playing cards and board games.

In the *PNAS* study, some of the activities that led to less brain stimulation and increased risk of Alzheimer's included watching television, listening to music, attending social clubs, talking on the phone, visiting with friends, and attending religious services. These were compared with reading books, studying a foreign language, and traveling.

They found that any type of stimulating activity was more beneficial than none. The more intellectual the activity, however, the better it was for strengthening your brain muscles. Whereas indoor activities were emphasized in the previous study on nuns, this report factored in the benefits of traveling, learning a foreign language, learning a musical instrument, and taking part in social and community activities.

It's a matter of engaging in life fully, having goals, having fun, and being interested in your surroundings, in other people, and in yourself. If you are a retiree who focused all your activities on your job, you just have to learn to reach out into your community of friends and family and see where your skills can be put to use. Sitting in front of the television set is not the best way to enjoy your retirement.

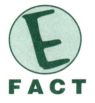

FACT

ABC TV reported on the *PNAS* study with the glaring title "Couch Potatoes Beware" and quoted Dr. Robert Freidland, the main author of the study, as saying that TV-watching may even be an Alzheimer's risk factor! Watcher beware. Dr. Freidland said that people who don't exercise their gray matter stand a chance of losing brainpower.

Before this study, researchers wondered if a sedentary lifestyle increased the risk of Alzheimer's or was simply a measure of the early stages of the disease, since most studies observed the elderly. By measuring younger adults, however, this study was able to conclude that it's wise to exercise your brain your whole life.

Mind Boosters

If watching TV is not giving your brain the stimulation it needs, here are some more ways to help flex your brain:

- Start a new hobby such as painting or gardening.
- Stimulate your brain with crossword puzzles, Scrabble, or books.
- If it's appropriate and you have backup help, get a pet.
- Keep a daily log. Write everything down; create routines; and use sticky notes to help keep you on track.
- Relax and de-stress to take the pressure off your mind and body.

Reading to the Elderly

Dr. Robert Griffith, who publishes wonderful articles on the Web site Health and Age (✒*www.healthandage.com*), reminds us of the importance of reading, not necessarily by the elderly, but to the elderly. He talks about the work of author Carolyn Banks.

When Ms. Banks worked at a day care center in Texas, she was tearing out her hair with the frustration of trying to find activities for her elderly clients, including people with Alzheimer's. This was not a day care of elderly people playing games and interacting with each other. This was a group that couldn't be left at home alone while their caregivers were at work.

Ms. Banks surveyed how other day care workers were meeting the challenge of keeping their clients interested in life. She found that many of them read books to the elderly, but they were usually children's books with lots of pictures and a very disjointed storyline.

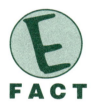

FACT

Two psychologists at Case Western Reserve University found that Alzheimer's and dementia patients can see and read better if the print is big and the contrast enhanced. In 1999 they began a five-year, $2.8 million study called "Visual Interventions to Improve Alzheimer Cognition." Just as hearing aids improve hearing, this research will develop ways for Alzheimer's patients to improve their visual and motion perception.

This led Ms. Banks on a search for suitable reading material for her special audience. It wasn't long before she realized that the act of reading was having a calming effect and seemed to bring a spark of life to her listeners; it even brought words from people who had been mute.

The next task Ms. Banks set for herself was to create an anthology of stories for the elderly day care population. She placed ads for short stories for the elderly but got back too much about death and dying. She had to place another ad, and as Dr. Griffith says, she asked for ". . . evocative stories with plenty of description and not much dialogue. Excess, schmaltz, and sentimentality were called for—just the things that fledgling authors should avoid!"

When she field-tested stories on her elderly listeners, she found that ones involving animals got the most reaction. She had already realized that the voice of the reader was important; she also realized that the enthusiasm involved in reaching a story's exciting conclusion was very well received by her listeners.

Ms. Bank sums up her experience and what she learned. "Being read to can be as welcoming as a touch, whether or not the listeners had been readers or the words have literal meaning any longer." Dr. Griffith concludes, "At an advanced age, to be touched, in any way, is often the high point of a day."

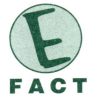

FACT

Dr. Patrick Byrd, in his "Keeping Fit" column for the University of Florida, says that because Alzheimer's does not initially disturb motor function, balance, or coordination, people can get physiological and psychological benefits from exercise. He adds that there is some evidence that exercise may improve the ability of Alzheimer's sufferers to communicate.

Exercise Your Body and Your Mood

According to author David Rakel, in his 2002 book, *Integrative Medicine*, over 10,000 trials have examined the relationship between exercise and mood showing that exercise may be just as effective in treating depression as psychotherapy.

Exercise stimulates circulation and increases blood flow to all parts of the body and brain, bringing extra oxygen, glucose, and nutrients. Exercise increases self-esteem and confidence, which makes you stand up straighter and look the rest of the world square in the eye. In animal studies, exercise helps increase healthy growth factors in the memory center of the brain.

It doesn't even matter what kind of exercise you choose. You can walk, jog, swim, lift weights, do yoga or tai chi—it all works. Even if you start sitting in a chair and doing stretches, that can help. Then you can hold 2-pound weights and flex your arms. After a while, you can graduate to 5-pound weights. For your hips and legs, just start by getting in and out of a chair about ten times. Slowly but surely, you can build up those weak muscles that are crying out for exercise.

How to Make Exercise Work

Everyone knows that exercise is beneficial for the elderly. Several nursing home studies have proven that exercise programs led by professionals improved physical function for even the weakest participants. A 2003 study published in the *Journal of the American Medical Association (JAMA)* was the first to show how to implement a workable program in the home.

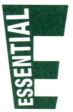

Dr. Byrd encourages people with Alzheimer's to become active in all forms of exercise such as bowling, cycling, dancing, golf, jogging, shuffleboard, skating, skiing, swimming, tennis, walking, and weight training. He does caution that supervision may be needed even when there is only mild dementia.

Health professional trainers in this study gave twelve hours of Alzheimer's education and training on exercise supervision to caregivers. Once they had the tools, the caregivers started their patients on a regular exercise program. With the necessary support and coaching, patients with moderate to severe Alzheimer's actually improved their physical and emotional health and shared a positive interaction with their caregivers.

Such a program described in *JAMA* can help to improve quality of life, create more independence, and keep Alzheimer's people healthier longer. The caregiver also benefits by learning more about the disease and also by doing the exercises themselves and staying healthy. What began as a study to help people cope and manage the disease became a report on how exercise could actually improve disease symptoms.

The Alzheimer's Association funded the study because caregivers had reported to them repeatedly that basic exercise had dramatic effects on Alzheimer's people by preventing challenging behaviors, enhancing independence, and even delaying institutionalization. With this study, what was first an observation became a scientific fact that should have an impact throughout the Alzheimer's community.

The *JAMA* study is important for many reasons, but one thing in particular that can be learned from this study is how important caregivers are in the Alzheimer's community. By expressing their concerns, needs, and observations to the Alzheimer's Association, they touched on an essential part of Alzheimer's care that can't be found in a pill.

A spokesperson for the Alzheimer's Association said, "These results from a well-conducted clinical trial provide solid evidence for the value of these nonpharmaceutical interventions and show us avenues for ongoing evidence-based research into similar therapeutic approaches."

JAMA Study Details

The study enrolled 153 patient-caregiver pairs assigned randomly to one of two groups. One group was the combined exercise and caregiver-training program, known as Reducing Disability in Alzheimer Disease (RDAD). The second group, or the control group, was the routine medical care group (RMC). The RDAD program was conducted over a period of three months in the homes of the Alzheimer's patients. The people with Alzheimer's disease ranged in age from fifty-five to ninety-three years old. The caregivers had an amazing age range of twenty-four to ninety-one.

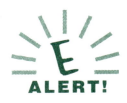
ALERT!

Before caregivers initiate an exercise program, they should have their Alzheimer's patient examined for heart disease or any contraindications to certain physical activity. This is sensible advice for any older person starting a new exercise program, but especially important for people with Alzheimer's because stroke and heart disease are risk factors themselves.

Healthcare trainers came to the home and taught aerobic exercises and endurance activities, along with balance, strength, and flexibility exercises. Trainers helped caregivers make the program easy and fun to do. They helped caregivers to find time in their schedule for thirty minutes of exercise a day. They also trained them in behavior modification techniques for motivation and how to handle conflicts that might arise in trying to implement the exercise program. Additional education about

Alzheimer's, its effects, and how to cope with challenging behaviors was shared with caregivers.

JAMA Study Results

After three months, the exercise groups were doing at least sixty minutes of exercise a week. The results were that people with Alzheimer's who participated in the home exercise program had much higher levels of physical activity on a daily basis, experienced lower rates of depression, and displayed better physical health and function than those who had routine care with no exercise.

Even more impressive was that Alzheimer's patients who exercised had a lower rate of nursing home placement for behavioral problems. Institutionalization is a big stumbling block for caregivers who really want to keep their loved ones at home. It also supports the economy because home care is often a less expensive alternative than a nursing home for both the family and the healthcare system. The benefits of the exercise program still persisted after two years.

Canadian Study on Exercise and Alzheimer's

In a study published in the *American Journal of Epidemiology* in 2002, Canadian researchers studied the topic of exercise and Alzheimer's. They followed a population of 4,600 men and women over the age of sixty-five to see how many would develop Alzheimer's over the course of the five-year study. None of the participants had signs or symptoms of Alzheimer's at the beginning of the study.

Information was obtained through detailed lifestyle questionnaires about their smoking, diet, exercise, and alcohol consumption habits. At the end of five years, 194 new cases of Alzheimer's had been diagnosed. Statistical data was then developed comparing those who succumbed to Alzheimer's with those who didn't. They found that those who didn't get Alzheimer's had the following associated behaviors:

- Regular physical activity
- Use of nonsteroidal, anti-inflammatory drugs

- Regular wine consumption
- Regular coffee consumption

It turned out that participating in regular physical activity contributed the most to lowering the risk of Alzheimer's. The percentage of lowered risk was 30 percent.

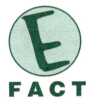

FACT

"If I had a medication that provided the same benefits that exercise does, I'd be a rich man," says Dr. Michael Gaziano, director of the Massachusetts Veterans Epidemiology Research and Information Center. Exercise helps with weight control, builds muscle, strengthens the heart, decreases tension, increases bone density, controls diabetes, improves sleep, increases energy, decreases back pain, improves posture, and makes you look and feel younger.

Exercise in a Bottle

Researchers are on the march to find out what it is specifically about exercise that caused these results. Perhaps they want to put it in a bottle. And, if they could, it would be a huge seller. In the meantime, they say the results are "intriguing" and "warrant further research."

There is no reason to wait for more studies to get those muscles moving. The U.S. federal guidelines for exercise say that getting at least thirty minutes a day most days a week will help prevent heart disease, osteoporosis, diabetes, obesity, and now, perhaps, Alzheimer's.

How Behavior Modification Works

We all know the saying, "You can lead a horse to water, but you can't make him drink." That's where the carrot comes in! According to the dictionary, behavior modification is an attempt to change somebody's behavior by rewarding new and desirable responses and making accustomed undesirable ones less attractive. It's also a matter of being nice to someone so they will be nice back.

In a situation where you want your loved one with Alzheimer's to participate in an activity, such as exercise, that you know they don't want to and always resist is where you can use behavior modification. Even though both of you know that exercise will be beneficial, it often ends up in a "tug of war" exercise with some vocal cord exercise thrown in. That whole "exercise" is called negative reinforcement because you are placing the activity of exercise in the middle of a war zone. Any time exercise is mentioned, the thought of a fight and a battle of wills comes up.

First, you have to turn around the negative reinforcement pattern that has been set up. How you do that may be very difficult at first; you have to ignore it completely. Ignore the fact that exercise is not being done and don't even bring it up for a while, several days, or even weeks.

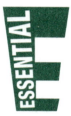

The WatchMinder (✐ www.watchminder.com) is a vibrating wristwatch that reminds people when to take their medications and when to exercise. It helps Alzheimer's patients to be more independent. It can also be used as a stimulus to relax and take a deep breath. The training mode is useful for behavior change and self-monitoring.

Even as you ignore the behavior you don't like, you are ready to reinforce any positive behavior that even remotely looks like exercise. The reinforcement doesn't have to be a million dollars; a kiss, a word of praise, a smile, or a hug is all that's needed. And if your patient wants more of that, he or she will do more of the behavior you are reinforcing. Actually, some people do want more reinforcement than that, like a mini-backrub.

Any extra body movement looks like exercise. Reinforce your patient's positive behavior when they pick something up off the floor—even if you put it there. Simply getting up in the morning, getting dressed, lifting, or carrying things is exercise. Even putting the dishes in the sink counts. It may seem like a lot of work, but taking the time to reinforce all positive behavior, not just exercise, will help everybody's health and mood.

Next, put hand weights in an accessible place and when they are picked up, reinforce that action. Before long, you will both be going for walks, doing stretches, and getting healthy together. Ⓔ

Chapter 11

Caregivers Coping and Caring for Alzheimer's

When it comes to Alzheimer's, we all must learn coping skills to deal with the disease. If you have been diagnosed with Alzheimer's, you've been told there is no cure. You must learn to cope with the finality of that statement and calmly come to peace with it. Your caregivers also learn to cope; they learn how to support you as they render care, especially if they put themselves in your place.

The Caregiver's Role

It's fascinating how a societal behavior such as caregiving is being so widely studied in the wake of chronic diseases like Alzheimer's, cancer, and heart disease. It has to do with the way our society has evolved. One hundred years ago, people with chronic diseases were nursed and cared for at home by an extended family. It was a time when grandparents and grandchildren all lived under the same roof, and everyone pitched in with the chores.

It's also true that there were fewer chronic diseases and maybe fewer elderly people in general, because they didn't live that long. All that has changed now, and as a society, we are forced to make the necessary changes to accommodate old age, chronic disease, and much smaller nuclear families.

ESSENTIAL

The Alzheimer's Association of Connecticut conducts a free five-part caregiver's course. The presenters include "registered nurses, social workers, elder law attorneys, therapeutic recreation directors, and physicians who are highly skilled in caring for people with chronic memory loss." They touch on the help available, hope for the future, the impact on the family, stress reduction, maintaining a safe and secure environment, and legal issues.

Caregiver status is not as valued as it should be, but it is slowly becoming recognized. There is the observation that caregiving is meeting a deep need in our society at great emotional, physical, mental, and financial costs to the caregiver. There is also the recognition that caregiving can be taught, and by so doing, caregivers can carry out their role a little more easily with the right tools and the right support. Your community may have a course going on right now.

The Gift of Caring

The great "vocations" in the world—the church, medicine, and nursing—have a major focus on helping people. It's the same with caregiving. And what many find out is that by caring for and helping others, you nourish your own soul. Giving the gift of caring to another actually allows you to reap many intangible rewards.

Many caregivers say they feel honored to participate in the deep intimacy of someone else's life. The skills learned in caring for someone with Alzheimer's are invaluable for any life challenge.

The Gift of Receiving

We often hear stories of community leaders who gave decades of service and then are struck down. Such a man is Reverend John Green, a Baptist minister who worked tirelessly for thirty-four years. In an article by Stacey Burling published in the *Philadelphia Inquirer* called "Working through Alzheimer's," Reverend Green talked about his "little joke" with parishioners. In the last year or so before his retirement, he would ask people as he greeted them at the door, "And your name is?"

They never knew he had a problem, even though he would often repeat a prayer a second time, and he did forget their names. Now, it's time for his church to give back to him and help him and his wife through the difficulties ahead. We give and we receive.

How to Be a Good Communicator

As a caregiver, you may take a special course in caregiving or just depend on your common sense and love to see you through. Please know, however, that there is a tremendous support system and network for you to tap into: support groups, books, articles, online support, and much more.

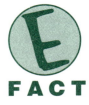

FACT

The Caregiver's Army supports people caring for loved ones. "Whether caring for a spouse, parent, or neighbor," it may be one of the greatest challenges a family can experience, and they are committed to helping you and your loved one. The number of family caregivers in North America has skyrocketed by 400 percent in the past ten years, affecting a quarter of all households.

Communication with an Alzheimer's sufferer means you have to get them to focus on you. Get rid of distractions first. We often spend our day at home with a TV or radio on in the background and tune it out. But someone with Alzheimer's may find such things very distracting when you are trying to talk with them.

Don't talk from across the room; get close enough to have eye contact in order to get and keep their attention. Don't give long-winded explanations of what you want to do; they may forget the first of it by the time you finish.

Just simply state what you want. Let's go for a walk. Let's brush your hair. Say sentences that ask for agreement rather than offering a choice, which may be confusing. And try not to sound reprimanding when you tell them not to do things. You must not speak down to them; just speak clearly and slowly with a lot of repetition.

Communication Tools: The Do's

One special Web site, Health and Age (✎ *www.healthandage.com*), features wonderful articles that give useful advice on many aspects of caring for Alzheimer's. A particularly helpful article, which was modified from a publication by the Alzheimer's Association, called "How to Talk to Someone with Alzheimer's," by Dr. Robert Griffith, helps us with the very first step of how to communicate.

In your relationship with an Alzheimer's patient, here are the tools you can apply to make your communication meaningful. Dr. Griffith says talking with someone with Alzheimer's is a skill that requires time and patience, but it all boils down to being a good listener. Dr. Griffith recommends several helpful do's:

- Approach from the front, make eye contact, and say your name if you aren't recognized.
- Speak slowly, calmly, and use a friendly facial expression.
- Use short, simple, and familiar words.
- Show that you are listening and trying to understand what is being said.
- Be careful not to interrupt; avoid arguing and criticizing.
- Ask one question at a time, and allow time for a reply.

- Make positive suggestions (e.g., "Let's go into the garden") rather than negative ones (e.g., "Don't go in there").
- Identify others by name, rather than using pronouns (she, he, etc.).
- Make suggestions if the person has trouble choosing.
- Empathize; have patience and understanding. Touch or hug, if it helps.

Communication Tools: The Don'ts

If your Alzheimer's patient is caught in a memory loop about their past, don't ask questions that they might not be able to answer. Instead, offer praise and support for whatever they have done in their life. The following are important don'ts:

- Don't talk about the person as if he or she weren't there.
- Don't confront or correct, if it can be avoided.
- Don't treat the person as a child, but as an adult.

Continuing the Conversation

Dr. Griffith wrote an update on his former paper about how to talk with someone with Alzheimer's; he gives more advice for the more serious or more challenging cases:

- Take your time and look for a response to your voice. A hearing disability may make it even harder for someone to communicate.
- When the person replies, show that you are listening and trying to understand.
- Give plenty of encouragement and reassurance—touching or hugging may help.
- Allow time for the reply—don't interrupt, argue, or criticize. Remember, you will never win an argument with an Alzheimer's person.
- If the person seems stuck for a word, you can offer a guess, but act like you have all the time in the world.
- If you aren't quite sure you understood what was said, repeat it back and ask if you've got it right.

- Try to understand the person's feelings and emotions, which may be hidden behind the words. You can ask whether the person is feeling angry or frustrated about a particular situation.
- Make allowances for digressions (reminiscences, backtracking, repetitions, etc.). However, if necessary, prompt the person gently, so they can get back on track.
- Choose a quiet time and place for your discussion, so that both of you are free from interruptions and distractions.
- Be aware that the person may want to point or gesture, if at a loss for words.

Communicating with Visitors

Nonverbal communication such as shaking hands is such a learned behavior that you can include the Alzheimer's patient in such a greeting; even if they don't remember the visitor's name, they can nod and shake hands. A friendly smile and "hello" with an outstretched hand will often elicit a handshake and a "thank you, just fine."

ESSENTIAL

The National Alliance for Caregiving is a good resource. It partners with dozens of elder groups such as the American Association of Retired Persons, medical associations, corporations, and pharmaceutical companies to provide support to family caregivers and the professionals who help them; this organization also increases public awareness of issues facing family caregivers.

You can make it much easier by introducing the visitor by name and give a little description so that the Alzheimer's patient can give a response; this will include them in the conversation and relieve the awkwardness and embarrassment of not remembering the visitor's name.

Caregiver Behavior Skills

There is a set of skills that may or may not come naturally to a caregiver, but from whatever place you start on your caregiving journey, you can certainly learn from others that have been there, and you will definitely learn from your Alzheimer's patient as well. Let's take a look at the various skills a caregiver needs to have in his or her arsenal.

Detachment

Learning to detach goes under the heading of "don't take it personally; don't react." Don't think that your Alzheimer's patient means disrespect or anger, or that his or her irritability is directed at you personally. It's usually the disease talking.

Misunderstanding, frustration, and confusion make many people with Alzheimer's very irritable. The usual human reaction to frustration is to blame someone else. And you, as the caregiver, are often that someone. Knowing that it's the disease talking can help you step back.

That being said, there are ornery people in the world, and Alzheimer's isn't going to make that go away; that behavior might get worse. In this case, you may need to learn to "turn the other cheek."

Patience

Some Alzheimer's patients become meek and very needy. They need constant reassurance and attention. This type of behavior can also be very frustrating, and this is where even more patience is necessary. Patience is important in every facet of Alzheimer's caregiving. Your patient is going to be very slow about every activity, and you must be willing to go slowly, too. Deep breathing, slow counting, and reciting poetry are all useful ways of developing patience and learning to slow down your normal pace. Especially if you work at another job during the day and are a caregiver at night, you need to switch off the fast-paced work mode and get into caregiver mode.

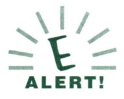

Alzheimer's caregivers are twice as likely to provide more than forty hours a week in caregiving as other caregivers. 61 percent of "intense" family caregivers (those providing at least twenty-one hours of care a week), however, have suffered from depression. Some studies have shown that caregiver stress inhibits healing.

Compassion and Empathy

When laypeople go to a religious retreat to gain greater spiritual depth and wisdom, they may be given the wise counsel to seek spirituality by unselfishly helping others. Some call it unconditional love. You feel it when you expect nothing back from the person you are caring for. By tapping into this unconditional love, you will feel greater empathy and compassion for your Alzheimer's patient and a very strong connection to your spirituality.

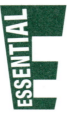

Since up to 80 percent of Alzheimer's patients are cared for at home, chances are that you will be called upon to give aid to someone with Alzheimer's one day. It's best to learn what you can about this condition and have a plan in place for the inevitable.

After all, when it all comes down to the question of life and death, you are ready to ask the important questions. What would I consider the most important thing in my life if I know I am going to die tomorrow? Most people answer that their family, friends, and loved ones are the most important thing. Material goods and societal accomplishments pale in comparison to a meaningful relationship with other human beings.

Scheduling Care at Home

Most people with Alzheimer's are taken care of at home by family and friends. The decision is often made immediately to have their loved one be cared for at home as long as possible. The family doesn't want to "abandon" their mother or father to an institution. There is a perception that care in nursing homes is not up to par, and they are often more than the family can afford.

Care at home means you need to create a schedule where four or five team members each cover a day and a half. Or, each team member may take one week on duty and rotate every month. Either way, it usually means that part of the team is working full-time and will have to make adjustments to their schedules.

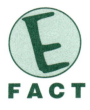

FACT

Caring for an Alzheimer's relative is a full-time and very stressful job. Previous statistics found that three-quarters of Alzheimer's caregivers are women, wives, daughters, friends, and paid caregivers. A survey taken in 2000, however, found that caregiving is no longer predominantly a woman's field. Men now make up 44 percent of the caregiving population.

If you are a professional, you may be able to schedule your appointments to allow time off to do "your shift." If you aren't in control of your schedule, you may find it more difficult to find time for your shift. That's when sick days, vacation days, weekends, and holidays all go into the caregiving pot. For all concerned, caregiving either means a loss of income or much more stress; often it is both.

The Sexual Reality of Alzheimer's

Alzheimer's also causes a huge shift in sexual relationships. If your spouse has Alzheimer's, then he or she may pull back from intimacy in the beginning because they have lost confidence in themselves in general. The sexual drive is very much affected by stress and anxiety. If and when depression occurs, that alone can cause a decreased interest in sex. Medications and physical problems can also interfere with intimacy.

As a caregiver, you may naturally experience changes in sexual feelings toward your spouse in your new role. It may be difficult to shift from your role as caregiver to a situation where you become sexually intimate.

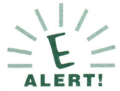

ALERT!

On August 27, 2001, Dr. Barbara Messinger-Rapport, on WebMD, said that sexuality has not been sufficiently studied as a component of Alzheimer's disease. But what we do know is that a combination of mood disorders, depression, and medications that cause sexual dysfunction is common. Alzheimer's dementia can also cause apathy that decreases interest in appearance, clothes, and friends, and may affect sexual function as well.

Who's Having Sex Anyway?

According to a survey on women's sexuality, only one in five older women is having regular sexual relations, and most of these women are married. They reach a peak of sexual activity in their thirties, and it's downhill from there. By age eighty or ninety, the rate of regular sex is only 2 percent.

But Dr. John Morley, a professor of gerontology at Saint Louis University, commented that there are many reasons why older women don't have sex, and it's not necessarily that they are opposed to the idea. Impotence in four out of ten men after age sixty, sick spouses, or no spouse, are the real reasons for the decrease, he says. (The study surveyed 2,000 women aged eighteen to ninety-four, in 1994, and the results were published in the March 2003 issue of the journal *Sexually Transmitted Diseases*. Viagra wasn't on the market in 1994. It would be interesting to repeat the survey to see if treatment of male impotence made a difference in the amount of sex older women had.)

Overtly Sexual Behavior

Behavior such as taking off clothes inappropriately may be just a reaction to feeling too warm and not a sexual display. Alzheimer's, however, may cause a person to have an increased sex drive. Try not to shy away from dealing with this behavior, which may be caused by anxiety and a need for reassurance. More hugging, a massage, stroking, or patting may be what's called for.

If your spouse actually forgets they are married, he or she may flirt or make advances on someone. This can be very distressing and requires you to be detached and to not take it personally. Either berating the person or making it into a joke is inappropriate. Distraction with another activity is the main way to deal with this type of behavior.

Care for the Caregiver

Taking care of someone who has Alzheimer's disease can be exhausting, frustrating, and overwhelming. Detachment is an easy word to say but very difficult to perform. Patience, compassion, and empathy also take their toll. Taking care of a loved one is hard work. You are responsible for their every need, but who's taking care of you?

Caregiver's Bill of Rights

As a caregiver for an Alzheimer's patient, you are often expected to be superhuman. The American Health Assistance Foundation understands the problems of caregiving, and through the Alzheimer's Family Relief Program, they make sure people know their rights. One of the first rights is the right to be human, to have human emotions and human needs.

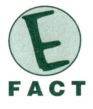

FACT

A 1999 report, "Economic Value of Informal Caregiving in the U.S.," found that $196 billion a year is contributed to the U.S. health-care system by an invisible health-care sector—families and friends who provide care at home for the chronically ill. In 2002, the value of the services family caregivers provide for "free" rose to $257 billion a year.

The Caregiver's Bill of Rights may seem like common sense, but it's necessary to keep the advice it gives utmost in your mind so you can maintain your mental and physical balance for yourself and your loved one. The Bill of Rights states that it's all right to have normal human emotions, but then make sure you turn that emotion into something more positive. It's okay to:

- **Be angry.** Work off this energy physically; take a walk, clean closets, talk it over with someone.
- **Be frustrated.** Count to ten and stop doing what is making you frustrated and do something else.
- **Take time alone.** Find a few minutes or hours to be alone.
- **Ask for help.** Canvas family, friends, and local Alzheimer's support groups for support.
- **Trust your judgment.** Trust that you are doing the best you can and realize you can't do more than that.

- **Recognize your limits.** It's of no use to you or your Alzheimer's patient to stretch yourself to your limit. You are a valuable person. Take care of yourself, too!
- **Make mistakes.** We learn through our mistakes. No one is perfect.
- **Grieve.** It's okay and perfectly normal to be going through a grief response for the loss of the way things were.
- **Laugh and love.** Laughter and love heal all wounds.
- **Hope.** Each new day may be better, may be easier, and a cure may be found.

Guilt

You may not know it, but you may be feeling guilty about your loved one's situation. You consciously or unconsciously may say, "Why should I feel fine if my loved one isn't?" And psychologically, people sometimes punish themselves when their loved one is ill. In some cultures, cutting off a finger when someone dies is normal. We don't go quite that far, but the tendency is there to try to take some of their burden by becoming ill ourselves. We need to guard against this.

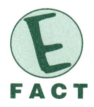

FACT

A June 2001 study by the Alzheimer's Association found that caregivers of family members with Alzheimer's disease feel that doctors aren't giving them all the information they need to deal with the challenges of caring for a loved one or dealing with caregiver stress. Most physicians interviewed for the survey said they do provide the information on those issues.

We also feel guilty if we find ourselves being happy or excited about something, and then feel like we are betraying our loved one and their suffering. But they wouldn't want your life to end because they are ill. We need to keep our perspective of life and death and realize that by our suffering, we aren't making their suffering less. If we can maintain a cheerful outlook and give a genuine smile, we can lift the spirits of our Alzheimer's sufferer and lift our own spirits as well.

The Caregiver Stress Test

This test is in a book called the *Caregiver's Handbook*, edited by Robert Torres-Stanovick and published by the San Diego County Mental Health Services in 1990. Caregivers are instructed to answer the following questions using the most appropriate word(s): Seldom, Sometimes, Often, Usually True, Always True.

1. I find I can't get enough rest.
2. I don't have enough time for myself.
3. I don't have time to be with other family members besides the person I care for.
4. I feel guilty about my situation.
5. I don't get out much anymore.
6. I have conflict with the person I care for.
7. I have conflict with other family members.
8. I cry every day.
9. I worry about having enough money to make ends meet.
10. I don't feel I have enough knowledge or experience to give care as well as I'd like.
11. My own health is not good.

Caregivers are further instructed that if they respond with "Usually True" or "Always True" in one or more of these areas, it may be time to begin looking for help with caring for the Alzheimer's patient and help in taking care of him- or herself.

Caregiver Respite

According to data about time spent by caregivers, you may be working about eighty hours a week in this role. You may hold down a full-time job and then come home to take over for an "elder sitter" or pick up your relative from an adult day care. It's a long, hard day with no breaks in the evenings or on weekends. There is no time to recharge your batteries or catch up on your own life.

What you need most is some time to yourself. Fortunately, there are caregiver support programs, counseling services, and respite opportunities. They are important aspects of Alzheimer's care because supporting the caregiver goes a long way in keeping Alzheimer's patients out of institutions.

Video Respite

One form of respite is provided by companies that produce videos especially for the elderly. One such company, called STB Productions, began in 1989 with "the goal of bringing the beauty and peace of our natural world back into the lives of people who, for whatever reason, cannot enjoy it on their own." For Alzheimer's patients and caregivers alike, these calming videos feature nature's beautiful sights and sounds as a wonderful stress release.

The founder of the company, Susan Beahan, in her former work as Secretary of Housing and Urban Development, was most interested in the plight of the housebound elderly. She says that "Our world is full of inspiring, uplifting, rejuvenating, and refreshing things, but you won't see them on the nightly news or network television! You have to *seek them out on your own,* and know where to look!" She provides people with "sparkling streams, deserted beaches, spring orchards, and peaceful farm fields we all long to experience and escape to, but simply don't have the time to visit and appreciate!"

Canine Respite

A wonderful service that gives caregivers a break is the Alzheimer's guide dog service called Okada Dogs. If you have ever been leaned on by a Great Dane or a Labrador retriever, or loved by a collie, you know what I'm talking about. Okada dogs are trained to help control wandering from home, eliminating the need for twenty-four-hour supervision by the caregiver.

When wandering occurs, the dog is trained to find the caregiver and take them to the Alzheimer's patient. Beyond safety, are the loving, therapeutic benefits of dogs in pet therapy programs. Dogs give unconditional love and are attentive and calming for both the caregiver and their Alzheimer's patient.

Respite Services Outside the Home

In the past, it was mainly Catholic convents and seminaries that made rooms available to people seeking solace and respite. Now, those services have grown along with the need for them. They are usually attached to an adult day care center, which is very often supported by the Alzheimer's Association. Such programs provide a stopgap when you just need temporary support, when you don't need a full homecare program, or while you are waiting for Medicaid to kick in.

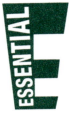

On November 22, 2003, the *News Journal* of Central Ohio filed a story on an Alzheimer's in-home volunteer respite program. Volunteers spend four or more hours per week giving caregivers a much-needed break. Such programs are flourishing around the country as an increasing need arises for these services.

Respite: A Growing Movement

Respite is part of a larger movement by Alzheimer's activists who see the need for home health aides, adult day care, private duty nursing, overnight respite, comprehensive caregiver assessment, homecare services, and home modifications. Additional services like counseling, Alzheimer's information and referral, and caregiver education and training are helpful but do not work if you are the only caregiver and can't find help with day-to-day care.

As these programs are being set up, the big chore is to make caregivers aware that these services exist. Caregiving can be such an isolated, and isolating, experience that you don't have a moment to spare to look outside the many tasks you are doing to even see if there is any help available. Ⓔ

Chapter 12

Caregiving at Home

Creating a safe and comfortable home environment for your Alzheimer's patient is doable, but it's important to enlist your family and friends. You'll have to tackle every room in the house and make sure it is safe for someone with Alzheimer's. It is a difficult process, time consuming, and tedious, but with the following plan in hand, it will make life much easier for everyone. First let's see who's going to be in charge.

Caring for Your Spouse

When your spouse receives a diagnosis of Alzheimer's, you are probably living independently in your house or apartment, in which case the task of caregiving falls on your shoulders. If the disease is in the early stages, then it's a matter of giving love and support, accompanying your spouse to doctor's appointments, meeting with the family, and eventually making appointments with your spouse's employer, your lawyer, and your financial advisor.

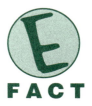

FACT

Heavy-duty caregivers, especially spousal caregivers, do not get consistent help from other family members. One study has shown that as many as three-fourths of these caregivers are "going it alone" and have great need for community support services.

Then you have to take stock of the home environment and see how to make things safe as your spouse's memory becomes more impaired. If you don't have family nearby to help, there are numerous organizations that can lend a hand. It's a matter of reaching out and asking for help. Nobody caring for someone with Alzheimer's should feel that they are alone.

When the task of caring for your spouse becomes too great, then you must rely on your family's support. If you don't have family, again, there are many agencies, foundations, and associations dedicated to helping those with Alzheimer's.

Family Choices

As a family, when you begin to see a problem with your relative, there is the conscious or unconscious shuffling about to see who is going to take charge of the situation. Temporary, and sometimes ineffectual, measures are often taken that make you feel better but don't really improve the situation. For example, you may feel the need to install safety locks or alarm systems, thinking that your elderly relative, who lives alone, needs to be protected. That can backfire because they can't remember the numbers for the alarm or figure out how to use the lock because their short-term memory is impaired.

Often, the next step is to find a housekeeper or caregiver to stay with your relative if that can be afforded. If not, then there is the inevitable move into one of your homes. Hopefully, this is decided in a family meeting where everyone agrees who should be the primary caregiver and what support the rest of the family members are offering.

Sibling Involvement

Even at the best of times, not all siblings get along. There is considerable stress involved with caregiving, and it's not unusual for tensions to become even more strained. It's important in communicating with your siblings to keep uppermost in your minds that it's not about you and not about them; it's about your parent. Regular meetings, in person or over the telephone, are important to keep open the lines of communication.

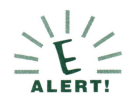

ALERT!

Be wary of a family member who selfishly puts their concerns above those of their Alzheimer's relative. To avoid helping, they may say, "I'm just so devastated by the news of this illness, I can't cope, and my doctor warned me that if I have any more stress, I'll get ill." Trying to force such a person to help is usually fruitless.

You may find that one of your siblings is more concerned about their needs than your parent's and draws away from involvement. If they are in poor health and under considerable stress, they may not be able to physically lend a hand. You can, however, keep them in the information loop and ask if they can help financially.

At some point, the family may want to sit with a trained Alzheimer's counselor to help with family communication and to help set priorities. Most families are not trained in either caregiving or communication, so it's an opportunity to learn how to deal with problems head-on, by keeping a level head, reining in your emotions, and communicating openly and honestly. Many issues have to be dealt with, and each one may need to be negotiated to achieve a consensus. Again, uppermost in your minds should be the comfort of your relative.

Sibling Concerns

It probably starts in the crib: "Who does Mum and Dad love best?" It's the perennial question, and it doesn't end when your parent is ill. If you are the primary caregiver, old rivalries and jealousies may make your siblings think you aren't giving the best care. They may be so uninvolved with the care that they haven't met with the doctor and might even deny the diagnosis or argue about the treatment.

If you are the appointed guardian and executor of your parent's will, then your siblings may feel you are going to cut them out. Or, maybe they are acting uncooperative so you won't ask them to help or contribute money. They could even be deliberately combative so that you will get mad at them, allowing them to feel justified in not helping. This all happens—and sometimes even worse things happen—when people feel they are being pushed into doing something they don't want to do.

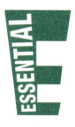

As an executor you will be responsible for settling your relative's estate and implementing their "last will and testament" once they have passed away. You will be responsible for creating an inventory, appraising and distributing assets, paying taxes, and settling debts owed by the deceased. You may be a family member or a family friend with expertise in law or accounting.

Part of the argument with your siblings may be that you feel you are doing all the work. But instead of complaining, just ask for help and make it specific. Create a list of things that need to be done and a schedule of where you need input. If your siblings don't respond to your requests, you have to move on to other family members, friends, and your church or community.

Some siblings may find that they just can't cope with another stress in their lives, and all they can think about is how to best protect themselves. These are the "it's all about me" people. Whatever the reason, primary caregivers often have to go it alone. But within your own nuclear family you may have more support than you realize.

When the Nuclear Family Is Involved

It appears that many nuclear families have no choice but to get involved. In a 1998 report called "Who Cares," the Alzheimer's Association and the National Alliance for Caregiving found that at least one in three families caring for Alzheimer's sufferers also cared for children under the age of eighteen.

We all know what happens if there are two or more children in the house—sibling rivalry. And with every new addition to the home, whether a child or an aging grandparent, there is a major shift in family dynamics. People who feel love and care is finite will be afraid that they won't get as much love and attention. Well, love isn't finite; it's boundless, but there will definitely be less time spent on other family members if the major caregiver is also taking care of someone with Alzheimer's.

Children's Concerns

Children living with an Alzheimer's patient can feel angry, jealous, sad, and even guilty, wondering, "Is Grandma crazy? Can I get Alzheimer's, or will my mom and dad get it?" They may display behavior such as withdrawing from the loved one, becoming impatient with the person, doing poorly in school, and complaining of headaches, stomachaches, or other minor ailments. (This information comes from ✑*mayoclinic.com* and ✑*cnn.com*.)

ALERT!

The Home Safety Council's 2004 report, the "State of Home Safety in America" stated that after motor vehicles, the home is the most common location of unintentional fatal injuries, accounting for more than 20 million medical visits and 20,000 fatalities at a cost of $379 billion in one year. Falls are the most common fatal home injury, followed by poisoning, fires/burns, suffocation, and drowning.

Caring for an Alzheimer's patient at home is even harder with very young children who don't know what Alzheimer's disease is and just think Granddad is acting weird or scary. If you are the primary caregiver and a mother as well, your children may be acting out in an attempt to get your attention. For some kids, negative attention is better than no attention, and acting out may be the only way they know how to get it.

Getting the Children Involved

To prevent the almost inevitable clash when dealing with the demands of caring for your relative, start having weekly family meetings and get everyone involved with the project of helping. Give the meetings a special name that everyone agrees on such as Granddad's Team Meeting, or Grandma's Club. In the meetings, ask everyone, even young children, for their advice. This approach can turn up incredibly helpful suggestions and elicit children's support. Being asked gives children a real "buy in" to the new situation.

Instead of trying to protect children from what you see as a very difficult situation, get them involved. Give young children chores such as giving five hugs a day to you and, if they feel comfortable, to their grandparent. If possible, try to "reframe" the task of helping your loved one as an adventure and not a burden. Kids can appreciate an adventure much more than a burden.

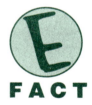

FACT

In 1995, the *Scandinavian Journal of Primary Health Care* did a survey to investigate the predictors for recurrent falls among elderly persons living at home. They found that previous falls, peripheral neuropathy, use of psychotropic medication, and slow walking speed were the main reasons for recurrent falling. They recommended review of medications by the doctor, proper footwear, and treatment for peripheral neuropathy.

Caregiver respite services, where a volunteer comes to the home once or twice a week for four hours or so, can give the family time for a much-needed outing and quality time together. You also need to build time together into your daily schedule. Maybe it's over breakfast or dinner or some other convenient time when everyone is together and your relative is sleeping. It's a time to catch up with what's happening at school or what's happening at your spouse's workplace.

Safeguarding Your Loved One

Considering all the ways an Alzheimer's patient can get into trouble, you'll find that protecting them is very much like protecting a child. Think of them wandering off unattended, grabbing a sharp knife by the blade, dropping an electric shaver in a sink of water or a full tub, or tripping on a loose carpet. You can protect them from all these things by following certain commonsense guidelines.

In case of wandering:

* Have your Alzheimer's relative wear an ID bracelet so rescuers, local police, medical staff, and others are alerted to his or her condition in the event of an emergency.
* Keep a recent photo and, better still, a video of your patient available.
* Use iron-on labels with the Alzheimer's patient's name, address, and phone number in his or her clothing to aid in identification.

In the home:

* Purchase rubber-soled shoes or slippers for your loved one to help avoid falls.
* Arrange furniture so he or she can move around easily.
* Eliminate or firmly tape down any scatter rugs, area rugs, or moveable carpets.
* Use nightlights to make finding the bathroom easier at night.
* Remove firearms and weapons from your home.
* Lock up over-the-counter medicines, prescription medicines, and cleaning fluids.
* Keep alcohol in a locked cabinet and away from your relative.
* Use bed rails or place a comforter or pillows on the floor around the bed in case of falling.
* Hide car keys and, if necessary, disconnect the car battery if the patient is not allowed to drive but refuses to stop.
* If the patient hallucinates or is bothered by his or her reflection, cover or remove all mirrors.

- Use a baby sound monitor in his or her room if you are in a different part of the house.
- Do not leave your relative alone in a parked car.
- Use safe plastic fans that won't cut the fingers if poked.
- If necessary, build a wheelchair ramp.

For the caregiver:

- Keep a working flashlight by your bed.
- Keep medical records on hand at all times.

Alzheimer's Safety in the Home

If you can remember a time when you felt spaced out and disoriented, such as after being up all night, or after surgery, or in the middle of a bad flu, you know how unstable you feel; you are constantly apologizing for bumping into things and forgetting things. Well, with Alzheimer's, that seems to be the pervasive feeling. Because of a very short attention span, problems naming and recognizing things, the inability to make decisions, and problems communicating desires, anything can go wrong.

ALERT!

Statistics from 1991 show that an average of 370 people of all ages are injured in and around their bathtub or shower daily in the United States. The Consumer Product Safety Commission documented 139,434 injuries in 1991. The elderly accounted for 20 percent of those injuries. More elderly people were injured in their bathroom than from potentially dangerous exercise equipment or cooking appliances.

The familiar act of boiling water on the stove can be forgotten as your Alzheimer's relative wanders away on some elusive task. The result is a burned kettle or, even worse, a fire or a severe skin burn when the white hot kettle is not recognized as dangerous. Candles left burning can be another danger, as can leaving the doors wide open for strangers to come in, or leaving the bathtub filling up with water until the house is flooded.

Supervision is the most important aspect of keeping your Alzheimer's relative safe, but you cannot be there all the time. So, it's important to make sure various rooms have simple safety features that help make your job easier.

Bathroom Safety

Safety in the bathroom is important for all members of the family but most important for the elderly. When injuries happen in a seemingly safe environment, such as a bathroom, it can serve to greatly erode confidence and can be a major setback even if there is no broken bone.

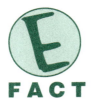

FACT

According to an article called "Bathing for Older People with Disabilities" from the Medical College of Cornell University, safety was never an important issue in the design of bathrooms. Bathtubs are no different than they were in 1700 B.C., except for the plumbing. Showers came about in the early 1800s, but their design has remained unchanged since the end of the first World War.

Starting with the tub, install safety bars on the sides of the tub; place a rubber bath mat or adhesive decals on the floor of the tub or shower; place a bath chair in the tub that is stable and secure; install a soap and shampoo rack on a level where standing and reaching are not required; install a handheld shower nozzle so the shower doesn't beat down on the head; and keep several bath mats on the side of the tub to prevent a severe head injury from an unexpected fall on the edge.

Next is the toilet. People call it the throne when they install a raised toilet seat with special side rails for holding onto while getting on and off the toilet. The faucets of the sink may need to be padded to prevent injury from a fall. Wrapping a facecloth around and securing with an elastic band may do the trick. Some people advise using permanent marker to label the taps with red for hot and blue for cold as a reminder. The bathroom medicine cabinet should be locked or else everything should be removed from it.

Lastly, a rubber-backed mat is important to have in the bathroom to prevent slips and falls on a floor made wet by a bath or steam from a bath. Throw out the fluffy bath mat that may trip someone who has a slow, shuffling gait.

Kitchen Safety

Whether it's gas range or electric, the stove is the most dangerous appliance in the kitchen. You can effectively neutralize the danger by removing the stove's knobs. When you want to use the stove, replace them; when you are finished, take the knobs off again and store them in a safe hiding place. While using the stove, if your Alzheimer's patient is in the kitchen, it's best to keep pot handles pointing to the back of the stove so your patient can't accidentally grab or bump them.

Many kitchen fires and house fires start with fat or oil that is left on the stove and forgotten about. It grows hotter, begins to smoke, and eventually bursts into flame, spraying oil and flames around the room. Another kitchen hazard comes from spilling water into a pan of heated oil, causing splashing oil that can catch fire on a gas cooking flame.

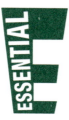

To prevent scalding, the temperature of the water heater for the whole house should be turned down to at least 120 degrees Fahrenheit. This is the temperature at which you can safely and comfortably hold your hands under hot running water without getting burned.

Drawers hold potentially lethal knives and scissors, which must be removed and safely stored. Kitchen cabinets under the sink usually contain unsafe cleaning supplies and must be padlocked. Even overhead cabinets can be unsafe; if your Alzheimer's patient tries to get something, cans and/or boxes can fall on his or her head. The kitchen is the place to keep the house fire extinguisher because most fires start in the kitchen. It's also the place for emergency numbers on a magnet pad on the fridge. And finally, mats in the kitchen should be avoided, as they can cause falls from being tripped over or slipped on.

Door, Window, and Stair Safety

Patient wandering is a common problem for Alzheimer's caregivers to deal with, so doors must be kept locked or equipped with childproof doorknobs. As extra protection you might have to install some sort of alarm or bell system on doors to the outside. There should also be locks on windows and patio doors.

For stair safety, what seems to work for children also works for wandering adults. This includes putting up a gate at the top and bottom of the stairs and locking the bolt. A handrail on the stair is a necessity; if you can put one on either side, so much the better. Bright duct tape across the top and bottom of each step can help to guide an Alzheimer's patient safely up and down stairs.

Fire and Electrical Safety

Fire safety is important because a match can be struck, electrical cords can be tampered with, paper can be stuffed around a radiator, a space heater can be knocked over, or the stove or fireplace can be turned on by someone who doesn't realize what they are doing. Keeping matches and lighters out of reach, removing electrical wires, covering radiators, using childproof covers on plugs, and not using space heaters are the first steps to preventing a fire.

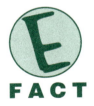

FACT

A 2000 *British Medical Journal* study on smoking and Alzheimer's showed that smoking doesn't protect against Alzheimer's. Another large study, performed in 1998 in the Netherlands, said the same thing. Over the years, however, several smaller studies have showed smokers may be diagnosed with Alzheimer's less frequently. A 2004 study found that nicotine can bind up certain brain proteins and partially block amyloid plaque formation, making this relationship worthy of research.

We already know there should be a fire extinguisher in the kitchen, but if there is more than one floor, each floor should have a fire extinguisher. Smoke detectors should also be installed on each floor and in your relative's bedroom. Fire drills are important so that you know the best ways out in case of a fire.

Smoking and Alzheimer's

An Alzheimer's patient who is a smoker presents a real challenge. This is the time to introduce the nicotine patch, acupuncture, hypnosis, or anything that can help them stop, for both health and safety reasons. We are all aware that falling asleep with a cigarette is the best way to start a fire.

Chapter 13

Alzheimer's Personal Care

We wake up in the morning and slip on our dressing gown, go to the bathroom, brush our teeth, take a drink of water, and start breakfast, seemingly without thinking about it. But if you have Alzheimer's, your brain may not allow you to remember what sequence of thoughts and actions are required to perform those basic steps. Eating, sleeping, and bathing all have to be thought through in a very organized manner when assisting your Alzheimer's relative. It's a matter of breaking things down into doable steps.

Dressing

The battle lines can be drawn over dressing. As a caregiver, you want to choose clothes that are loose-fitting, which often translates into baggy; comfortable, which translates into dowdy; and with zippers instead of buttons, which means you've dressed your mother in a housecoat! At least dads are easier to dress—shirts and pants.

But think of the last time you were in the hospital, what did they make you wear? An easy-to-remove johnny that left you feeling pretty demoralized. In every instance of helping your Alzheimer's relative, go back to the guiding principle of a caregiver: Offer comfort, dignity, and respect.

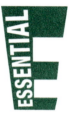

Comfortable, easy-to-fit shoes are extremely important for an Alzheimer's patient. Find running shoes with Velcro fasteners. Nothing is more demeaning than being forced to watch someone tying your laces. Fortunately, these days there are many fashionable styles of shoes to choose from that won't make them seem so utilitarian.

If your mother had a particular style or flair, you want her to keep that for her confidence and a semblance of everything being all right with the world. It's easy in the beginning; the clothes are in the closet, and she helps to choose what to wear. Of course, as the dementia worsens, she may need more help in dressing.

Dressing Tips

Try to allow your parent to make their own choice of what to wear as long as they can, to give them a feeling of independence. Give them lots of time to choose and then to dress. If you are frustrated with waiting, use that time to have a conversation, reminisce about the past, pick up about the room, or even sit and relax. This will put less pressure on your patient than if you are hovering about waiting for the next button to be done up.

Various Alzheimer's groups advise the following to help with the process of dressing:

- Make sure the room is warm and the blinds are shut.
- Lay out clothes in the order the patient will put them on—underwear first, socks last.
- Remove dirty clothes from the room at night; otherwise they will seem to be among the next day's choices.
- Casually remind the patient what to put on next or hand it to them.
- If your patient exhibits confusion, walk them through what to do: "Put your foot through the pant leg."
- If they become agitated because they can't do something themselves, try to distract them with another activity, and then go back to dressing.
- Never tell your patient they are doing it wrong or berate them, but be willing to laugh or cry about it.

The Difficult Part of Dressing

In the beginning, you are there to help choose the clothes; people with mild and even moderate Alzheimer's can usually manage themselves. Dressing is such an intimate activity, most people aren't used to someone being there to help them put on underwear, for example. It can be very embarrassing and uncomfortable, perhaps for both of you, and especially for a daughter helping her father. Even so, it must be done and here's how.

Usually your relative is sitting down on the side of the bed. If the patient is your father, first help him put on his shirt so it will cover his genitals. Then place his underwear on the bed, and as he takes off his pajama bottoms, you just turn your back. If he seems to be grunting and groaning and having a struggle with his underwear, approach from behind and see if you can lend a hand without being right in his face. You can avert your eyes if his seem to be looking at you to see your reaction.

With your mother, you can stand behind her while she puts on her bra and you can clasp it from behind. Then comes her shirt or sweater, which will cover her genitals while she puts on her panties and then her skirt or slacks.

You will find that your presence beside your patient as they dress will become routine and soon seem comfortable and almost normal. And as time goes on and you are needed to do most of the dressing, you'll be quite ready to do it and, truth be told, they might not even realize they are naked in front of you. With severe Alzheimer's, dressing is mostly changing nightshirts, and the inevitable johnny is very useful.

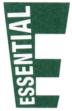

Clothes do make the man, and the woman. If your relative stays in their nightgown or nightshirt all day, they will feel more like an invalid than if you help them dress in their normal clothes. And dressing up for a party or to go out to dinner is all part of the excitement and helps distract them from their burdens.

A Day at the Spa

A day at the spa—that's what you call the manicure, pedicure, backrub, and hand or foot massage. Who had time for any of these when working day and night to survive and bring up a family? But now, with all the time in the world, your Alzheimer's patient can have a spa day. Just calling it a spa day sets a nice relaxing and fun tone.

You probably have all the tools right at hand, too. Nails have to be trimmed anyway, so add bright nail polish for your mom or clear for your dad and make it a treat. For the massage, use some mildly scented massage oil. You don't have to do the regulation one-hour professional massage. Even ten minutes is enough. It's the touch that's important; it's soothing and reassuring, and can be comforting, especially for someone with Alzheimer's. Keep your manicure tools and massage oil together in a basket within easy reach. Then you can declare a spa day at any time you feel your patient needs an enjoyable distraction and your undivided attention.

Eating

Meals and snacks are very important for keeping your parent or spouse healthy. You'll find, however, that with various mood changes such as depression and apathy, with medications, and with memory problems, food is not a priority. Planning and making nutritious meals can be a full-time job in itself and when they aren't eaten, it can be very frustrating.

Make a list of the patient's favorite foods including a wide variety from the four food groups: grains, dairy, protein, and fruits and vegetables. And keep the kitchen well-supplied. One of the members of your support team could do the weekly shopping as his or her task.

Make Use of a Slow Cooker

The easiest way to prepare meals is to use slow cookers. In fact, you may call them a small miracle once you start using them. They can help you free up valuable time that you can spend on other activities or even allow you to get a bit of rest.

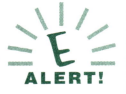

ALERT!

You may be concerned about the possibility of your Alzheimer's patient starting a fire if either of you use the stove. There is much less danger for your relative with the use of a slow cooker, a toaster over, and an electric kettle. If you use these appliances, you can cover the top of the stove and remove all the knobs for the burners.

You can get a small, one-quart, electric slow cooker and cook grains in it overnight and have wonderful cooked cereal for breakfast. Dinner can be cooking from early morning in a three- or four-quart slow cooker. You can throw in poultry or meat and vegetables all at the same time and find a delicious meal at the end of the day.

Breakfast Recipes

Mix together half a pound each of rye, oats, millet, pumpkin seeds, and sunflower seeds in a large canister. Every evening, for each person, measure 3 ounces of the grain and seed mixture into the slow cooker and add a little more than twice as much water. In the morning, if the cereal is too dry, just add more water and stir well. Cut up a banana and put some flax oil on it for your essential fatty acids, and you have a filling and incredibly nutritious breakfast.

When the grain canister is empty, buy some more grains. You can even experiment with different varieties with weird-sounding names that you find in the health store such as kamut, spelt, quinoa, and amaranth.

You may find that mixing two different canisters a day gives you even more variety. If you need milk on your cereal but are allergic or sensitive to dairy milk, with gas, bloating, or diarrhea, use rice milk, soymilk, or almond milk found in health stores.

Dinner Recipes

In the morning, place whole lamb chops, whole pork chops, cut up chicken or turkey breast or thigh (without the skin), or cut up beef in the bottom of the slow cooker. Add several types of root vegetables cut up in big chunks (carrots, potatoes, yams, turnips, parsnips, etc.). Then add about 3 cups of water, plug in on high, and leave all day.

The delicious smells will permeate the house and by dinner, everyone's mouths will be watering. Tear up some romaine lettuce; cut up some tomatoes and celery; and add avocado, olives, cilantro, endive, or arugula for variety, and you have a fresh raw salad along with the cooked dinner. The meal is complete.

Lunch Recipes

Take the extra stew stock from last night's dinner and make a quick and nutritious soup. It will be different every time, and if there are leftover vegetables, so much the better. But first heat up the stock, add more water to make about 2 quarts, then add rice—brown rice has the most nutrients. Bring to a boil and then put to simmer for about forty minutes. Set a timer so you won't forget.

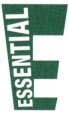

A smoothie is probably one of the easiest and most nutritious meals you can prepare. Take ½ cup of apple juice or orange juice and ½ cup of water, 1 banana, ½ cup of frozen blueberries, and 3 tablespoons of protein powder (rotate the following protein powders—whey, egg, and soy), and blend until smooth.

Add water if some has boiled away and add the leftover vegetables, or frozen ones, to finish off your soup. Adding a can of coconut milk and some curry can give it added zest. You can start the soup midmorning if you are adding rice; otherwise, it only takes a few minutes to prepare. Make a quick salad or serve some raw vegetables along with it, and there is your fast and nutritious lunch.

Don't Forget the Water

Dehydration is a common factor in the elderly, especially if there are memory problems. You just don't remember you need to drink. Actually, very few people remember to drink enough. It's important to drink two quarts of water a day. To remember to do that, fill up two one-quart containers with water—filtered or bottled water is best. Put one in the fridge and let the other one sit by your chair or bed and pour yourself a glass of water. Make sure that the two quarts are gone by the end of the day. Do the same for your Alzheimer's patient, making sure that he or she drinks both quarts each day.

The Bathing Ritual

Bathing is an even more challenging task than dressing for both you and your relative with Alzheimer's. Emotionally and physically, it's a challenge. Emotionally, your patient may be very embarrassed to be seen naked and have to be scrubbed in intimate parts by a family member. The only advice is to keep in mind the big picture—millions have done it before you, and millions are doing it along with you. Physically, your patient may find it difficult to get in and out of the tub unassisted. This is why it's very important to install bath chairs and bath railings.

Depending on his or her level of functioning, your patient may feel the bathing experience is either just uncomfortable or actually threatening, which may make them agitated. In severe Alzheimer's, your patient may actually not know why they have to have a bath, and fight against you.

Go about the bathing process at a slow pace. To keep dignity intact, some patients might want to cover themselves with a towel both in and out of the tub. With time, however, that modesty will give way to familiarity as you become a part of the process. In some cases, you might even be part of the shower. In order to hold someone up in a bath chair and help them wash their hair with the shower hose, you might have to step in behind them. That alone can lead to a lot of hilarity. Sharing such an experience is not only fun, but a moment of bonding.

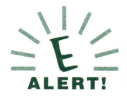

ALERT!

Skin care begins with regular washing and bathing. Unless you look at your patient's skin every day, you may miss the beginnings of a bedsore, a scratch that can become infected, or a wound that isn't healing. Use only a small amount of neutral pH soap, because it can dry out the skin. Use body oils and lotions to seal in moisture.

Bathing and Showering Tips

Intersperse bath and shower days with sponge baths. As Alzheimer's advances, however, your patient should take a shower sitting on a bath chair and using a showerhead on a hose.

Keep the following checklist of how to prepare the bathroom so that everything can go as smoothly as possible.

- ❏ Adjust the temperature in the bathroom.
- ❏ Warm a bath towel; do this by spinning it in the dryer just before you need it.
- ❏ Make sure the temperature of the bath or shower is not too hot.
- ❏ There should be a nonslip carpet on the floor, not a thick bath mat, and safety bars on the bathtub.
- ❏ Remember whose bath it is; make them in charge and guide them through the steps.

Bathroom Dangers

Never leave the room, even for a second, with your patient lying in the bathtub. It doesn't take long for them to try to get up by themselves, fall and hit their head, and drown. Even though you installed all the other aids in the bathroom, you really have to be there to make sure they are used. If your patient is not used to the bathtub safety rail or the rails on the toilet, he or she may have to be encouraged to use them.

Sleeplessness in the Elderly

There are a number of causes of sleeplessness in Alzheimer's patients; one of them is the simple fact of age. According to Dr. David Neubauer of the Johns Hopkins Sleep Disorders Center, elderly people in general have a harder time with sleep than younger adults. A full spectrum of symptoms can include difficulty falling asleep, less time spent in the deeper stages of sleep, early morning awakening, and less total sleep time. Napping during the daytime and sleeping in to all hours can reinforce poor sleep habits.

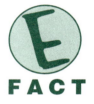

FACT

Researchers at the National Institute on Aging published a report in 1995. They surveyed over 9,000 persons aged sixty-five years and older and found that more than 50 percent reported that they suffered from at least one chronic sleep complaint such as difficulty falling asleep, waking early, restless sleep, and daytime sleepiness.

Eating late, taking medications, and drinking coffee and alcohol can all interfere with sleep. Physical conditions such as hiatus hernia, acid reflux, restless legs syndrome, and periodic limb movement disorder can disrupt sleep. Sleep apnea, which occurs with increased age and increased weight, can lead to excessive daytime sleepiness. These factors must be ruled out in anyone with a sleep disorder.

It is generally accepted that an average of eight hours of sleep is required in a twenty-four-hour period for the best daytime alertness. Sleep deprivation causes increased sleepiness and may cause cognitive impairment. Normally the body clock causes nighttime sleepiness and daytime alertness with a midafternoon dip in alertness, which can result in a desire to nap.

Sleeplessness in Alzheimer's

Dr. David Harper says, "Sleep disturbances are actually more disturbing to the caregiver and is often cited as the primary factor behind the decision to institutionalize." He reported in *The Harvard News* on April 20, 2001 that Alzheimer's sufferers have a different wake-and-sleep cycle. They have a lower body temperature in the morning that doesn't reach its peak until later in the day.

That's only one of the things going wrong in the Alzheimer's sleep pattern. According to a German research study published in the January 2004 *Proceedings of the National Academy of Sciences*, low levels of acetylcholine, a brain messenger, are crucial during sleep to form long-term memories. Higher levels are important during the day to enhance wakefulness and to learn new tasks or information. Researchers say giving drugs to Alzheimer's patients that keep acetylcholine levels high during sleep should be re-evaluated.

What Works?

A study published in the *Journal of the American Geriatric Society* in October 2003 sought to train caregivers to change the sleep hygiene practices of patients with dementia. It was called the NITE-AD project. Twenty-two Alzheimer's patients and their family caregivers were given written materials describing age- and dementia-related changes in sleep and standard principles of good sleep hygiene.

A group was given special recommendations about setting up and implementing a sleep hygiene program for the dementia patient. Steps in the program included maintaining a consistent bedtime and a consistent rising time, napping less during the day, and taking a daily walk. With these simple rules, caregivers were able to help patients change sleep scheduling, napping, and walking routines. On this regimen, Alzheimer's patients can improve their quality of sleep.

ESSENTIAL

Elderly persons tend to have less total nighttime sleep than younger people and wake several times during the night. This causes increased daytime sleepiness and the need for naps. The deepest stages of sleep are frequently reduced or nonexistent in elderly persons, causing less satisfying and less restful sleep.

Sundowning

One of the most distressing aspects of sleeplessness in Alzheimer's is a symptom called sundowning. As the sun goes down, restlessness increases and sometimes continues through the night until morning. Many reports indicate that up to 20 percent of people with Alzheimer's will go through an episode of sundowning with symptoms of increased confusion, anxiety, agitation, and disorientation.

Factors contributing to sundowning include:

- Less need for sleep, which is common among older adults
- Circadian (day/night) rhythm imbalance, which causes a mixup between day and night
- Reduced lighting and increased shadows, which adds to confusion and paranoia
- End-of-day exhaustion, both mental and physical
- Disorientation due to the daytime hallucinations, which seem like dreams
- Medication
- Eating a large meal late at night
- Coffee and sweets in the evening

Sundowning Tips

Reducing episodes of sundowning requires a concerted effort. The following tips will reduce agitation and restlessness and help promote a more balanced sleep:

- Encourage more physical activity during the morning and early afternoon, especially if the problem is wandering.
- Encourage more mental activity during the later afternoon and evening.
- Discourage afternoon napping; take a walk instead.
- Limit soda, sweets, and coffee to the morning hours.
- Make lunch the larger meal and serve a light dinner and a snack at bedtime.

- Keep a small lamp on in the bedroom to avoid darkness and shadows.
- Keep the house quiet in the evening to prevent overexcitement and agitation.
- Consider a bedside commode or urinal if the problem is frequent trips to the bathroom.
- Consult with your doctor. A bladder infection or incontinence problems can cause frequent waking.

Experts say that sundowning peaks in Stages 4 and 5 of Alzheimer's but lessens as the disease worsens. Unfortunately, sundowning means your patient is awake at night when you need to get your sleep. And there is a chance that they may wander and hurt themselves. Motion sensors can sound an alarm in your bedroom when wandering occurs. Just make sure the house is safe, with everything locked away and doors and windows locked and secure.

Confronting a Sundowner

Once the person is awake and upset, experts suggest that you approach them calmly. They may need to go to the bathroom or be hungry or thirsty. Then, gently guide them back to bed, offering reassurance. If they are agitated and seem confused, turn on more lights in case the darkness is disturbing them. Offer a reclining chair or a couch to sleep on if they resist going back to bed.

Repetitive words or behaviors are common at the stages of Alzheimer's when sundowning occurs. Take advantage of this by offering an activity that you have observed to be calming. This could be something as simple as holding or stroking a fur fabric pillow or stuffed animal, or manipulating a net bag of marbles or coins.

Keep in mind that the individual with Alzheimer's has no idea that their behavior is annoying. Several nights with sundowning, however, will have you down for the count. You must call in reinforcements. Have another member of your support team sleep in the room with your relative for a few nights to make sure they are safe so that you can get some rest to take care of the next day's activities. Ⓔ

Chapter 14

A Day in the Life Inside and Out

Scheduling of an Alzheimer's patient's day is very basic: arising to greet the day, morning face wash, breakfast at the table, morning activities, preparing lunch, lunch at the table, afternoon activities, preparing dinner, dinner at the table, evening activities, bedtime snack, and lights out. But it's what is infused into the routine schedule—the love, the bonding, and the sharing—that can make a little magic. This chapter gives the caregiver a look into some activities to make use of when caring for someone with Alzheimer's.

An Alzheimer's Log

It's quite an experience to follow a day in the life of an Alzheimer's patient on the Web. Some individuals in the early stages of Alzheimer's disease, with mild to moderate memory loss, are writing Web logs to help them keep track of their daily lives.

Chip Gerber was a social worker who worked with senior citizens just before he was diagnosed with early-onset Alzheimer's at the very young age of fifty-four. Five years after his diagnosis, he testified before the House of Representatives on the need for more research on Alzheimer's.

In his online journal, called My Journey (*www.zarcrom.com/users/ alzheimers/chip.html*), Chip invites the reader to come along with him on his journey as he explores his feelings and tries to gain insight into what has happened, and is happening, to him—his dreams and goals, his successes and failures. He tells readers, "Perhaps you will find something along the way that you can relate to, something of interest, something to help you through a troubled time in your life. I share with lots of everyday experiences, laughter, and hope in tomorrow. Please join me on My Journey. Come and travel with me as I enter a place that has a long goodbye."

ESSENTIAL

Sheryne Hanson at BellaOnline (*www.bellaonline.com*) offers you online journaling for emotional catharsis! Several other sites provide a similar service. On BellaOnline, you can also find a list of other sites that host journaling; some of these sites offer public journal space, which provides instant feedback from other writers, or private journal formats, which can help you collect your thoughts.

We can learn a lot from reading Chip and his good-natured wisdom and self-effacing humor as he pokes fun at his own situation. There are the sad times, too, like when he's on the phone with his elderly mother who also has Alzheimer's and sometimes she just stops talking and hangs up the phone. Chip imagines she's off on her own journey, and he'll catch up with her another time.

Up and At 'Em

On January 7, 2003, Chip wrote about waking up that morning: "I'm breathing and that counts for something! The buzzards aren't circling yet, and I haven't given up. I may just be occupying space for the moment, but tomorrow, I may be moving a little more. Don't give up on me. It's not over until it's over."

You've got to smile at that attitude, and hopefully you can foster it in your own life, whether you have Alzheimer's or you're caring for someone with the disease. Greet the new day and look for that silver lining wherever you can. You can help to create a silver lining in the day by keeping fresh flowers in the house. Open the blinds and let the morning light in, and keep the air fresh by opening the windows.

Flowers growing in the window boxes and birdfeeders outside the window help brighten up the morning and put a smile on everyone's face. So, up you get, put on your dressing gown, and you're off to the bathroom. This could all be at a very slow pace, of course.

Morning Hygiene

Usually, first thing in the morning, there is time for a quick face wash and brushing of teeth. A bath or shower takes time and can be done after breakfast. You can accompany your Alzheimer's patient to the bathroom and be there to help out if they need something. But it's important that you let them perform these simple tasks alone as long as they are able.

Breakfast Time

Breakfast is what most people want right away. The seventy-to-eighty age group seems to eat by the clock and depend on regular mealtimes. Try to have breakfast in the kitchen or at the dining room table. Some Alzheimer's patients feel low in the morning and might ask for breakfast in bed. That just reinforces the illness. Usually, if you can encourage them to get up and come to breakfast, they will feel much better and more independent.

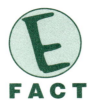

FACT

Dr. Roy Walford and Dr. Richard Weindruch report in their various studies and papers that caloric restriction is a proven method of promoting longevity. Caloric restriction research has produced over seventy years of data confirming in all animal species studied that less food means more health and more longevity. Anecdotal human case studies confirm this research.

If you've taken the suggestion about a Crock-Pot cereal, your breakfast is waiting for you. Just cut up half a banana into the cereal and add a tablespoon or two of flax seed oil and some milk and away you go. If you don't want cereal, eggs and toast, yogurt and fruit, or a protein drink will all give you a good nutritious start for the day.

Chip says that he usually wakes up in a fog, and coffee is the best thing to clear his head. Coffee is not great in the evening because it's a stimulant; too much coffee in the daytime can act like a diuretic and you lose too much water. But one cup in the morning can be just the medicine you need, as long as you make sure to drink plenty of water during the day.

Morning Activities

We've talked about bathing and dressing in Chapter 13; they usually come after breakfast. Then the morning has to be filled up with activities that keep your relative occupied but not bored or overstimulated. Ask for their help with the morning chores such as clearing the table, washing and drying the dishes, sweeping floors, dusting, and folding clothes. These are all tasks that aren't too difficult and can make your relative feel they are useful.

After the chores are done, if the weather is nice, spend some time outdoors. Sitting on the porch, puttering around in the garden, or going for a walk in the fresh air can be very calming and relaxing. An Alzheimer's patient has a lot of internal anxiety because the disease is causing confusion most of the time, so it's important to choose calming activities as much as possible. Sharing time together, linking arms when you walk, and just enjoying each other's company can be very special.

A rest time is usually important after the morning physical activity. Sitting in a reclining chair or rocker is probably better than going back to bed. You don't want to encourage daytime sleeping—that can throw off the nighttime sleep clock and keep your patient, and you, up at night.

Time for Lunch

Preparing lunch together can mean sharing simple tasks of buttering bread, cutting up vegetables, and setting the table. Remember, most people in the Alzheimer's age group are used to being busy and being useful. As a caregiver, you may become impatient because you know you can do something much faster. But that's not the point. The point is to foster independence and confidence.

ESSENTIAL

Most people interpret dehydration and the need for water as hunger. Since water is vital for health, think of offering a fresh glass of spring water before a snack or instead of a snack. Water is important for all the metabolic processes in the body; it helps flush out toxins, decreases constipation, and keeps the skin healthy.

Lunch, like breakfast, should be at the kitchen or dining room table, if possible. Fresh flowers on the table are sure to be remarked upon and really lift the spirits. Cloth napkins instead of paper, good silverware, and china all help to make mealtime a treat. When someone has the apathy of Alzheimer's, they do need encouragement to eat.

After lunch, a rest may be in order. As a caregiver, you know the signs of early fatigue and know it's important to avoid exhaustion because it can lead to agitation. Also, if you wait for exhaustion to declare a rest period, then your Alzheimer's patient will probably fall asleep. A short, relaxing break will give them an energy boost but won't interfere with their nighttime sleep.

Criteria for Alzheimer's Activities

Researchers and caregivers have given a lot of thought to what constitutes a beneficial Alzheimer's activity. Alzheimer's activities should draw on past memories and not force new learning; promote confidence and self-esteem; compensate for lost abilities; and provide contact with others and enjoyment. (Elizabeth Wright gives advice on activities for people with Alzheimer's on the Web site Alzheimer's Outreach ✎ *www.zarcrom.com/ users/alzheimers.*)

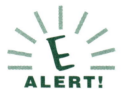

ALERT!

Scrabble is probably not the best activity for someone who is having trouble remembering words. Basket weaving will not go over very well for someone who spent their life in a machine shop. And don't expect your grandmother to suddenly take up playing cards if she never touched them in her life.

Knowing your patient's history is very helpful in choosing appropriate activities. As a family member, you will know about their previous work, hobbies, recreational and social interests, travel, major life events, religious affiliation, and sense of humor. All of these will help to create appropriate activities. Just as important is to find out what they don't like and to make sure to avoid these land mines.

Build on Past Memories

Retracing old tasks can actually help trigger the memory. Because we have done things like washing and drying dishes, watering plants, and sweeping the floor a million times, when an Alzheimer's patient starts to do one of these tasks, often the old memory kicks in and away they go. It's a boost for them because they have remembered something, and for you, the caregiver, it keeps them occupied for a time. For instance, if your relative played a musical instrument, encourage that activity.

Promote Confidence and Self-Esteem

This doesn't have so much to do with the task, but rather to the extent that you, the caregiver, offer praise for the help you are getting. These tasks can be simple things such as unpacking groceries from the car, carrying packages, pushing the shopping cart, feeding the pets, and all the other household chores. We all know what a simple and sincere thank you can do to buoy our spirits.

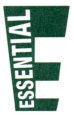

Help your Alzheimer's patient compensate for lost abilities. For instance, for a person who is losing the ability to do intricate carpentry, offer projects that are precut with predrilled holes that you can get from an occupational therapist. For someone who used to sew and knit, you can offer projects of a more simple nature.

In the case of an Alzheimer's sufferer, life is filled with a sense of frustration and the failure to communicate due to deteriorating brain function. A nonsufferer can only imagine how frightening it must be to be unable to interpret everyday happenings. The aim of positive activities is to counter the sense of failure your patient feels every time he or she attempts a word, a thought, or an action, with something they can do.

Experiential Activities

Activities such as sightseeing, music, and dancing do not require memory but are more along the lines of entertainment. Even though a person may enjoy an experience but forget it soon after, they will still have enjoyed that moment for the time they had it.

Contact with babies, children, and animals can provide pure joy. The unconditional love of an animal, the hug of a child, and the babblings of a baby all go straight to the heart.

Sensory experiences include the spa day, smelling fresh flowers, incense, or aromatherapy. Elizabeth Wright says that the sense of movement and rhythm is retained longer than most other abilities. Therefore, sitting in a rocking chair or gently swinging in a hammock provides enjoyable outlets.

Pets Provide Companionship

You may be fortunate enough to already have a pet as a member of the family. Pets, especially dogs and cats, live to be loved. In return, they give undivided attention and unconditional love, and greatly reduce stress. You don't have to talk to them and feel embarrassed because you can't remember what you were going to say. They don't care. They just want to be petted and fussed over. They also know when someone is emotionally upset. A golden retriever will crawl right up on the lap of someone who is crying and offer a hug.

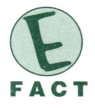

FACT

Pet Therapy, Inc. was inspired by a visit to a nursing home. In 1996, when Kathy Alexander took her little dog to visit her father-in-law at his nursing home, he was an instant celebrity. Kathy made it her goal "to take her cuddly dogs to nursing homes all over the county to 'honor our elders through consistent, unconditional love.'"

Activity Ideas

Within your schedule, you will want to incorporate activities that meet the above criteria. Some such activities are included here. Feel free to get creative and come up with some activities that are best suited to your Alzheimer's patient. While these activities can be done in the morning, afternoon, or evening, it seems the more physical activities and exercise are best done in the morning or early afternoon; activities requiring less physical exertion are better suited for the afternoon and evening.

If some of these activities can be done outdoors, weather permitting, so much the better. Activities include familiar pastimes such as listening to music—on radio, CD, audiotape, or record. Have a selection available that you can turn to at any time. Your relative may have a list of favorites, and as a caregiver, you will become accustomed to what type of mood you want to create with music. Toe tapping, singing, and dancing are all encouraged.

What about Television?

Watching TV, as we mentioned earlier, is not equated with enough brain stimulation to make it a therapeutic activity, so be careful not to rely on it too much. Use the TV for nature shows, biographies, fun movies, and sports. You can order videos from companies that specialize in subjects for Alzheimer's patients. In other words, watch shows that make the brain work a bit, not mindless sitcoms.

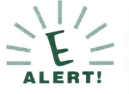

ALERT!

Americans spend an average of thirty hours each week watching TV, yet complain that they don't have enough time to exercise. Harvard University researchers published a study in *Archives of Internal Medicine* in August 2001, following 40,000 men for ten years. The 1,000 men who developed diabetes watched the most TV, over forty hours a week. Those who exercised had a 50 percent lower risk of developing the disease.

Card games have an element of mental activity that's important to encourage. Picture puzzles and crossword puzzles are real brainteasers, but if they are too difficult, they might make a patient feel more frustrated and inadequate. Reading books or being read to can be very soothing; this activity can also trigger the imagination as you fill in the pictures for the spoken words. Looking through old photos can help retrace memories and is a wonderful way to share.

Reminiscing in Alzheimer's

Author Carmel Sheridan, in her book *Reminiscence: Uncovering a Lifetime of Memories,* explains the power of reminiscing. She says that in Alzheimer's disease, memories of the past usually remain much clearer than memories of recent events. It's the short-term memory connections that are damaged first. Therefore, she says, it's no surprise that reminiscing can have profound value, especially in the early stages of the disease.

Many people may think it might be too sad to bring up the past when the future looks bleak, but it's quite the opposite. Bringing up the good parts of the past can infuse a patient with the confidence of that time that can spill over into their present circumstances.

Ms. Sheridan says that there are few activities that have as calming an effect on Alzheimer's patients as speaking about pleasant experiences from the past. The process of remembering also helps to stimulate memory function and may keep the mind active for longer periods of time.

Tips for enhancing the reminiscing experience:

• Make it a one-on-one activity.
• Use a photo or souvenir as a memory prop.
• Keep memory props around to stimulate silent reminiscing.
• Don't push for stories but encourage the experience.

Planning an Outing

Having Alzheimer's should not restrict a patient from going on day trips. If properly organized, they can provide companionship, exercise, mental stimulation, and relaxation all at the same time. Many types of outings are appropriate, but the success of an outing is all in the planning and organization.

Depending on the level of functioning of your Alzheimer's patient, you will decide on whether the outing should take one hour or several. Even difficult issues such as incontinence can be handled with adult diapers, and if your relative has an episode of agitation at the thought of going out, then you don't go. The key is flexibility and compromise.

The main rule is not to overstimulate your Alzheimer's patient. Large crowds with lots of noise and bustle such as at a sports or music event or a shopping mall at rush hour would be too much. When you choose to go to a public place or event, make sure it is during slack periods when there is less noise and stimulation.

Trips to a park, zoo, or museum are worth a call ahead to see if there are wheelchairs available. You might even have already rented your own wheelchair for times when your relative gets tired on an outing.

Types of Outings

You'll probably want to begin your adventures outside with shorter trips to make sure you are organized and to make sure your Alzheimer's patient feels comfortable. Shorter trips can be taken to a pet store or a flower shop; or they can consist of a walk in a local playground or by the waterfront. An hour or two on a Saturday morning visiting garage sales can be a lot of fun, especially if you are able to find some treasures. The most important aspects of these trips are that your Alzheimer's patient and you are sharing time together and enjoying being out of the house.

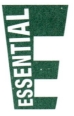

Walking the family dog is the best way to combine companionship, fresh air, and exercise. The benefits of the whole experience include a lighter step, more confidence, better digestion, and better health in general. If your relative can go alone, especially if the dog is trained to follow a particular route, so much the better.

Going to a restaurant, zoo, aquarium, the public gardens, or a park; walking barefoot along the beach; having a family picnic; or visiting an art exhibition or a museum might take a longer time, but can be curtailed if your Alzheimer's patient is not enjoying themselves or becomes agitated.

How about a Cruise?

In the past decade, cruises have become *the* vacation destination, and they are perfectly suitable for someone with mild Alzheimer's and several companions. Perhaps the family could plan a trip together with everyone sharing in the fun and the care. A "dry run" on a ferry might be a good idea to make sure water and being confined to a boat is not a problem. The cruise ships that are sailing the high seas these days, however, are as big as cities, and if you aren't on the deck or near a porthole, you won't even know you are sailing. (E)

Chapter 15

Daily Health Check and Common Ailments

A health journal is crucial for the daily health check. If you can't find one, make your own by listing the various parts and functions of the body that you want to check on the left side of a sheet of paper. The list should include: skin, eyes, ears, nose, mouth, lungs, digestion, bladder, extremities, and acute symptoms. Draw several lines down the page so that each box represents one day, and each page represents one week. Make several copies, and you have a health journal.

Routine Medical Visits

Most doctors following the care of someone with Alzheimer's schedule regular three-month or six-month checkups. It will be up to you, the caregiver, to keep these appointments on a calendar, accompany your Alzheimer's patient to the appointment, help describe his or her current state of health to the doctor, and then explain the doctor's recommendations to your patient. It's the "nurse's aide" hat that you will be wearing—one of many.

Your Alzheimer's patient and the doctor both depend on you. The doctor should appreciate this fact and make you feel that he or she is available to answer any questions you have. When it comes to agreeing to medical tests and prescription medications, it will be difficult for your Alzheimer's patient to make a decision, and it may be up to you and the doctor to make the best choice. If there are other family members around, however, it is important to have a family meeting to decide.

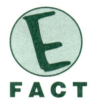

FACT

According to the Office of Medical Informatics at the University of Florida, older patients don't always report all their symptoms. Therefore a good doctor must ask about the following five areas: 1) Iatrogenic (side effects of medications); 2) Impaired Homeostasis (blood sugar problems); 3) Instability (arthritis); 4) Impaired intellect; and 5) Incontinence.

When you go to a doctor's appointment, it can be very helpful to bring a medication journal—this is a journal that lists drugs and the dosage schedule and has an area to check off when the drug has been taken. It is also helpful to bring your relative's health journal, which will indicate what symptoms may be evolving or demonstrate concerns you may have.

The medication journal will also help your pharmacist to assess any drug interactions. Many elderly people take several medications, so it is important for all doctors to be aware of what prescription and over-the-counter drugs and supplements patients are taking.

A medication journal should include:

- The name of the medication
- A sample of the medication taped beside the name
- The reason for taking the medication
- The dosage
- The times during the day the medication is taken
- A daily chart with medication times blocked off to be checked when taken

Some experts suggest that if several medications are taken at three or four different times a day, then a chart can be made that marks out the time of day to take medications and lists all the medications to be taken at that time. A date can be entered when the medication is taken to keep track.

Skin and How to Treat It

As we age, our skin has a tendency to become drier and even thinner and less elastic, with less ability to heal if injured. When caring for the skin, consider the general environment. For example, if the air is too dry in the winter, you notice how rough and dry your hands get. The same is happening to the rest of your skin, leading to flakiness and itching. It's important to use humidifiers to the point where there is a small amount of moisture on the windows.

To prevent dry skin, take baths, not showers. Showers can strip away the natural acid mantle of the skin, whereas with baths, you have a chance to use simple remedies that can nourish the skin. Some of the products for dry, itchy skin use oatmeal. You can make your own by putting ¼ cup of oatmeal in a cloth bag and squeezing it into a bath. A few tablespoons of apple cider vinegar can restore acidity to the skin. And a few drops of bath oil can help oil the skin. You can use even more oil if your relative doesn't want you to rub cream on their skin after a bath.

What you ingest is also important for how your skin behaves. Drinking plenty of water is extremely important. Eight glasses of water a day should help keep the skin hydrated and more healthy. Essential fatty acids found in flaxseed oil and fish oils, or from eating fatty fish, are necessary for strong and healthy skin. The mineral zinc is important for wound healing and healthy skin and nails.

Bruising

With less layers of skin cells covering more fragile blood vessels that seem to be much closer to the surface, the elderly skin is more susceptible to bruising. If you have thin skin and bump into the corner of a table or chair, a big bruise can form. The best thing to do is immediately put pressure and ice on the area. Often, however, you may only be momentarily aware that you've hit yourself and not notice the bruise until much later.

ESSENTIAL

A homeopathic medicine called Arnica is a valuable treatment for any sort of injury, pain, or bruising. It can be found in health food stores in small tubes containing white pellets. Twist the pellets into the cap and put three to five pellets under your tongue to melt.

Bruising can increase with the use of several medications that interfere with blood clotting. These include aspirin, usually given for pain relief or as a blood thinner to protect the heart; warfarin (Coumadin), which is a blood thinner for people who have had blood clots; and nonsteroidal, anti-inflammatory drugs such as ibuprofen (Advil), Nuprin, and naproxen (Aleve), often given for arthritis. Cortisone drugs like prednisone and cortisone creams encourage bruising by increasing the fragility of the tiny blood vessels in the skin.

In August 2003, the *Journal of Drugs and Dermatology* described a number of natural substances that are used to treat aging skin. They include retinoid derivatives of vitamin A, beta and alpha hydroxy acids, antioxidants, and vitamin E. Other studies show that vitamin E, vitamin C, and bioflavinoids prevent skin damage from the sun and help heal sun damage that is already present. Adequate intake of vitamin C prevents scurvy, and the first signs of vitamin C deficiency are skin lesions and bruising.

Bedsores

The skin, especially covering bony prominences, should be inspected and felt daily for evidence of bedsores. If your patient is sitting or lying on one area of his or her body constantly, the skin can break down. Once that happens, it's often very difficult to heal. Most at risk are people who are confined to a bed or wheelchair and can't change their position without help. This can occur in the later stages of Alzheimer's.

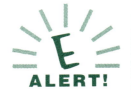

ALERT!

When the National Decubitus (pressure ulcer) Foundation was launched in 1998, its press release said that "one in ten hospital patients, one in eight home-care patients, and one in four nursing home patients suffers from bedsores. Hospital stays are increased five times the average, a huge waste of funds and resources. Patient suffering is immense, and death can result."

Pulling or dragging someone to a sitting position instead of lifting them can scrape the skin and further the process of a bedsore that has already started. Bedsores begin because the pressure of sitting or lying has cut off the capillaries in that area, leading to cell death and then tissue death.

Stages of Bedsores

A stage-one bedsore is defined by a persistent pink or red area that does not blanch (turn white) when you press on it with your finger; it also can feel hard or spongy, definitely different from the rest of the skin. Even at this stage, the area may feel painful or itchy.

Stage two is an abrasion with a blister or a broken blister with a shallow depression. Stage three is a skin lesion that extends through all layers of the skin. The skin ulcer is deep and very difficult to heal. Stage four extends into muscle and bone, exposing underlying tendons, organs, or joint space.

Stage one can be healed readily by taking pressure off the skin. A person should not be in one position for more than two hours.

If incontinence is an issue, frequent changing is necessary to prevent moisture from breaking down the skin. Stage two requires the same plus an antibiotic cream and soft bandages and should be discussed with your doctor. Stage three often requires hospitalization and may take up to a year to heal and will only get worse and become infected if not treated medically. Stage four is the most serious stage; in this stage, the ulceration goes right through to muscles, tendons, and bone. The wound is excruciatingly painful, usually infected, and almost impossible to heal. Pain, dehydration, and infection are the preludes to death.

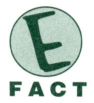

FACT

According to an August 2002 Medicare report, the average percentage of nursing home residents with bedsores in the United States is 9 percent. The standards of individual nursing homes, however, can vary greatly. For example, the percentage of residents with bedsores in Greater Hollywood Area nursing homes ranged from 0 percent to 49 percent.

Prevention of Bedsores

All the experts in the treatment of bedsores say that the best treatment is prevention. For years sheepskin pads and rubber egg-crate mattresses were recommended. They are superior to standard mattresses, but they only offer minimal protection. They do not do anything to change the pressure on the skin. People on standard mattresses or sitting in a chair should have their position changed hourly.

Air-filled medical mattresses have been studied and do relieve pressure on bony prominences. The heels, however, are at additional risk and may require elevation with a pillow under the lower leg, not under the knee, which can cut off circulation. A doughnut cushion is not recommended because it can increase pressure and cut off circulation.

Other recommendations for prevention include diet and exercise. In order to heal a pressure ulcer, protein and nutrients are required. Perhaps the same could be said for preventing them. If your relative is not eating properly, perhaps a balanced nutrition powder is in order. Check labels, however, because some products have an excessive amount of sugar in them, which delays wound healing. Water intake is also very important—eight glasses a day. Exercise is important to increase blood flow and speed up wound healing. Even people confined to bed are able to do some basic exercises.

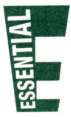

Pressure ulcers are easier to prevent than to cure. Risk factors include general physical condition, nutrition, activity, mobility, friction, sensory perception, incontinence, skin moisture, level of consciousness, and mental status. Even after a pressure ulcer has healed, the skin does not fully recover, and future risk is significantly increased.

Eye and Ear Care

Failing eyesight that goes unrecognized can lead to increased confusion in an Alzheimer's sufferer. Regular checkups with an eye doctor should be made to rule out cataract, glaucoma, macular degeneration, and diabetic retinopathy.

Most Alzheimer's patients are probably wearing some form of eyeglasses, whether for distance or for reading. Care should be taken to keep these in good shape and regularly cleaned. Having a backup pair of glasses on hand is probably a good idea considering that one pair might be misplaced, lost, or broken. If you can provide an alternate pair immediately, you can prevent disorientation and confusion in your Alzheimer's patient.

Eye Disease Study

The Age-Related Eye Disease Study (AREDS), completed in 2001, was a major clinical trial sponsored by the National Eye Institute, one of the federal government's National Institutes of Health (NIH). AREDS studied the natural history and risk factors of age-related macular degeneration and cataracts and also evaluated the effect of high doses of antioxidants (like vitamins A, C, and E) and zinc on the progression of these diseases.

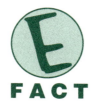

FACT

Age is the biggest risk factor in vision impairment and blindness in the United States. Cataracts affect nearly 20.5 million American seniors. About 2.2 million Americans have been diagnosed with glaucoma, and 2 million more don't know they have it. Advanced macular degeneration impairs the vision of more than 1.6 million Americans over age sixty.

Promising results from the AREDS showed that high levels of antioxidants and zinc significantly reduce the risk of advanced age-related macular degeneration and its associated vision loss. Since no one knows why macular degeneration appears, it may be wise to ask your eye doctor how much of these vitamins to take to lessen your chances of getting this condition.

Ear Care

Aging itself is a risk factor for hearing loss, and hearing loss is the third most common chronic condition of the elderly. About 2 million Americans are deaf and more than 28 million have some degree of hearing loss due to an ear disease, a middle ear disorder, or an inner ear problem. The middle ear could be infected, have a wax buildup, or an eardrum perforation, all of which can impede the mobility of the three small ear bones (the hammer, anvil, and stirrup), which move the eardrum to create sound.

Nerve deafness occurs when the sensory cells in the inner ear or cochlea are permanently damaged. Damage occurs due to aging, overexposure to loud noise, or a side effect of certain medications. Regular hearing exams are important for someone with Alzheimer's since diminished hearing can add to the confusion. A properly fitted hearing aid can be of great help to the whole family.

Nasal Passages and Sinuses

The sinuses can become blocked with mucus and interfere with sound sleep and also cause snoring. If they become severely blocked, this can lead to facial pain, headaches, and sinus infection. The most common cause of sinus mucus is too much dairy and sugar in the diet. Cut out dairy and sugar for two weeks and see if there is a change. Add back a lot of these foods on one day and see the result. You may find that offering these foods only every three days keeps the sinuses clear.

Colds and Flus

Colds and flus can occur any time of year, but they seem to increase as the weather gets colder. But it's not so much the weather as people getting together in larger crowds in confined spaces passing their germs around that causes colds and flus. If there are young children in the house going to day care or school, they can bring colds and flus into the house. Keeping everyone healthy is the key here. There are a host of natural remedies that you can use as a preventive or as a treatment to decrease duration of colds and flus.

E ALERT!

Oscillococcinum, a homeopathic medicine found in pharmacies and health food stores, is the number one flu medicine of France. In clinical trials it decreased the duration and intensity of flu symptoms including fever, chills, and body aches and pains. It is safe to use with any existing medical condition or medication. There are no known drug interactions and no side effects.

Vitamin C, zinc lozenges, herbal Echinacea tincture, homeopathic Oscillococcinum, herbal elderberry, and herbal Astragalus are but a few of the remedies that you might ask about at your local health food store. Most of them work as well as over-the-counter cold remedies and have none of the side effects. Some parents rotate several of these remedies and give their children a dose of one of them every morning during cold and flu season.

What about the Flu Vaccine?

Hugh Fudenberg, M.D., past chairman of the Department of Basic and Clinical Immunology and Microbiology at the Medical University of South

Carolina, has about 850 papers in peer review journals. He reported at a National Vaccine Information Center conference in Arlington, Virginia, in September 1997 that in a study conducted from 1970–1980, individuals who had five consecutive flu shots in those ten years had a ten times higher risk of getting Alzheimer's than someone who had one, two, or no vaccinations. Dr. Fudenberg stands by his findings. The increased incidence of flu appears to be due to mercury and aluminum ingredients in every flu shot that can cause cognitive dysfunction.

Mouth, Teeth, and Dentures

Oral hygiene is very important for healthy teeth. And teeth are very important to chew food properly and begin the digestive process. A visit to the dentist is in order if there are gaps between teeth, decayed teeth, or gum disease. If the teeth or gums are infected, the taste of decay can certainly make eating unpleasant. If teeth have to be filled, do not allow mercury fillings but request white composite fillings.

If your relative wears dentures, be aware that weight loss that may occur during Alzheimer's due to apathy about eating may actually cause shrinkage of the gums and loose-fitting dentures. Dentures that don't fit can cause problems with cankers on the gums.

ESSENTIAL

According to the American Dental Association, it's hard to smile, eat, or speak properly without teeth, and your facial muscles sag, making you look older. Even with dentures, you still must brush your gums, tongue, and palate every morning with a soft-bristled brush before you insert your dentures to stimulate circulation in your tissues and help remove plaque.

Using the blender to create purée and liquefy foods is one way to get food past teeth that don't work. But make sure you serve meals with proper nutrition. For example, lack of proper vitamin C in the diet can actually cause sub-clinical scurvy, which presents as bleeding gums. Unhealthy gums are an indication of poor nutrition in the rest of the body.

Lung Disease

Pneumonia occurring after a cold, flu, or bronchitis is very common in the elderly. The best protection against pneumonia is to prevent colds and flus. Another cause of lung disease is due to aspiration of stomach contents. This can happen if your loved one goes straight to bed after eating and lies flat. Food from the stomach can reflux into the esophagus and be inhaled into the bronchial tube and into the lung when you cough and choke on the food being regurgitated. To prevent this from happening, keep the bed propped up after meals; don't eat big meals before lying down, and don't drink a lot of liquids with meals.

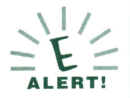

ALERT!

The CDC's National Center for Health Statistics reported that in 1999 and 2000 1.5 percent or 20,300 homecare patients, at the time of the survey, had pneumonia; 2.5 percent or 46,000 nursing home patients were diagnosed with this condition. The total number of deaths from pneumonia in 2001 was 61,777.

Digestion and Bladder Infections

Nausea, gas, bloating, and constipation are common symptoms in the elderly in general, and more so in Alzheimer's patients. The low level of anxiety or the mild depression that may come with an Alzheimer's diagnosis can make food seem unappetizing and lead to nausea. Some people when they are upset eat more, but the majority feel a lump in their throat, which may be anxiety, and when they eat feel queasy.

You may have a tendency as a caregiver to try to encourage your loved one to eat by tempting them with tasty treats. Tasty usually means sugary or fatty foods. Both of these foods can cause more queasiness and are not healthy. The B vitamins are necessary for food digestion, and they help enhance mood. They can be used alone or in a good multivitamin and mineral supplement. Encourage slow and thorough chewing; do not allow a lot of liquids with meals, and if food is not properly digested, you might ask your doctor for a prescription for a digestive enzyme or pick one up in the local health food store.

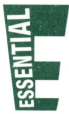

Lots of water between meals and lots of fiber in the diet help prevent constipation. If it is still a problem, psyllium seed powder or capsules help to bulk up the stool, but you have to drink extra water if you are using psyllium. Regular exercise can also keep the bowels moving. Stool softeners or senna capsules may be required.

Bladder infections are more common in women than in men. It has to do with the anatomy and bathroom hygiene. If bacteria from the colon are wiped near the urethra, the opening of the bladder, then these bacteria can migrate into the bladder and cause an infection. A bidet would be a great asset to ensure that the whole perineum is washed after every bowel movement.

To prevent bladder infections, encourage your patient to drink eight glasses of water a day and offer diluted pure cranberry juice, which is a proven treatment for mild bladder infections. Giving "probiotics" called acidophilus, which are normal intestinal flora, can build up the beneficial bacteria in the intestines and help colonize the perineum with good bacteria.

Extremities

Examine the feet for coldness and red or blue mottled skin. Poor circulation in the extremities can be due to underlying heart and blood vessel disease that is related to a poor diet and lack of exercise. The obvious solutions are to cut down on refined carbohydrates and fats and encourage exercise. If your Alzheimer's patient is a diabetic, you must pay particular attention to any cuts or abrasions on the feet, especially those on the heels from rubbing against the sheets.

Chapter 16

Community, State, and National Support

Since approximately 80 percent of people suffering from Alzheimer's are cared for at home and the primary caregiver is usually the spouse, a vast array of support structures have been erected in America to help keep the caregivers healthy and support them in their task. Caregiving is very difficult in the beginning and the difficulty increases as the disease progresses, so it's important to know where you can turn for financial assistance, reassurance, support groups, literature, and practical strategies for coping.

Small Beginnings

In Chapter 1, we learned how the Alzheimer's Association began in 1979. Spearheading that national group, however, were a number of people who had formed Alzheimer's support services in their communities. People only need to know that someone else shares the same experience, and they want to get together and talk about it. Then, they want to make sure the others don't feel alone, and a support group is born. Those simple beginnings have resulted in Alzheimer's groups and organizations that span the globe.

Alzheimer's Disease International

Formed in 1984, Alzheimer's Disease International (ADI) is a federation of over sixty-six national Alzheimer's associations around the world. Their role is to help create and support Alzheimer's associations, particularly those in developing countries that depend on the aid of the ADI. They work along with the World Health Organization and other organizations with similar interests. ADI began in the United States but is now based in the United Kingdom. Among its organizational tasks are an annual international conference, a World Alzheimer's Day, lobbying for research, providing information, and an Alzheimer's University.

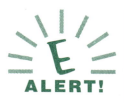

The pool of family caregivers is dwindling as the population ages. People over eighty-five years of age are the fastest growing segment of the population. Half of them need some help with personal care. In 1990, there were eleven potential caregivers for each person needing care. In 2050 that ratio will be four to one.

Alzheimer's U

The Alzheimer's University provides training in a series of three-day workshops that instruct how to build an organization and run an Alzheimer's association. Participants come from all over the world and learn how to direct their resources toward raising awareness about Alzheimer's, educating the public, and training caregivers.

The process of identifying aims, fundraising, recruiting volunteers, running support groups, raising awareness, and providing information can all seem overwhelming if not put into a specific structure. ADI financially supports participants to attend this program, which is held in London, and provides ongoing support after the course. Further training is held at ADI's annual international conference.

Community Resources Abound

From small beginnings, Alzheimer's awareness is spreading around the world, and it has probably reached your community already. There are dozens of agencies and organizations that are available to Alzheimer's sufferers and their families. There are government agencies that can direct you to federally funded services and nonprofit associations that provide information on everything from caregiving to financial planning.

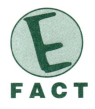

FACT

One half of the U.S. population has a chronic condition. Of these, 41 million were limited in their daily activities. Twelve million are unable to go to school, to work, or to live independently. Elderly caregivers with a history of chronic illness themselves who are experiencing caregiving-related stress have a 63 percent higher mortality rate than their noncaregiving peers.

With so many caregivers stretched to the point of breaking, it is necessary to reach out to community support groups for help. As you will see, these organizations have been operating for decades, and usually you can just pick up the phone or go online to find help. Beyond helping individuals with Alzheimer's, many of these organizations also lobby local, state, and national government to increase funding for Alzheimer's care and research.

Alzheimer's Disease Education and Referral Center

In 1990, the U.S. Congress created the Alzheimer's Disease Education and Referral Center (ADEAR) under the National Institute of Aging (NIA) within the NIH and the U.S. Department of Health and Human Services. Their mandate is to "compile, archive, and disseminate information concerning Alzheimer's disease" for health professionals, people with Alzheimer's disease and their families, and the public. The NIA conducts and finances health research for seniors and works closely with ADEAR.

ADEAR provides information and materials about the search for causes, treatment, cures, and better diagnostic tools for Alzheimer's that are carefully researched and thoroughly reviewed by NIA scientists and health communicators. It supplies patients, caregivers, and professionals with a large national database where you can access state, regional, and federally funded services available in your community. ADEAR's toll-free number is ✆ 800-438-4380. You can access their Web site at ✍ *www.alzheimers.org/adear.*

ESSENTIAL

Keeping up with the times, the Alzheimer's Disease Education and Referral Center has designed a beautiful Web site that won the Mature Media gold award in the Government category for "superlative quality of information on this site as well as ease of use and visual appeal." Their online ordering section also won "best e-commerce site," and allows visitors to order publications, most of which are free.

ADEAR's Information Specialists can provide you with answers for questions about Alzheimer's; free publications about Alzheimer's symptoms, diagnosis, related disorders, risk factors, treatment, caregiving tips, home safety tips, and research; referrals to local support services and centers that specialize in research and diagnosis; information on clinical trials; training manuals; and a newsletter for health care professionals and caregivers.

The Alzheimer's Association

Founded in 1979, the Alzheimer's Association is the foremost Alzheimer's organization in the United States. Its home base is in Chicago. It has a public policy office, however, in Washington, D.C., and eighty-one chapters throughout the United States. Branching out from the chapters are 180 Regional Centers and forty-eight Points of Service for a total of 309 sites nationwide.

All Alzheimer's Association chapters are able to offer five core programs and services in the surrounding area. The core services include care consultation, information and referral, support groups, education, and Safe Return/Safety Services. Individual chapters also offer programs and services based on specific community needs. These could entail assistance for people with Alzheimer's who live alone, plus outreach to rural and multicultural populations. Some Association chapters provide funding for local researchers.

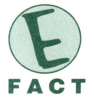

FACT

The Alzheimer's Association does not enumerate all their many volunteers. Any one of the eighty-one chapters, however, can have thousands of volunteers for programs, services, and events held throughout the year.

The Alzheimer's Association provides callers with information and support twenty-four hours a day, seven days a week, in more than 140 languages, from professionals who understand the disease and its impact. Beyond information about Alzheimer's treatment and links to community programs and resources, professionals can also provide confidential care consultation with master's level clinicians. These consultations may provide decision-making support, crisis assistance, and education on issues people with dementia and their families face every day.

Safe Return

Wandering behavior is common in Alzheimer's disease. Safe Return is a national, government-funded program of the Alzheimer's Association. It was developed to assist in the identification and safe return of individuals with Alzheimer's disease and related dementias who wander off and become lost. This is a unique nationwide program that began in 1993. Since that time nearly 110,000 individuals have registered in Safe Return nationwide and more than 8,000 individuals have been safely returned to their families and caregivers.

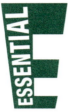

With a registration fee of $40 and $5 for the identification jewelry, a person with dementia or their caregiver fills out a simple form, presents a photograph, and selects the most suitable identification product. The cost of the Safe Return registration may be covered by your local Alzheimer's Association chapter.

The program utilizes identification products including wallet cards, jewelry, clothing labels, lapel pins, and bag tags. It supports a national photo database and a twenty-four-hour, toll-free emergency crisis line, and offers wandering behavior education and training. Quite simply, when the Alzheimer's patient is found, the finder calls the Safe Return number on the identification products, and the family is alerted. And when the individual goes missing, the family can notify Safe Return, which in turn supplies local law enforcement with the missing person's photo and information.

The American Health Assistance Foundation

The American Health Assistance Foundation (AHAF) is a nonprofit, charitable organization founded in 1973. For over thirty years, this organization has funded research on age-related and degenerative diseases and educated the public about these diseases. AHAF has awarded more than $55 million in grants to sponsor medical research on Alzheimer's disease, glaucoma, macular degeneration, heart disease, and stroke. Thirteen of twenty-seven research efforts underway are focused on Alzheimer's disease.

AHAF also provides cash grants up to $500 to needy caregivers through its Alzheimer's Family Relief Program. Since 1988, the program has given more than $1.9 million in emergency financial assistance to families in need in forty-nine states.

AHAF also provides a variety of published materials about Alzheimer's disease for patients and family caregivers. It has a national toll-free line that provides information, support, and referrals (✆ 800-437-AHAF, 9 A.M. to 5 P.M. Eastern Standard Time, Monday to Friday). Its community outreach works with community organizations to distribute information and educational material, making its presence known by exhibiting at national conferences and meetings and sponsoring conferences on Alzheimer's.

The American Health Care Association

The American Health Care Association (AHCA) has been in operation since the 1940s. It is a nonprofit federation of affiliated state health organizations, which together represent nearly 12,000 nonprofit and for-profit assisted living, nursing facility, developmentally disabled, and subacute care providers. In total, they care for more than 1.5 million elderly and disabled individuals nationally.

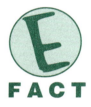

FACT

AHCA established National Nursing Home Week in 1967. In 2004 it coincided with Mother's Day, May 9, with a theme called, "Embracing Our Heritage." Activities were designed to foster intergenerational relationships, collect and preserve patients' reminiscences, strengthen relationships with family members, and celebrate quality. Each year the AHCA offers a planning guide to help facilities develop their own program.

AHCA is the main representative of the long-term care community for the United States and promotes ongoing improvement in the field. AHCA provides information to caregivers on how to choose such a facility and how to pay for it. From its Washington, D.C. headquarters, the association maintains staff working on legislative, regulatory, and public affairs, as well as member services working both internally and externally to assist the interests of government, the general public, and member providers. Their toll-free number is ✆ 800-555-9414. You can access their Web site at ✍ *www.ahca.org.*

The AHCA's established tenets are:

- To improve the standards of service and administration of member nursing homes.
- To secure and merit public and official recognition and approval of the work of nursing homes.
- To adopt and promote programs of education, legislation, and better understanding and mutual cooperation.

The AHCA is a very important organization for families coping with Alzheimer's because so many Alzheimer's patients in the last stages of the disease are cared for in nursing homes. The AHCA says their "ultimate focus is on providing quality care to the nation's frail, elderly, and disabled, who are served by the long-term care professionals who comprise AHCA's membership. These providers believe that the individuals whom they serve are entitled to a supportive environment in which professional and compassionate care is delivered."

The National Association of Area Agencies on Aging

The National Association of Area Agencies on Aging (N4A) is the umbrella organization for 655 state Area Agencies on Aging (AAAs) and more than 230 Native American aging programs in the United States. N4A is located in Washington, D.C., where it is a strong advocate for necessary resources for its local aging agencies. The fundamental mission of the AAAs' programs is to help older individuals to remain in their homes and maintain their independence and dignity.

Local AAAs coordinate and support a wide range of home- and community-based services, including information and referral, home-delivered meals, transportation, employment services, senior centers, adult day care, and a long-term care ombudsman program. Each state has a government Agency on Aging office located in the state capital. The state agency will connect individuals with the nearest local agency in their community. Referrals include meal delivery, home health workers, transportation services, and caregiver support groups.

ESSENTIAL

The N4A also publishes the *National Directory for Eldercare Information & Referral*, which includes a listing for all Area Agencies on Aging, Native American grantees, and State Units on Aging. N4A holds an annual conference in July, an annual spring Legislative Briefing in Washington, D.C., and regional advocacy training around the country.

N4A operates the Eldercare Locator, a toll-free, nationwide telephone service offering information and referrals for many helpful services for older people in their communities. These include adult day care, respite for caregivers, transportation, home health care, meals on wheels, assistance with housing, and other services available locally. Their toll-free number is ☎ 800-677-1116. You can access their Web site at ✍ *www.aoa.dhhs.gov.* This service is supported by a cooperative agreement with the U.S. Administration on Aging.

Health Care Professionals

Health care professionals provide important links to community health resources. Your first contact about Alzheimer's will likely be your family doctor or neurologist. The neurologist, especially, should be able to connect the family with local Alzheimer's resources. Your primary contact for support services will usually be through a doctor's referral to a social worker who will enlist home health care and make recommendations for other services such as meals on wheels.

The social worker will likely make an appointment to come to your home and make an on-site assessment of the Alzheimer's sufferer's needs and what the caregiver needs for support. Most social workers will have a working knowledge of what is available in your community, but it doesn't stop you from getting all the available information about assistance that you can. There is a wealth of information and support on Alzheimer's, but often it doesn't reach the individual. The cost of direct advertising for these services would take up the whole budget. So, you can read about these services here and do your own research as well.

Government Information

There are many government resources available to seniors. Some of them overlap with other services, and some of them are difficult to find without guidance. Besides providing direct services, various government branches support Alzheimer's organizations and foundations and direct funds to Alzheimer's medical research.

Resource Directory for Older People

This is a free directory accessed through a toll-free number (✆ 800-222-2225) coordinated by the National Institute of Aging and the Administration on Aging. The directory is designed to help older people and their families locate national organizations offering health information, legal aid, self-help programs, educational opportunities, social services, consumer advice, or other assistance. The directory lists over 200 federal agencies, professional societies, private groups, and voluntary programs.

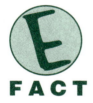

FACT

More than one-quarter (26.6 percent) of the adult population has provided care to a family member or friend during the past year. Based on current census data, that translates into more than 50 million people.

The directory provides information to health and legal professionals, social service providers, librarians, and researchers, as well as older people and their families. It lists federal agencies, Administration on Aging resource centers, professional societies, private groups, and volunteer programs. Some of the organizations listed deal mainly with older people and their families, while others serve professionals who work with older adults, and still others target people of all ages.

HealthFinder

HealthFinder is a government Web site providing health care information for all ages and includes access to online journals, libraries, an encyclopedia, and medical dictionaries. Specifically for seniors, there is the pension search directory. The site can be accessed at ✐*www.healthfinder.gov*. It has a health library covering prevention and wellness, diseases and conditions, and alternative medicine. There are selected health topics organized for men and women, by age from kids to seniors, by race and ethnicity, and for parents, caregivers, health professionals, and others.

Under the heading, "health care," it provides information about doctors, dentists, public clinics, hospitals, long-term care, nursing homes, health insurance, prescriptions, health fraud, Medicare, Medicaid, and medical privacy. It provides a directory of HealthFinder organizations and health information, as well as Web sites from government agencies, clearinghouses, nonprofits, and universities.

The National Family Caregivers Association

The National Family Caregivers Association (NFCA) is a grass roots organization of caregivers "created to educate, support, empower, and speak up for the millions of Americans who care for chronically ill, aged, or disabled loved ones." It states that it is "the only constituency organization that reaches across the boundaries of different diagnoses, different relationships and different life stages to address the common needs and concerns of all family caregivers." NFCA is funded by pharmaceutical corporations, health care corporations, and charitable foundations.

ALERT!

The National Family Caregivers Association is supporting the Lifespan Respite Care Act of 2003 (H.R. 1083), which is before the 2004 Congress. It would fund development of respite programs at the state and national levels, provide emergency respite, and train and recruit respite workers.

One NFCA project is dissemination of the IDentify Alzheimer's Disease (IDAD) free Resource Kit, which includes important information about how to distinguish Alzheimer's disease warning signs from normal aging, resources for caregivers of loved ones newly diagnosed with this illness, and much more. The kit includes "Alzheimer's Disease: What Everyone Should Know," an educational video featuring TV personality Linda Dano; "Caregiving: What Everyone Should Know," a brochure written by Linda Dano; "IDentify Alzheimer's Disease Early," an educational brochure; "Detecting Early Stage Alzheimer's Disease," a questionnaire; and an educational brochure "Improving Caregiver/Doctor Communications."

Starting an Alzheimer's Caregiver Support Group

It is possible that in your small town there is, as yet, no Alzheimer's caregiver support group. So why not start one yourself? Alzheimer's Disease International offers a booklet called "Starting a Self-Help Group" so you won't have to reinvent the wheel. We will summarize it briefly here. The booklet was created by experienced caregivers who work with support or self-help groups around the world.

The purpose of a self-help group is to meet with people who are sharing the same experience that you are and to offer mutual support. In such a group, you don't have to spend a lot of introductory time explaining what you do, how you feel, or what your stresses are. A few key words like wandering or sundowning, and phrases like "my mother is there but not there," speak volumes to those who are in the same position. The purpose of the group is to:

- Share feelings and experiences.
- Learn more about the disease and giving care.
- Give caregivers an opportunity to talk through problems they are facing or choices they have to make.
- Listen to others who share similar feelings and experiences.
- Help others through the sharing of ideas and information and providing support.
- Gain satisfaction from sharing with and helping others.
- Offer caregivers a break and a chance to get out of the house.
- Encourage and give permission for caregivers to take care of themselves in order to safeguard their health and well-being.
- Remind caregivers that they are not alone.

You must acknowledge for yourself before embarking on this new project whether you have the time and energy for it. Do you have support from family and friends? Can you cope with the additional demands of organizing a support group? Can you bear to hear about other people's difficulties?

You may have the idea to create a support group because you need other caregivers to talk to. Perhaps you met one or two other caregivers at a doctor's office and enjoyed the companionship and the fact that you shared a common bond. Maybe starting to have a regular meeting with one or two other caregivers could be a beginning point for you. By word of mouth through the doctor and friends you can start building a network.

Support Group Details

If you want to create a larger group and offer it to other caregivers who need support, then you will need to create a "to do" list. For example, new people will want to know the aim of the group, such as meeting for mutual support, to share feelings and experiences, or to learn more about Alzheimer's and caregiving.

Will you announce your meetings in doctors' offices, at church, in the local newspaper, or as a community event on the radio or local TV? This immediately brings up the question of how many people you can accommodate. You may need to find a large place—a church hall or local community center, or a room at your local library.

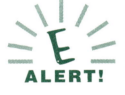

It is important that everyone knows a support group is not there to fix and solve all the problems that people have. Much of what caregivers have to cope with is something that cannot be changed. Medical and health problems will invariably be discussed, but the group should not offer medical advice that is not supported by a doctor or health professional.

Meetings can be weekly, bimonthly, or monthly; it's the group's decision. But the meeting dates and times should be on a regular basis so if someone misses one meeting, he or she just shows up at the same place on the next scheduled date. The group also needs to decide if the meetings are for support or information or both. Will you invite speakers to share information? By information, this doesn't mean just didactic statistics on Alzheimer's; you can also invite psychologists and social workers who can teach coping skills and behavior modification skills.

Group Dynamics

One or two group leaders are essential for good group dynamics. If you started the group, it doesn't mean you necessarily want to be or should be the group leader. Group leaders must first have the time to coordinate and organize the group; he or she should be a good speaker and be able to make everyone feel that they belong without judging. But don't forget that group leaders are also caregivers and need support, too.

Group rules should be set up early on. These rules are basic to all support groups and help establish a trusting environment:

- All information about members and discussions within the group is kept confidential.
- Members of the group listen and support each other without criticizing or making judgments.
- No one is expected to be the "perfect" caregiver.
- Each member is respected, and all are made to feel equal in the group.
- Each member has a chance to speak if he or she wishes.
- Each member's situation is respected. What is right for one person may not be right for another.

How to Run a Meeting

The duration of the meeting should be set and then the group leader will give each item on the agenda specific times. The group leader greets everyone, welcomes new members, and states the purpose of the group. The rules of the group, including confidentiality, are spoken, especially if there are new members.

Each meeting can have a topic as the focal point of the discussion. It could be about finding caregiver support; medical, financial, or legal problems; or about the larger experience of dealing with Alzheimer's. The group leader opens the discussion and guides it to make sure everyone has an opportunity to speak. At the end of the meeting, the group leader can ask for people to share their thoughts about the meeting and then give a summary of the discussion points. The date and time of the next meeting are announced and the meeting is adjourned. Most groups will have a time for refreshments and mingling at the end of the meeting. Ⓔ

Chapter 17

Insurance, Financial, and Legal Issues

These are tough subjects to write about and tough subjects to read about, especially if you don't have insurance, have limited finances, and can't afford to ask a lawyer legal advice. It's by focusing on these issues, however, that the real planning for Alzheimer's care takes place. When you know what your resources are, then you can make decisions.

Types of Insurance

The United States does not have a nationalized health care system but makes everyone responsible for his or her own insurance. Many layers of health insurance and disability coverage exist. Some people don't even realize what they have until they go over a checklist: health insurance as part of an employee package, union health coverage, veteran's benefits, TRICARE for Life covering military retirees and their spouses and survivors, prescription drug program, disability insurance, long-term insurance, and life insurance.

You may have private health insurance that covers all your needs. If not, and you decide to add insurance or change your insurance, make sure you don't have to wait for coverage to be effective. Many insurance policies will not allow coverage for an existing condition for one year after purchase. You must have a person knowledgeable about insurance review your health insurance very carefully to make sure Alzheimer's is covered and to find any possible loopholes in coverage. If you have no insurance, there are several government plans in place, but it's a minefield of information that has to be negotiated carefully, and you may need some help.

Employee Benefits

Many workers underutilize their health coverage because they do not read the details of their coverage. Your policy may entitle you to sick leave with pay or short-term disability benefits. Pension plans usually pay full benefits for a disabled worker even before retirement age.

COBRA Coverage

A federal law protects workers' health insurance if they are diagnosed with a condition like Alzheimer's and have to either leave work or cut back on work. It is called the Consolidated Omnibus Budget Reconciliation Act of 1985 (COBRA). It allows you to keep your employer group health care coverage if you have to stop work or cut back to a part-time position.

You must apply for COBRA within sixty days of change in job status. And it may be extended up to three years. The only drawback is that you must pay the full premium; your employer does not participate. COBRA provides stopgap insurance until you find other coverage or are accepted for Medicare under their disability clause or become of age.

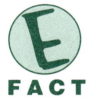

FACT

COBRA is a law; it is not an insurance plan or company. COBRA generally covers group health plans maintained by employers with twenty or more employees in the prior year. It applies to plans in the private sector and those sponsored by state and local governments. The law does not, however, apply to plans sponsored by the federal government and certain church-related organizations.

Union Health Coverage

A member or former member of a union who has health coverage will usually continue to be covered after retirement or if they have a disability. In January 2003, however, 17,500 unionized workers at General Electric went on a two-day strike to protest new health insurance deductibles, which will cost GE workers at least $28 million. "Until we take some of the profit out of health care and start serving the needs of people, this crisis will not get better," said Stephen Tormey, spokesman for the United Electrical, Radio and Machine Workers of America.

Veterans' Benefits

According to U.S. Representative Thomas M. Reynolds, "Under the current [Veterans Administration (VA) system], many veterans suffering from Alzheimer's are not receiving the specialized care required to deal with this devastating disease . . . Hundreds of memory care facilities around the country are equipped to help these veterans. Yet they are not able to receive such important treatment because the VA does not currently contract with specialized memory care facilities."

In June of 2003, Mr. Reynolds introduced new legislation in the House of Representatives to direct the Secretary of Veterans Affairs to conduct a pilot program that will determine the effectiveness of contracting private Alzheimer's facilities for veterans. Such facilities would provide specialized services and housing specifically tailored to the needs of those suffering from Alzheimer's disease or related memory disorders.

TRICARE For Life

TRICARE For Life is a permanent healthcare benefit. In October 2001 the most sweeping changes in thirty years took place in the Department of Defense's health care system. The changes were legislated by the National Defense Authorization Act. Expanded medical coverage known as TRICARE For Life was given to uniformed service members aged sixty-five and older who are eligible for Medicare, and who have purchased Medicare Part B.

Prescription Drug Programs

Health insurance may or may not cover prescription drugs. If it does, there is often a co-pay that you have to pay for each prescription. There is much debate over covering the cost of drugs to seniors because so many can't afford the escalating prices. Medicare has agreed to cover prescription drugs by 2006, but the costs are higher than were first proposed.

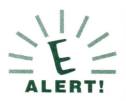

ALERT!

One in four patients suffered side effects from the 3.34 billion prescription drugs taken in 2002 (*New England Journal of Medicine (NEJM)*, April 2003). "With these 10-minute appointments, it's hard for the doctor to get into whether the symptoms are bothering the patients," said one researcher. *NEJM* editor William Tierney said, "Given the increasing number of powerful drugs available to care for the aging population, the problem will only get worse."

Disability Insurance

This can be a private or a work-related policy. Most policies are sold on the basis of providing you with between 60 and 70 percent of your income. If it is a private policy, you may have opted to pay for a higher amount. Employer-driven policies are tax deductible. Personal disability policies are tax-free.

Long-Term Care Insurance

This is a specific type of policy intended to cover nursing home or extended-care institutions. It usually also covers home care, adult day care, and assisted living care. If you have this policy already in place, you are covered for life. It will probably be difficult, if not impossible, however, to buy such coverage once you have the diagnosis of Alzheimer's.

Life Insurance

An existing life insurance policy can provide an important source of income specifically to be used for health care costs. Most companies allow you to borrow against the value of the policy to use for long-term care expenses.

Getting Answers

We'll give you some details below, but your State Health Insurance and Assistance Program (SHIP) can provide answers to your questions about Medicare Plus Choice plans and Medigap policies. (These will be discussed in detail later in this chapter.) Fortunately, they can also provide free one-on-one counseling to help you make the right choice about your health care insurance. SHIP numbers can be accessed through the government Medicare Web site (✑*www.medicare.gov*) or by contacting the following agencies.

Local/state health or social services departments can tell you what services in your state are covered by Medicare and which providers are Medicare and Medicaid certified. These agencies should be able to provide information about support and respite services available to Alzheimer's patients and caregivers in your area.

The National Council on the Aging has created an online service that identifies federal and state assistance programs for older Americans. Every day, thousands of people over the age of fifty-five find cost-saving programs for prescription drugs, health care, utilities, and other essential items or services. Just go to ✑*www.BenefitsCheckUp.org.*

The Social Security Information Hotline answers questions about social security payments or eligibility; this hotline will direct you to the proper office or department. Their toll-free number is ☏ 800-772-1213.

The American Association of Retired Persons (AARP) is a nonprofit membership organization that provides information to retired persons and seniors regarding long-term care options, caregiving, legal and financial planning, Medicare and Medicaid, and legislative issues affecting the elderly. Their phone number is ☏ 202-434-2277.

Medicare

Medicare is a federal health insurance program that provides coverage for people age sixty-five or older who are also receiving social security retirement benefits. You have to have paid into the social security system for ten years to be eligible. Some people under age sixty-five who have disabilities and people with permanent kidney failure on dialysis or awaiting kidney transplant are also accepted. The criterion for someone under sixty-five with disabilities is to have been on social security disability for two years before applying.

Medicare: Part A and Part B

There are two parts to Medicare. The first, called Part A, covers hospitalization, nursing, hospice, and some home health care. Part A is an automatic free benefit at age sixty-five to individuals if they or their spouse paid Medicare taxes while they worked. Those who did not pay Medicare taxes while working may be able to purchase Part A coverage.

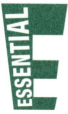

Medicare operates a toll-free hotline to answer questions about coverage and to get information about a patient's claims. Their toll-free number is ☏ 800-772-1213. Their Web site can be accessed at ✐ www.medicare.gov.

Part B is medical insurance that covers medically necessary doctors' services, outpatient hospital care, some specialty services such as physical and occupational therapists, and some home health care. The cost of Part B is about $66 per month in 2004, which can be deducted from your monthly social security check or is billed to you every three months.

What Does Medicare Cover?

According to the Fisher Center for Alzheimer's Research Foundation at the Rockefeller University, Medicare covers 80 percent of certain medical services for the treatment of Alzheimer's disease. Before the March 2003 announcement and change of policy, Alzheimer's patients were denied coverage for mental health services, hospice care, and home health care. The services Medicare now covers include "reasonable and necessary" doctors' visits; physical, occupational, or speech therapy; psychotherapy or behavioral management therapy by a mental health professional; and skilled homecare services (such as skilled nursing and speech or physical therapy).

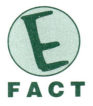

FACT

The Washington Post reported on January 31, 2004, that the new Medicare drug coverage plan will cost taxpayers $534 billion over the next ten years. This enormous price tag is one-third higher than the amount agreed upon by Congress in November when the bill was enacted.

The new policy reflects recent scientific evidence indicating that people with Alzheimer's can often benefit from mental health services and specialized types of therapy. This policy change emphasizes the need for ongoing research on Alzheimer's. Alzheimer's experts confirm that the new benefits will allow Alzheimer's sufferers to stay at home longer by providing access to services that help improve activities of daily living and help people with the disease maintain a better quality of life. A gap in Medicare was filled in November 2003 when a new Medicare drug law came into effect. Medicare will now cover prescription drugs.

Medicare does not cover the expense of adult day care, room and board at assisted-living facilities, or supervised care in a nursing home. It will pay for medically necessary skilled-care services at assisted-living facilities or nursing homes.

Medicare Coverage of Long-Term Nursing Care

The criteria to be considered for long-term nursing care coverage by Medicare are very strict. An Alzheimer's patient must have had a minimum three-day hospitalization, entry into a nursing home within thirty days of hospital discharge, and have the same diagnosis on admission to long-term care as the hospitalization diagnosis. Having met these requirements, the first twenty days may be paid in full by Medicare, and days twenty-one to 100 are covered with a co-payment of about $100 per day. Most patients, however, do not meet the above qualifications. In these cases, the Medicare program only pays about 2 percent of long-term care costs. Medicare will pay for home or inpatient hospice care for persons who qualify during the last six months of their life.

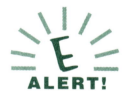

ALERT!

On October 24, 2003, ABC News presented "Spreading the Pain: How Uninsured Americans Affect Your Care." The Institute of Medicine found that 18,000 Americans die annually because they are uninsured, with a loss of $65 billion to $130 billion every year in wages and benefits. But, if insurance was provided to the 46 million uninsured Americans, it would cost $39 billion to $69 billion a year.

Medicare Health Plans

Now it gets even more complicated. There are three different ways to receive Medicare benefits. The first is the Original Medicare Plan. Because this plan doesn't cover all eventualities in a health crisis, however, you may need to add Medigap, which supplements Medicare. Or your former employer could still be providing supplemental coverage.

The other two plans, which add on to the original Medicare Plan, are sold by private companies. They are called Medicare Plus Choice plans and include Medicare Managed Care Plan and Medicare Private Fee-for-Service plans. Medicare Managed Care is a Medicare HMO, or health maintenance organization. It may provide the additional benefit of prescription medication coverage, but it usually restricts access to its own list of doctors and hospitals.

Private Fee-for-Service plans are called Medicare + Choice health plans. They are offered by private insurance companies, which are under contract to the Medicare program. Medicare pays the Private Fee-for-Service organization an agreed upon amount of money every month to arrange for the extended health care coverage for Medicare beneficiaries who have enrolled in these plans.

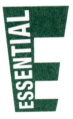

On September 30, 2003, the Census Bureau announced that 2.4 million people were added to the ranks of those without health insurance in 2002, making a total of 43.6 million Americans. The American Medical Association expressed grave concern that without insurance, many Americans do not seek medical care until their health problem reaches crisis proportions.

These plans entitle beneficiaries to go to any eligible doctor or hospital anywhere in the United States that is willing to provide care and accepts the member's Private Fee-for-Service plans' terms of payment. These plans, however, usually charge for the above Medicare benefits with a co-payment, or co-insurance, and added premiums for prescription drugs. Some of these charges will change since Medicare is now legislated to cover prescription drugs by 2006.

In dealing with Alzheimer's, you need to be aware of your possible long-term needs, visits with specialists, costly medications, home care, hearing aids, eye examinations, and nursing home care. To cover all these possibilities, the cost may be higher, but you may save money in the long run.

Medigap

Medicare may not cover all the expenses incurred by an Alzheimer's patient. Medicare coverage, however, can be supplemented with Medigap.

This is a private insurance that charges premiums to cover co-payments and deductibles required by Medicare. There are policies that are more expensive that also cover prescription drugs. If you are in a Private Fee-for-Service plan, however, or if you are covered by Medicaid you won't need a Medigap policy.

Medicaid

Medicaid is a government program run jointly by local, state, and federal agencies and administered by each individual state's welfare agency for people with limited incomes and little or no assets. Criteria for eligibility and benefits vary from state to state, but it can be used by people who have exhausted their own resources. Medicaid covers all or a portion of nursing home costs, and that's where most of Medicaid dollars are spent. Some states, however, are developing home care and community care options. A person with Alzheimer's can qualify for long-term care under Medicaid only if he or she has minimal income and cash assets. Such people will also be covered for hospice care if not covered by Medicare.

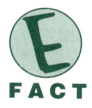

FACT

In 1998 the Alzheimer's Association established a Medicare Advocacy Project with the American Bar Association's Commission on the Legal Problems of the Elderly. The goal of this project was to promote and encourage improvement in Medicare coverage of care and in treatment for beneficiaries with dementia.

Financial Issues in Alzheimer's

A diagnosis of Alzheimer's comes with the crushing reality that you might not be able to continue working for many more years. Immediately, your thoughts spiral out to concerns about how you can afford your future care. You wonder how expensive Alzheimer's care is and how long you will live with the disease. And will you have to depend on your family for financial support? These are very scary issues, but when you start talking about them with your family and friends and find support networks, you will be able to make financial plans for the future.

You may have disability insurance that gives you some regular income. You may have planned for retirement and have income either through your workplace or through individual retirement accounts (IRAs), annuities, investment assets (stocks and bonds, savings accounts, real estate, etc.), and personal property (jewelry and artwork). If you own your home, money from the sale of your home can be invested, or a new mortgage can be taken out on your home. If your assets are limited, financial resources are available through government assistance or community-based organizations.

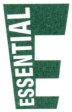

There is a special option for people over age sixty-two. It's called a Reverse Mortgage; it's a home equity loan where you can convert home equity into cash but still retain ownership.

Your banker, the person handling your retirement savings, or a financial planner along with a knowledgeable family member or friend, can help to create a financial picture of your future. With their support, you will need to look at the following health-care expenses: ongoing doctor visits, prescription medications, home care services, and possible future nursing home care. You will also need to decide who will manage your finances when you no longer can.

Finances Are a Private Matter

You may have never shared confidential information on your finances with your children before, and this can make you feel more vulnerable and less in control. But, if you have already sat with your family and told them about your diagnosis and begun to discuss the future, the next obvious step is discussing finances. Your children may rise to the challenge and reassure you that they will support you during your illness and take good care of you.

After a general discussion about finances with the family, the next step is to sit with one designated person and go over all your financial paperwork. Bankbooks, your income tax return from the previous year, retirement savings bonds, insurance policies, pension benefits papers, social security information: hopefully, are all in one place. If not, they all need to be gathered together and assessed. You may even uncover treasures that you had long forgotten, such as deeds to property or stocks that may be worth a tidy sum. A review of all this paperwork will help sort out what you have and what needs to be put in place.

A Financial Advisor

Once you and a family member have tackled the financial paperwork, it's time to sit down with a financial professional who works in eldercare. A financial planner, estate planner, or your banker will have information about financial support for people with Alzheimer's. Your banker will also be able to advise about direct bill payment and direct deposit of incoming money including your social security checks.

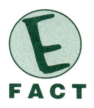

Disability is a special circumstance under which you may be able to withdraw money from your IRA or employee retirement plan before the requisite age of fifty-nine without the penalty of 10 percent for early withdrawal. You will be required, however, to pay taxes on these withdrawals. Social security benefits can be accessed before age sixty-five if you become disabled.

Financing Long-Term Housing

The mostly costly aspect of Alzheimer's will be your future housing. With Alzheimer's, one thing we know is that you will not be able to live alone. Usually the family does what they can to meet your needs as long as they can with home care support. Then it's a matter of finding out about the expense of residential care and nursing home care and planning appropriately.

A knowledgeable financial consultant will advise you on what to do about family assets. If titles are transferred or wealth given to family members, you may not be entitled to Medicaid if you need it in the future. One rule is that anything you give away up to three years before applying to Medicaid is still part of your income. These legal issues, and also tax issues, need to be investigated before making any decisions.

Tax Deductions and Alzheimer's

Long-term care costs, including nursing homes, assisted living facilities, group homes, day care centers, respite care, home care, adult diapers, and home installations for a disabled person, may all be deductible medical expenses. And they may also be deductible on another family member's tax return. The criteria are that the deductible medical expenses must total more than 7.5 percent of adjusted gross income.

Federal Assistance

Supplemental Security Income (SSI) is a federal income supplement program funded by general tax revenues. It does not come from social security taxes and is not the same as social security disability income. It was set up to help people over sixty-five who are blind, or disabled people with little or no income. Needy Alzheimer's sufferers are eligible. It guarantees a minimum monthly income that provides cash to cover basic needs for food, clothing, and shelter. Immediate application at the time of diagnosis is important because payments may be retroactive to that date.

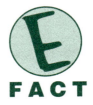

FACT

Workers who are disabled and under the social security benefit age of sixty-five can apply for social security disability. Eligibility requirements are having worked a minimum of five years in the past ten years and medical documentation of disability. In the case of Alzheimer's, your neurologist will be able to sign papers for you.

The National Council on Aging provides a service called Benefits Checkup that matches the financial statistics of an elderly person with available state and federal assistance programs. Benefits Checkup responds to thousands of requests every day to find programs for people over the age of fifty-five that may pay for some of their costs of prescription drugs, health care, utilities, and other essential items or services.

Benefits Checkup is linked to over 1,100 federal, state, local, and private programs. They include: prescription assistance (over 250 public and private patient assistance and prescription savings programs), health care programs, nutrition programs, property tax programs, veteran's assistance, housing assistance, and financial assistance. Their Web site is located at ✎ *www.benefitscheckup.org.*

Legal Issues in Alzheimer's

While organizing your financial paperwork, you will also want to put your legal paperwork in order. Legal papers include your will and a living will and directives on how you want your care to evolve.

Elder law is a growing field, and you will want to choose a lawyer who is familiar with issues related to Alzheimer's. The family member who is helping you sort out your financial and legal affairs should be present at any meetings with your lawyer. If you can't afford an attorney, you can obtain free legal advice through your local Legal Aid Society, Area Agency on Aging, or nonprofit legal assistance organizations. The AARP or your local chapter of the Alzheimer's Association may be able to give you appropriate referrals for legal advice and services.

Planning for the Future

Planning for care begins to evolve once you start gathering insurance, financial, and legal papers. Legal and financial planning should begin as soon as possible after a diagnosis has been made. Exploring care options early will give you the comfort and security of knowing what lies ahead in terms of health care and living arrangements.

According to Joseph Jackson of ElderCare Advisors, Inc., because Alzheimer's is becoming the most disabling chronic illness in the United States, it is putting an incredible strain on all available social services. This means people with Alzheimer's and their caregivers will need to be much more resourceful in their planning for Alzheimer's care. Jackson outlines a new practice model for planning care called Community Life-Care Planning (CLCP) and four basic steps in the Alzheimer's CarePlan.

1. Advance Directives
2. Estate Inventory
3. CareNeeds Assessment
4. Defining the Options

Advance Directives

Advance directives are legally binding documents that allow you to state your preferences regarding ongoing and future treatment and care. Jackson says that being able to execute advance directives is one of the best arguments for early diagnosis. The chief symptom of Alzheimer's is losing your memory and ability to reason and make appropriate decisions. Taking the time to create your advance directives allows you to make your own decision about how you want your care to evolve and who will be in charge of your care and your finances.

Jackson describes five advance directives:

- A power of attorney
- A health care proxy
- A will
- A living will
- A Do Not Resuscitate (DNR) order

Power of Attorney

A power of attorney is a document in which you empower someone to legally act on your behalf whose actions are deemed to be your actions. You will need to appoint such a person who will be called your agent. You will have to decide, sooner or later, whom you are going to appoint. This will usually be a trusted family member or friend. It's best, however, if the whole family agrees who this person will be to prevent rifts in the future. And getting the whole family involved from the beginning can be important for the family dynamic and also to make sure everyone shares responsibilities for both decisions and support of your care.

ALERT!

Your oldest child or oldest male child may feel that they are "entitled" to be your power of attorney and be in charge of your finances. If they do not have a history of making the best or the most intelligent financial decisions, however, then they aren't the person you want.

The term *durable power of attorney* means that your agent can continue to act on your behalf when you are no longer able to make decisions for yourself. This is very important in Alzheimer's because you don't want your resources to be cut off if no one is there to sign the checks or deposit your income. A durable power of attorney for health care will allow your agent to make all decisions regarding your health. In order to make a power of attorney durable, it must be stated in the terms that the power of attorney remains in effect when you become incapacitated.

Health Care Proxy

Someone who makes health care decisions for you when you are unable is called a health care proxy. It is someone you legally appoint to perform this service when you are still competent and is usually a family member. There is a standard health care proxy form signed in front of two witnesses where you designate your choice and also note specific health care choices you would like them to make for you. For example, if you do not wish to have any surgery, intravenous feedings, a respirator, or CPR, you can note that choice. If you didn't have a health proxy, your doctor may be obliged to give you medical and surgical treatments that you would have rejected if you were able to.

The health care proxy only comes into effect when your doctor finds that you are no longer able to make decisions. It differs from a power of attorney, which is an authorization for someone to make financial decisions for you. A living will is another way of making your health care wishes known by writing and signing a document that declares your decision about resuscitation, life supports, and other heroic measures at the end of your life.

Wills and the Do Not Resuscitate Order

You may want to change your will if it's old and since your circumstances have changed. A will is a document you create that names an executor to manage your estate after you die, and also names beneficiaries that will share your estate according to your wishes. The executor is usually known before the will is read after your death and is often the same person who helps you manage your ongoing finances.

A living will is a more formal advance directive that states your preferences for future medical care decisions, especially the use of artificial life support systems. If it is your decision not to be put on life supports, you have the legal right to limit or forgo the use of mechanical ventilators, cardiopulmonary resuscitation, antibiotics, feeding tubes, and artificial hydration.

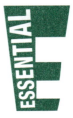

Increasingly in our society, we have come to equate the end of life with nursing homes, hospitals, and life supports with tubes running in and out of every orifice. But it doesn't have to be that way. An enlightened combination of hospice care, living wills, health care proxies, and Do Not Resuscitate directives give people choice at the end of life and dignity in dying.

A Do Not Resuscitate directive states that you do not want "heroic measures" taken to save your life in the event of a heart attack or stroke. By making these decisions early on, your family will not have to make them for you or go against your wishes. Copies of these documents can go to your doctor, lawyer, family, and caregiver.

Estate Inventory

Knowing what you have to work with is important at the outset of planning for care. An estate inventory gives a picture of available and dependable resources for ongoing care. This includes:

- Health insurance, including long-term care insurance
- Income and assets: social security, pension, and other retirement income; savings; investments; equity in the home
- Community resources: local, state, and federal programs
- Family and friends
- Home environment
- The Alzheimer's patient's capacity for self-care

A CareNeeds assessment is usually implemented by social services through a doctor's referral. A home care nurse will assess the Alzheimer's patient's capacity for self-care, the suitability of the home environment, and the resources of family and friends. In the beginning, the care needed may be minimal, but with time more will be required and the plan must reflect that.

Defining the Options

The actual planning for care begins once the advance directives are in place, the estate inventory organized, and care needs assessed. Jackson recommends a short-term and long-term approach to planning. This approach only makes sense because you have to deal with immediate needs now while planning for the future. And the future will evolve and change over time. Jackson also suggests that it's helpful to "hope for the best but plan for the worst." Alzheimer's disease is progressively debilitating.

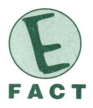

FACT

Second Wind Dreams is a national nonprofit organization that helps grant seniors' wishes. With the help of individual and corporate donations, the Georgia-based organization has fulfilled the dreams of seniors in more than 400 centers in thirty-eight states. One eighty-five-year-old Atlanta fire captain with Alzheimer's remembered what his life was like when firefighters brought their fire trucks to the nursing home and turned on the sirens.

In planning for the "worst," you acknowledge that you may have to place your loved one in a nursing home at some point in time. The cost of nursing homes can be subsidized, but private ones can cost several thousand dollars per month. Knowing these costs can help you focus on finding the solutions to keep your loved one at home as long as possible and use family and community support.

Chapter 18

E

Choosing Care Outside the Home

The goal of most families with an Alzheimer's relative is to keep their loved one at home as long as possible. As the disease progresses, however, it's possible that you will need to have round-the-clock care. Physically, emotionally, and financially, you just may not be able to meet that challenge. And you shouldn't have to. Planning now for long-term care can be a great relief to everyone and relieve your loved one of thinking that they are going to be a burden or wondering how they will spend their last days.

The Long Road to Long-Term Care

The chronic care involved with Alzheimer's disease precedes long-term care. From the beginning of caring for your loved one, you have been delivering chronic care, and it has become more and more time-consuming. Occasionally, that chronic care has been interrupted with acute episodes of illness either requiring a doctor's visit or even hospitalization. Bladder infections, pneumonia, or a bad fall will all require immediate attention. The majority of time is spent, however, as we have outlined in various chapters, on daily personal care, support, companionship, supervising activities and exercise, giving medication, and daily household tasks of meal preparation, shopping, cleaning, and laundry.

Adult Day Care

Along the caregiving path, you may have become involved with adult day care, placing your relative in a day care facility that had a specialized dementia-care program, while you worked. You may have home care services, meals on wheels, visiting homemakers, and visiting nurses that help share the burden of care and responsibility. Even coordinating these services calls for planning and organization in your busy day as a caregiver.

The ARCH National Respite Network and Resource Center, funded in part by the U.S. Department of Health and Human Services, produced an important information handout on adult day care in 2002. They call it "One Form of Respite for Older Adults."

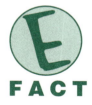

FACT

In 1978 there were only 300 adult day care centers nationwide. By the 1980s there were 2,100 centers, and in 2002 there were about 4,000 centers nationwide, according to the National Adult Day Services Association (NADSA). NADSA reports that the need for such centers has "jumped sharply to keep pace with the mushrooming demand for home and community based services."

Adult day care has grown because of Medicaid waiver programs that find it cost effective to support alternatives to institutional long-term care.

Mary Brugger Murphy, director of National Adult Day Services Association (NADSA), reports that "many of the people served by adult day centers would have been institutionalized just ten years ago."

Adult day care centers provide an opportunity for a person with Alzheimer's to socialize with friends while offering respite to their caregiver. Some caregivers, however, have to use adult day care in order to continue to work at their full-time jobs. Just as they do their children, adult children with an Alzheimer's parent will drop them off at day care and continue on to their job, picking them up after work and taking them home to continue their care.

In an adult day care, participants can also obtain health services and therapeutic services according to their needs. Some adult day care centers have specific services for dementia, which means they can offer activities and exercise that help improve cognitive skills and their patients' physical conditioning. Other day cares serve the broader population and may not be as sensitive to the needs of an Alzheimer's sufferer.

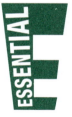

Approximately 80 percent of adult day care providers are non-profit; 10 percent are for-profit; and 10 percent use only public funds. Fees range from $25 per day to $70 per day, often on a sliding scale. Most adult day care centers provide transportation. Half the centers provide this service free of charge; others charge a fee. Full-time nursing services are in place at most sites.

A typical day at an adult day care center can include all the following according to needs and abilities:

- Supervised care
- Activities such as reminiscence, sensory stimulation, music, and art
- Intergenerational activities with visits from children and teens
- Nutritious meals
- Transportation
- Case management
- Recreation and exercise
- Nursing care

- Education
- Family counseling
- Assistance with activities of daily living
- Occupational, speech, and physical therapies

Assessing Proper Placement

Sometimes you can keep your loved one at home until nursing home care and attention are required. But usually it's not like that. Usually there is a sequence of care and care facilities that meet the needs of your relative at a particular stage of their disease but not at another. A suitable and reputable facility that matches financial resources and location may be difficult to find and will require the help of health professionals.

A CareNeeds assessment by a qualified professional helps avoid the mistake of an inappropriate placement. If your loved one is still mobile and social, they will not be happy in a nursing home with no interaction with other residents. If they are not able to take care of themselves, they will not be properly attended to in a limited-care facility.

An assessment of safety is another issue in choosing long-term care. An Alzheimer's patient who smokes is at high risk for physical injury, as are patients who wander, and who are at the stage where they can't use a stove safely. For people with safety risks, more supervision is required, even to the point of round-the-clock care.

Referral Agencies for Alzheimer's Care

Eldercare locator at ☎ 800-677-1116 runs a service during regular business hours. Your local Area Agency on Aging can provide information, and your local library will carry the National Directory of Retirement Facilities. For example, one such state referral agency is called California Registry. It's a licensed free referral agency for seniors and their families. Since 1939 this agency has been providing senior housing information, counseling, referrals, and facility evaluations at no charge. They provide clients from all income levels with the best possible information and referral for their needs.

Reviewing the options given by the California Registry to their clients, we can see how difficult it can be to find housing for your loved one without assistance. For example, in California alone, there are over 7,500 facilities to choose from. Calling a facility directly may not be appropriate when they are trying to sell their services, as they may not meet your needs.

American Association of Homes and Services for the Aging

American Association of Homes and Services for the Aging (AAHSA) is a national nonprofit organization representing 5,600 not-for-profit retirement communities, senior housing facilities, assisted living residences, community service organizations, and nursing homes. They have been operating since 1961 and have state representation in most states. They provide consumers and family caregivers with important information on all types of facilities and a listing of places accredited by the Continuing Care Accreditation Commission.

ALERT!

There is no standard definition and no yardstick to measure it; quality in long-term care is multidimensional and complex. Assessing quality in long-term care requires different types of measures than those used in acute care, where stays are short and clinical outcomes paramount. In long-term care, quality of clinical care and quality of life are equally important.

AAHSA's mission is to advance the vision of healthy, affordable, ethical aging services for America. One million elderly are served every day by AAHSA's member facilities. Member facilities in the organization make a "Quality First" pledge to achieve excellence in aging services and to earn public trust. Members work in partnership with consumers and government to create an environment in which consumers can feel confident that they are receiving the high quality care and service they deserve. Check out their Web site at *www.aahsa.org*.

In analyzing the quality of available housing for seniors, AAHSA sees a widening gap as the population ages. Presently many seniors live in poverty, struggling to afford decent housing. There is a tremendous additional burden to seniors who have Alzheimer's disease. AAHSA reports tremendous growth in assisted living care in the past decade.

Continuing Care Retirement Communities

A new level of care called Continuing Care Retirement Communities (CCRC) is an innovative answer to an aging retirement population by offering continuing care in their community. Previously if a retired person became disabled, or as in the case of Alzheimer's, developed progressive symptoms, they would have to move to an extended care facility. Now CCRCs can meet their needs.

The future cost for long-term care facilities cannot be handled by Medicare and Medicaid alone. Financing for home and community based services must be found in order to meet the escalating need for services.

Assisted Living Federation of America (ALFA)

ALFA claims to be the largest association exclusively dedicated to the assisted living industry and the population it serves. ALFA represents over 5,000 for-profit and not-for-profit providers of assisted living as well as a diverse range of organizations involved in the assisted living industry. It has forty-one state affiliates nationwide and promotes the philosophy of consumer choice and quality of life for seniors. It provides consumers with a selection of information sheets on assisted living, a list of questions to ask when considering a facility, and a directory of providers to identify facilities in a particular area.

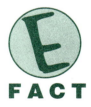

FACT

Assisted living communities are springing up all over America such as Silverado Senior Living: A Specialty Alzheimer's Community. It has communities in several states and established the Silverado Foundation, funded by donors who give in appreciation of the special care offered to Silverado Senior Living residents. The foundation also helps to fund research and provide education and financial and emotional support to caregivers, individuals, and families who serve those afflicted with Alzheimer's.

Volunteers of America

Volunteers of America is a nonprofit provider of quality, affordable housing for seniors, operating ninety-three senior housing communities, as well as fourteen nursing homes and seven assisted living facilities. In 2002, Volunteers of America Elderly Service programs assisted about 182,000 seniors nationwide.

Volunteers of America has a commitment to the elderly and lobbies for a decent standard of living through a strengthened social security system; access to affordable, safe, age-appropriate housing; affordable, comprehensive health care and long-term care; accessible supportive services along a continuum of care; and helping seniors contribute their knowledge and experience to their communities in both paid and voluntary activities.

Facilities for Alzheimer's Care

The types of facilities in the sequence that you may need for your relative include retirement homes with assisted living programs, licensed residential care homes, dedicated Alzheimer's care facilities, and nursing homes. As mentioned earlier, the Alzheimer's sufferer will go through different stages in which he or she will need different levels of care. The facility you choose must be able to provide that particular level of care needed at that time.

Retirement Homes with Assisted Living Programs

This type of residence will likely have licensed personal care programs that are suited to people with early stage Alzheimer's and symptoms of confusion and short-term memory loss. It may also be the most appropriate choice for a couple where the spouse is independent and taking care of a loved one with early Alzheimer's. CareNeeds assessment will determine whether a residential facility will be safe and appropriate at the outset. As symptoms progress, the residential care facility may not be suitable.

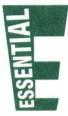

The cost of retirement homes is broken into two parts: the apartment rental and the assisted living services. Assisted living costs range from $200 a month to over $1,000 a month depending on level of care required. This fee is far below the cost of most private nursing homes and meets the needs of many elderly people.

If you and your partner wish to enter a retirement residence, you have to be sure the program is integrated for both independent and assisted living residents. The accommodations are usually a small apartment where you have all the amenities. You may have a choice of signing up for dining room privileges, and there are usually ongoing group activities.

Some retirement homes have a separate section dedicated to assisted living residents, but in other residences, there is no segregation. It appears, however, that most retirement residences have some kind of assisted living programs available, which adds to their appeal to disabled seniors or families trying to place their relative.

Care Offered

You will have to carefully assess and ask questions about what their care covers. We have all heard the stories of someone being allowed to stay in a facility as long as they are not incontinent, and then having to find another facility. As itemized by the counselor, such as the California Registry, what you are looking for is assistance with bathing and dressing, supervision of medications, assistance with going to the bathroom, management of incontinency care (both bladder and bowel incontinency), and special dietary requirements.

Skilled nursing services are not covered or even allowed to be offered by a retirement residence. If acute or chronic care of a colostomy or necessary injections of medication are required, this has to be prescribed by the resident's doctor and administered by an outside licensed home health agency as needed. Otherwise, the resident would have to immediately be admitted to a nursing home to receive nursing care. Allowing the two systems to intersect, retirement residence and home health care, allows a measure of independence.

Assisted Living Facilities

An assisted living residence combines housing, personalized supportive services, and health care designed to meet the changing needs of people who require help with activities of daily living. Health-care workers who understand wandering behavior and can supervise several people at one time make these facilities an important phase in the sequence of caregiving facilities.

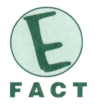

FACT

Currently, more than a million Americans live in an estimated 20,000 assisted living residences. A typical resident is a woman in her eighties and is either widowed or single. Residents may suffer from Alzheimer's disease or other memory disorders. Residents may also need help with incontinence or mobility.

Usually smaller than retirement homes, assisted living facilities are organized to provide a broad range of services for dependent seniors who can no longer live alone. They are often individual apartments but modified with special adaptations for disabilities. They will have wide doors for wheelchairs, tiled floors, walk-in showers, and emergency call pull cords.

The ALFA describes the following services customarily provided in assisted living facilities:

- Three meals a day served in a common dining area
- Housekeeping services
- Transportation
- Assistance with eating, bathing, dressing, going to the bathroom, and walking
- Access to health and medical services
- 24-hour security and staff availability
- Emergency call systems for each resident's unit
- Health promotion and exercise programs
- Medication management
- Personal laundry services
- Social and recreational activities

When nuclear families, with a mother and father both working, could no longer afford to have someone at home to take care of parents or grandparents, retirement residences began to gain momentum. With the increase in numbers of seniors and seniors' disabilities, assisted living became another added on feature to retirement homes.

The Assisted Living Federation of America members strive to adhere to the following 10-point philosophy of care:

1. Offering cost-effective quality care that is personalized for individual needs.
2. Fostering independence for each resident.
3. Treating each resident with dignity and respect.
4. Promoting the individuality of each resident.
5. Allowing each resident choice of care and lifestyle.
6. Protecting each resident's right to privacy.
7. Nurturing the spirit of each resident.
8. Involving family and friends, as appropriate, in care planning and implementation.
9. Providing a safe residential environment.
10. Making the assisted living residence a valuable community asset.

Costs and Who Pays for Assisted Living?

The cost of assisted living, according to the ALFA, naturally varies with the residence, room size, and the types of services needed by the residents. The range across the nation, however, is from $450 to $6,000 per month. Residents usually pay the cost of assisted living from pensions, insurance, social security, or from family support.

Some residences have their own financial assistance programs. But, be warned, government assistance for this type of care has been limited. Some state and local governments offer subsidies for rent or services for low-income elders in the community that they obtain from various sources.

Licensed Residential Care Home

This is a type of assisted living facility that offers care for moderate to severe stages of Alzheimer's. They are in a home setting, usually have a maximum of six residents, and provide round-the-clock care. For example, in California, there are over 5,100 licensed residential care facilities for the elderly. Residential care is defined as a nonmedical service by caretakers in either a single family residence, retirement residence, or nursing home. Most residential care, more than 90 percent in California, is in single-family dwellings.

As with retirement homes, residential care facilities are not permitted to provide skilled nursing services, but they provide all other caregiving assistance including help with bathing, dressing, going to the bathroom, and urinary or bowel incontinency care. Since Alzheimer's is not a disease with physical disabilities per se, skilled caregivers meet most needs, and patients don't require nursing assistance. The only drawback might be for those people who require more activities and stimulation. This can be overcome, however, by linking with community resources that have adult day care programs.

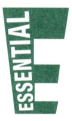

States regulate residential care. For example, the State of Vermont's Agency of Human Services, Department of Aging and Disabilities Residential Care Home Licensing Regulation protects the rights and welfare of residents and assures that they receive an appropriate quality of care, a level of personal independence, and a home-like environment. Homes must provide room and board, assistance with personal care, general supervision, and/or medication management.

The costs of residential care run about half that of nursing home care. In California, the range is from $850 to $4,000 a month, with an average cost of $1,500 to $1,900, depending on the amount of care needed, the size and quality of the accommodations, and the location of the facility. Few smaller homes will accept Supplemental Security Income (SSI), and if they do, they will require an additional several hundred dollars a month on top. Larger facilities may accept SSI, but only if the resident does not require full-time care.

Alzheimer's Dedicated Care Facility

Because of the growing need for Alzheimer's care, more Alzheimer's facilities are opening. Because they are few at present, the cost for care appears higher than other facilities. This type of facility, which specializes in dementia care, may be what is required for someone in the severe stage of Alzheimer's with aggressive behavior. These facilities are not nursing homes, but rather are licensed as residential care facilities. They are much larger than residential homes with an average of sixty residents. Staff in these facilities have more experience in working with dementia patients.

Nursing Homes

The final resting place, when your loved one is bedridden, may in fact be back at home. Their care is still challenging but perhaps less so than the wandering and aggressive or dangerous behavior. Otherwise, the final stop for many Alzheimer's patients is a nursing home. The most appropriate facility for someone with advanced and terminal stages of the disease would be a nursing home with a dedicated Alzheimer's care program.

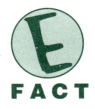

FACT

According to the Alzheimer's Association, half of all residents in nursing homes have Alzheimer's disease. And the National Citizens' Coalition for Nursing Home Reform, in June 2000, found that at any one time in the United States, approximately 1.6 million elderly are confined to nursing homes. By 2050, that number could be 6.6 million.

Hospice Care

A hospice is an end-of-life compassionate care service for people who are terminally ill. It is most often a small residential facility where treatment focuses on well-being rather than a cure. Medications are given for pain management and symptom relief. Hospice services, however, can be provided in the patient's home, in a hospital, in a nursing home, in an assisted-living facility, or wherever the patient resides.

The goal of hospice is to keep the patient with Alzheimer's as comfortable as possible in the final stages of disease and to provide emotional and spiritual support to the dying relative and his or her family. The hospice team may include a medical director, the patient's attending physician, nurses, social workers, counselors, clergy, and home health aides. Regular team meetings ensure the best care is given to each patient. A member of the team is usually always on call to family members.

By definition, hospice services are only for people who are terminally ill. To be accepted into hospice care, the following criteria should be met:

- A doctor's diagnosis of end stage Alzheimer's with six months or less to live must be presented.
- The family must consent to hospice services.
- The family must provide a health care proxy or living will signed by the person with Alzheimer's.
- If no proxy or living will is available, the family must provide clear, convincing evidence that the wishes of the person with Alzheimer's are known regarding extraordinary treatment such as resuscitation or tube feeding.

National Hospice Foundation

The National Hospice Foundation, founded in 1978, changed its name to the National Hospice and Palliative Care Organization (NHPCO) in 2000. NHPCO is the largest nonprofit membership organization in the United States and represents hospice and palliative care programs and professionals in the United States. Its commitment is to improve end-of-life care and expand hospice services to enhance the quality of life for people dying in America. Palliative care was defined in 1990 by the World Health Organization as addressing not just physical pain but also emotional, spiritual, and social pain.

Its headquarters are near Washington, D.C., in Alexandria, Virginia, where it advocates for the terminally ill and their families. For its membership, it develops public and professional educational programs and materials to enhance understanding and availability of hospice and palliative care. NHPCO hosts meetings and seminars on hospice issues, provides technical informational resources to its membership, conducts research, monitors Congressional and regulatory activities, and works closely with other organizations that share an interest in end-of-life care.

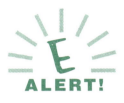

ALERT!

Hospice care costs are more, not less, than regular hospital costs according to a new RAND Corporation study in the February 17, 2004 *Annals of Internal Medicine*. The Medicare costs for about 250,000 hospice patients were compared with similar patients who received regular medical care. Hospice costs were 11 percent higher for people who died from illnesses other than cancer.

NHPCO represents 80 percent of hospices nationwide. According to its statistics, NHPCO estimates that more than 90 percent of the 885,000 hospice patients in 2002 were cared for by its members. More than seven million patients have been served by hospice since 1992. NHPCO helps family members of terminally ill patients locate either in-hospital care or home hospice care. Their toll-free number is ✆ 800-658-8898, or you can visit their Web site at ✎ *www.hospiceinfo.org*.

The Hospice Foundation of America

The Hospice Foundation of America is a not-for-profit organization that provides leadership in the development and application of hospice and its philosophy of care. It was chartered in 1982 to help provide fundraising assistance to needy hospices operating in South Florida. This was prior to passage of the Medicare hospice benefit.

In 1990, the Foundation grew to a national level in order to provide leadership and advocate health care for the entire spectrum of end-of-life issues. The Foundation offers professional development, research, public education, and information to assist those who cope either personally or professionally with terminal illness, death, and the process of grief. It offers information on locating a hospice, what questions to ask when interviewing for a hospice, and resources related to hospice care and grieving. The Hospice Foundation of America is supported by contributions from individuals and corporations, grants from foundations, and gifts from associations and civic and fraternal groups.

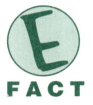

FACT

Research shows that 70 percent of Americans would prefer to be at home with loved ones in their final days, yet only about 25 percent die at home. Where people die—in a hospital, a nursing home, or at home—depends largely on the state or community where they live and the health care resources available there.

Last Acts

Last Acts, whose honorary chair is former First Lady Rosalynn Carter, is a broad-based national coalition whose vision is "to improve care and caring at the end of life." The Last Acts coalition of 1,205 group members is said to include virtually every major relevant national interest group, including the American Medical Association, the American Nurses Association, the American Hospital Association, the AARP, and the NAACP, as well as many local organizations and media personalities. You can visit their Web site at ✑ *www.lastacts.org.* The goals of Last Acts are:

- To improve communications between dying people and their loved ones, and between dying people, families, and health professionals.
- To reshape the medical care environment to better support high-quality end-of-life care.
- To change American culture so that people can more comfortably face death and the issues raised by care of the terminally ill.

Last Acts sponsors a Palliative Care Resource Center, which provides practical guidelines to improve the practice of palliative care in hospitals, nursing homes, hospices, and long-term care facilities. Their palliative care experts offer workable solutions to overcome barriers and make palliative care operational in clinical practice, institutional life, and public policy.

ALERT!

Not enough hospitals offer pain management programs and hospice services. It has been reported that nearly half of the 1.6 million Americans living in nursing homes have persistent pain that is not noticed and not adequately treated. All states have laws addressing the use of controlled substances. Some are effective, but others create formidable barriers to good pain management.

On November 18, 2002, Last Acts released a report that informed America that it was doing a mediocre job of caring for its most seriously ill and dying patients. The report was the nation's first state-by-state "report card" on end-of-life care. Most states earned Cs, Ds, and even Es on the majority of the criteria. Another survey showed that a significant number of Americans, including those who have recently lost a loved one, are dissatisfied with the way the country's health care system provides care to the dying. The survey found that 93 percent of Americans believe improving end-of-life care is important. **E**

Chapter 19

Preventing Alzheimer's

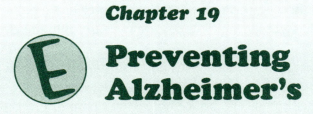

Researchers at Yale and Miami Universities studied people over fifty and their views on aging. Those who viewed aging as a positive experience lived an average of 7.5 years longer than those who did not. This wasn't a study specifically on Alzheimer's, but it probably holds true for everyone. Simply looking on the positive side of a negative experience seems to help us cope by giving us access to more energy, fewer physical limitations, less pain as we age, and also increases lifespan.

Making Choices

We have a choice to be pessimistic or optimistic. Researchers in the Yale study didn't conclude that optimism is the magic pill. What they did say was that optimists are also motivated to do positive things for their health. That means they exercise more, eat a healthier diet, seek out and follow sound medical advice, and take better care of themselves than pessimists.

Speaking of choices, in January 2003, Surgeon General Richard H. Carmona made the following statement: "As I see it, we can no longer, as a society, afford to tolerate the poor choices that have given us this huge disease and injury burden and huge costs. We have a health care crisis now, in terms of cost. Everyone's trying to decide how we pay for diagnosis and treatment. We are a treatment-oriented society. We wait for people to get sick. We reward caretakers for doing extraordinary things that are very costly to save somebody who largely could have made decisions years before that would have prevented that from occurring."

Dr. Carmona asks how we are to bridge the cultural divide from a treatment society to a prevention society. And he also says we better find out soon because 15 percent of the U.S. gross national product is gobbled up by health care and the current $1.5 trillion health bill will be $3.1 trillion in the next decade. He warned that even though we spend much more than most prosperous countries, our outcomes are no better than some of the poorer countries. Is that acceptable? Absolutely not. Dr. Carmona, however, believes that all the American people need to make healthy choices is the right information and the incentive.

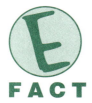

FACT

In a 2000 *JAMA* paper, Dr. Barbara Starfield reported on thirteen countries that were compared on sixteen health indicators. The United States ranked an average of 12th (second from the bottom) for 16 available health indicators. Countries in order of their average ranking were Japan, Sweden, Canada, France, Australia, Spain, Finland, the Netherlands, the United Kingdom, Denmark, Belgium, the United States, and Germany.

James S. Gordon, M.D., the first chairman of the White House Commission on Complementary and Alternative Medicine Policy, in his book *Manifesto for a New Medicine*, describes a growing health care movement. He says that millions of Americans are being drawn to more effective, less toxic, less expensive health care "through self-awareness, relaxation, meditation, nutrition, and exercise—as the true 'primary care.'"

Dr. Gordon says the new medicine "is a synthesis of modern technology and perennial wisdom, of powerful and definitive treatment and compassionate care, of Western and Eastern, high technology and indigenous and folk healing traditions." It's probably how Dr. Carmona envisions people taking more responsibility for their health and making better choices.

Awareness of Alzheimer's

The Alzheimer's Association, on February 12, 2004, released results from a national survey measuring baby boomers' awareness of Alzheimer's disease. This is the first analysis ever done of baby boomers' perceptions about the future of Alzheimer's. The survey is part of the Alzheimer's Association's "Maintain Your Brain" campaign to help energize and motivate Americans. But the campaign won't work if people don't have an awareness of Alzheimer's in the first place.

ESSENTIAL

> The Alzheimer's Association recommends eating right and keeping yourself mentally and physically active. Advocate for more government funding of Alzheimer's research. And if you can, give generously of your time and money to the Alzheimer's Association. Help them continue leading the way toward new discoveries, better treatments, and care.

Even though about 50 percent of Americans by age eighty will have Alzheimer's, only 26 percent of adults say they have any personal concerns about the disease. It's not that they didn't know about Alzheimer's, because half of those surveyed personally knew someone with the disease.

The Denial

There seems to be an element of denial at play here. And it's only understandable—why worry about something that you know you can't change? The Alzheimer's Association, however, is trying to bring the message to Americans that you can "Maintain Your Brain." How do they break through the denial to make people, first, aware of Alzheimer's, and second, aware that there are proven actions that you can take to prevent Alzheimer's or lessen your risk?

There is, however, one major contradiction present in modern medicine versus lifestyle intervention. While medicine "promises" the "magic pill" that will cure disease, there is the increasing knowledge that we have to take more care of our physical body because there really is no "magic pill." Maybe in 200 years there will be a "magic something," but not today.

The Reality of Our Lifestyle

The reality is that we make our bed and we lie in it. We all know the "bad" things we do in our life: not enough exercise; too much sugar; too many soft drinks; too many pastries, cakes, cookies, and candies; too much fried food; too much weight. Then why are we surprised when we have too much cholesterol? But why worry about cholesterol? Instead of finding the solution to the problem of lack of exercise and an unhealthy diet, we are given a "magic pill."

E ALERT!

Dr. J. Frey in a 2001 French journal, *Annales De Biologie Clinique*, asked the important question, "Is There Sugar in Alzheimer's Disease?" His answer was, yes; sugar may not cause Alzheimer's, but it does contribute to the symptoms that we see in Alzheimer's such as dizziness, lowered immune resistance, hypoglycemia, irritability, skin rashes, shakiness, and impaired hormonal function.

For an increasing number of people, the side effects of the magic pill create symptoms that require . . . another magic pill. And so it goes, and so it will go, until you realize that the solution is in the problem. And the problem is lifestyle. An unhealthy lifestyle impacts Alzheimer's as well as most of the chronic diseases in our country.

Is Alzheimer's Prevention Possible?

Dr. Majid Foruhi, a neurology consultant at the Alzheimer's Disease Research Center at Johns Hopkins Hospital, wrote *The Memory Cure* in 2003. Dr. Foruhi presents a ten-step memory protection plan for better memory in your seventies.

1. Take control of your blood pressure.
2. Lower your cholesterol.
3. Check your B_{12} and homocysteine levels.
4. Eat a diet rich in fruits and vegetables and add some wine.
5. Protect your brain from injury.
6. Check your eyes and ears; sharpen your senses.
7. Exercise.
8. Jog your brain; use it or lose it.
9. Socialize; become a more interesting person.
10. Beware of depression and stress; be happy.

The American Federation for Aging Research

The American Federation for Aging Research (AFAR) is dedicated to promoting healthier aging through biomedical research and helps scientists begin and further careers in aging research and geriatric medicine. AFAR reports on "the latest research on lifestyle and habits that may delay or prevent Alzheimer's disease." They list the factors that may predispose to Alzheimer's. They remind us that some of these we can change, such as diet and leisure activities, and some, like our genes, we cannot:

- Moderate alcohol—1–6 drinks per week, 50 percent less risk.
- Excess alcohol—14+ drinks per week increases risk.
- Tobacco consumption—increases risk.
- Education—increased education lessens risk.

- Marital status—married people have less risk.
- Diet—high-fat diet increases risk; high fruit and vegetable diet decreases risk.
- Hobbies and leisure activities—the more active, the less risk.

The Alzheimer's Prevention Foundation

The Alzheimer's Prevention Foundation (APF) thinks the prevention of Alzheimer's is possible. APF is a nonprofit organization dedicated to reducing the incidence of Alzheimer's disease. The organization conducts clinical research and provides educational outreach. Its founders believe that chronic, unbalanced stress is a major cause of cognitive decline and that an integrative medical program can prevent and reverse memory loss.

APF is undertaking the research of natural and alternative therapies since conventional researchers largely ignore these areas. They are seeking funding for several research projects: the effect of medical meditation on stress reduction and memory loss; the effect of different nutritional regimes on the prevention of Alzheimer's disease and other dementias; and the effect of nutrition, stress control, lifestyle factors, and hormone balancing on the prevention and treatment of early-stage Alzheimer's disease.

ESSENTIAL

The Alzheimer's Society's preventive tips to reduce risk are: don't smoke; reduce salt and saturated fat; participate in regular exercise; drink alcohol in moderation; eat plenty of fruit and vegetables; eat oily fish once a week; have a General Practitioner check your blood pressure and cholesterol levels; avoid head injuries; and have an active social life, with outside interests and hobbies.

In fact, APF believes that nutrition, stress control, lifestyle factors, and hormone balancing are the keys to preventing memory impairment and Alzheimer's disease. Through their research and clinical experience, they believe that MCI (minimal cognitive impairment), AAMI (age associated memory impairment), and Alzheimer's disease are conditions that are connected along a continuum and are not separate disorders. APF also believes that MCI, AAMI, and Alzheimer's are caused by a host of factors interacting with each other (multifactorial) and never from one single cause. The suspects are poor diet, lack of essential nutrients, chronic stress, lack of mental and physical activity, and genetics.

The Alzheimer's Prevention Program designed by APF appears to be a commonsense approach that could be applied to most chronic diseases. It does not depend on one drug or therapy. They say it is designed to affect as many of the causative factors as possible. Each of the four components in their program is equally important.

1. Diet
2. Nutritional supplementation
3. Stress reduction and optimal mental and physical activity
4. Pharmaceutical drugs and hormones

Let's take a look at each of these in depth.

Diet

We've already mentioned that the brain is only a fraction of the total weight of the body, about 2 percent, but requires 20 percent of the body's blood supply, utilizes 20 percent of the body's total oxygen supply, and 65 percent of its glucose. Along with the rich supply of glucose comes a host of nutrients that are needed by the brain. If those necessary nutrients are not included in the diet or in supplements, the brain becomes nutrient depleted and can develop symptoms.

Fats

The most important nutrients in the brain are essential fatty acids; our diet, however, is sorely lacking in the essential fats from flaxseed oil, olive oil, and fish oil, but is overabundant in saturated, hydrogenated, and partially hydrogenated trans fats found in all commercial baked goods, margarines, and processed foods. According to the APF's Alzheimer's Prevention Program, the first dietary recommendation is to reduce fat intake to about 15–20 percent of your total calories. But, they also say that even more important is the quality of the fats that you eat.

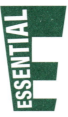

In November 1999, top nutrition experts at Harvard School of Public Health and the Department of Medicine at Brigham and Women's Hospital advised that "By our most conservative estimate, replacement of partially hydrogenated fat (trans fat) in the U.S. diet with natural unhydrogenated vegetable oils would prevent approximately 30,000 premature coronary deaths per year, and epidemiologic evidence suggests this number is closer to 100,000 premature deaths annually."

Trans fats are artificially produced solid fats created by heating liquid vegetable oils in the presence of metal catalysts and hydrogen. This process, called partial hydrogenation, causes carbon atoms to bond in a straight configuration and remain solid at room temperature. Naturally occurring unsaturated fatty acids have carbon atoms that line up in a bent shape, resulting in a liquid state at room temperature. Trans fats may be even more harmful than saturated and hydrogenated fats. They disrupt the production of energy in the mitochondria (the energy factories) of brain cells.

Antioxidants

Fifty percent of the brain is composed of fat, making it vulnerable to "rancidity" or the more scientific "oxidation." This fact makes antioxidant fruits and vegetables the next most important thing on an Alzheimer's prevention diet. Antioxidant is the term used to describe a class of organic substances, including vitamins C and E, vitamin A (converted from beta carotene), selenium, and the carotenoids. Carotenoids, of which beta carotene is the most common, are pigments that add color to many fruits and vegetables. Together as antioxidants, these organic substances may be effective in helping to prevent cancer, heart disease, and stroke.

Within the body, the job assigned to antioxidants is to neutralize certain particles called free radicals. Free radicals are atoms or groups of atoms with an odd (unpaired) number of electrons that can be formed when oxygen interacts with certain molecules in the body. Once formed, these highly reactive radicals can start a chain reaction, much like dominoes. They are dangerous because they can damage DNA, cell components, or cell membranes. Cells may function poorly or die if this occurs and over a long period of time, lead to diseases such as cancer.

Free radicals are the natural by-products of many processes within and among cells. They are also created by exposure to various external environmental factors such as tobacco smoke and radiation. A number of drugs can increase the production of free radicals including the antibiotic nitrofurantoin, steroid therapy, various cancer drugs, and sulfasalazine (a sulfa drug that treats bowel inflammation). Inhalation of mineral dust (asbestos, quartz, silica) can lead to lung injury that is partially mediated by free radical production. In addition, a wide variety of environmental agents including photochemical air pollutants—pesticides, solvents, anaesthetics, exhaust fumes, and the general class of aromatic hydrocarbons—also cause free radical damage to cells.

Vitamin E

Vitamin E is the most abundant fat-soluble antioxidant in the body. It is also one of the most efficient antioxidants available. It defends the body against oxidation and lipid peroxidation (rancidity). This fat-soluble vitamin is present in nuts, seeds, vegetable and fish oils, whole grains (especially wheat germ), fortified cereals, and apricots.

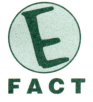

FACT

Tufts University estimates that 75 percent of adults do not get their 15 milligrams (for men) or 12 milligrams (for women) recommended daily allowance (RDA) for vitamin E. Men get 10 milligrams a day and women, 7 milligrams a day. Here are some counts for your reference: 24 almonds: 7.4 mg; 20 hazelnuts: 4.3 mg; 1 cup cooked broccoli: 2.6 mg; 1 tablespoon olive oil: 1.7 mg; 1 cup red bell peppers: 1 mg; 1 kiwi fruit: 0.9mg; 5 large olives: 0.7mg; 1 cup of cooked spinach: 0.6 mg.

There are eight forms of vitamin E, four tocopherols and four tocotrienols. Researchers used to think only the alpha tocopherols were beneficial to the body. Now we know that all forms are active, especially a mixture of the tocopherols. Current recommended daily allowance is only 15 milligrams per day for men and 12 milligrams per day for women. Studies show, however, that therapeutic levels of vitamin E, around 400 milligrams daily of mixed tocopherols, are the most beneficial to the body.

Vitamin C

Vitamin C is the most abundant water-soluble antioxidant in the body. It acts primarily in cellular fluid and is of particular note in combating free-radical formation caused by pollution and cigarette smoke. It also helps return vitamin E to its active form. Ascorbic acid is the chemical name of vitamin C. It is a water-soluble vitamin present in citrus fruits and juices, green peppers, cabbage, spinach, broccoli, kale, cantaloupe, kiwi, and strawberries. The RDA is 60 milligrams per day.

Beta Carotene

Beta carotene is a fat-soluble antioxidant. It is a precursor to vitamin A (retinol) and is present in liver, egg yolk, milk, butter, spinach, carrots, squash, broccoli, yams, tomatoes, cantaloupe, peaches, and grains. Because beta carotene is converted to vitamin A by the body, there is no set requirement.

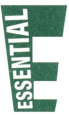

The best way to get vitamins and minerals is through a healthy, well-balanced diet! Eat a diet rich in fruits, veggies, and whole grains. Buy organic produce if you possibly can. That way, you will avoid the chemical herbicides and pesticides that cover commercially grown fruits and vegetables and create free radicals in the body.

Sugar and the Brain

The brain uses 65 percent of the body's glucose, but too much or too little glucose can have a detrimental effect on brain function. When you drink a can of soda, which contains ten teaspoons of table sugar, that sugar is absorbed into a blood stream that only contains a total of four teaspoons of blood sugar. The blood sugar level rockets to an excessive level, setting off alarms in the pancreas, and a large amount of insulin comes out to deal with the excess blood sugar. Some sugar is quickly ushered into the cells, including brain cells, and the rest is put into storage or into fat cells. When all this is done, maybe in about one hour, the blood sugar may fall dramatically and low blood sugar occurs. These rapid swings in blood sugar produce symptoms of impaired memory and clouded thinking.

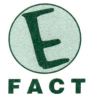

FACT

University of Virginia researchers demonstrated that performance of the brain is impaired in the short term when a patient has too much blood sugar. At a blood glucose level of about 270, the brain starts to show evidence of slowing down. A similar thing happens when you get to a level of less than 80. The brain works optimally between those levels.

The body does a much better job of keeping the blood sugar balanced and not overusing insulin with a diet high in complex carbohydrates, such as whole grains, root vegetables, legumes, and small amounts of organic animal protein, than with refined and processed foods.

The Prevention Diet

The Alzheimer's Prevention Foundation's Prevention Program recommends the following foods to feed your brain:

- Omega-three fatty acids found in fish, flax oil, and spinach
- Colorful vegetables that are rich in antioxidants
- Whole foods such as brown rice, whole wheat bread and pasta, and legumes
- Clean protein from organic meats, fish, soy, and legumes

They advise a limit on foods that may harm the brain:

- Excess saturated fat (meat, cheese, and fried food)
- Trans fat (margarines, baked goods, chips, and fast food)
- Excess calories
- Refined carbohydrates like white rice, white bread, chips, pasta, and cookies

Nutritional Supplements

The Alzheimer's Prevention Foundation advises optimal levels of essential nutrients to allow the brain to operate at peak performance with proper protection from oxidative damage. They recommend a good multivitamin supplement containing B vitamins: thiamine (B_1), riboflavin (B_2), niacin (B_3), pantothenic acid (B_5), pyridoxine (B_6), and cobalamin (B_{12}). This multi should contain at least 50 milligrams of B vitamin, except B_{12}, which is needed in smaller amounts (400–1,000 mcg). There should also be 400 micrograms of folic acid.

Next, they recommend brain specific nutrients. The first one is called Co-Q10. This is a powerful antioxidant and is important for the production of energy in the mitochondria of your brain cells. You should take at least 100 milligrams a day. They recommend vitamin E in doses of 400–800 international units (IU) to prevent and treat early memory loss. They also recommend docosohexenoic acid (DHA). DHA is one of the essential omega-3 fatty acids. The best food sources are cold-water fish. The dose range is 100–1,000 mgs.

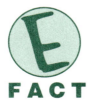

FACT

A study in *Archives of Neurology*, July 2003, found that increased blood levels of DHA, and fish three times a week caused a 48 percent reduction in the risk of Alzheimer's. "These dramatic results show how older adults can play a significant role in their neurological health. This study suggests that low dietary intake of DHA may be a risk factor for Alzheimer's Disease.

Ginkgo biloba is an antioxidant that also works by increasing blood flow to the brain. Ginkgo is an herb that has been shown to improve short-term memory in only a matter of a few hours. The Alzheimer's Prevention Foundation recommends a starting dose of 120–240 mgs, divided throughout the day.

Stress Reduction and Mental and Physical Activity

In Chapter 10, we talked about the importance of exercise in weight loss, increasing physical strength, and reducing stress. Physical exercise increases the blood flow to the brain, bringing oxygen and nutrients and taking away waste products. The APF says that brisk walking for thirty minutes a day is all that is needed for brain health.

An October 2000 *Brain Research Bulletin* study confirmed what has been known since the mid-1980s: Cortisol levels are high in Alzheimer's. This study also showed that high levels of cortisol correlated with a more rapid deterioration of the Mini-Mental State Examination (MMSE) over a forty-month period in a group of elderly women. It is well known that chronic stress elevates cortisol levels, which is one of the main causes of brain cell death. Popular stress reduction techniques include regular prayer, meditation, and self-hypnosis. We also talked about the need for mental exercise as being essential for brain health. Crossword puzzles, taking courses, writing, and reading all keep your brain cells healthy.

Hormones and Pharmaceutical Drugs

Three-quarters of the Alzheimer's Prevention Program can be done on your own. The final one-quarter, however, should be measured and monitored by your medical doctor or naturopathic doctor. A growing number of doctors are aware of the need for balanced hormonal levels in treating any brain disease. Pregnenolone, dehydroepiandrosterone (DHEA), estrogen, progesterone, testosterone, thyroid, and melatonin are all hormones that are essential for brain health.

Decrease in Hormone Levels

Measurements of hormone levels show that from about thirty years of age the levels of most of these hormones begin to decline. Research links the signs of aging to diminishing levels of hormones, DHEA in particular. Blood and saliva levels of hormones should be tested before supplementing with any of these hormones.

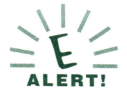

A nineteen-year study of 574 men, published in the January 27, 2004, issue of *Neurology,* showed that men who developed Alzheimer's had about half the amount of testosterone compared to men who didn't. For some, a drop in testosterone was noted a full ten years before diagnosis.

The APF Alzheimer's Prevention Program recommends the natural compounds huperzine A and galantamine as the first line of acetylcholinesterase inhibitors before moving to pharmaceutical drugs. The natural acetylcholinesterase inhibitors have fewer side effects than the commonly prescribed prescription drugs, Exelon and Aricept. Deprenyl is another drug that is recommended for Alzheimer's. It increases levels of brain neurotransmitters, particularly dopamine, and also prevents oxidation of the brain neurons. It has been shown to prevent the progression of Alzheimer's disease.

Hormone Replacement Therapy

For many years, drug companies have been telling women that hormone replacement therapy will protect against osteoporosis, heart disease, and dementia. The Women's Health Initiative Memory Study (WHIMS) was designed to find out if hormones do preserve our memory. WHIMS was part of the larger Women's Health Initiative (WHI) government-funded, fifteen-year study to address the most common causes of death and disability in postmenopausal women.

In July 2002, the investigators stopped the estrogen-plus-progestin part of the WHI study after finding that the associated health risks outweighed the benefits. The results of the study were tabulated, and in an October 2003 issue of *JAMA*, the osteoporosis part of the study showed that there was increased benefit derived from taking estrogen plus progestin, even in women considered to be at high risk of fracture. A February 2004 issue of *Circulation* published the report that among generally healthy post-menopausal women, estrogen with progestin did not confer protection against peripheral arterial disease.

As for the question of prevention of memory loss and decrease in dementia, which many said would be a result of taking estrogen and progestin, the May 27, 2003, issue of *JAMA* published the WHIMS results, which showed that the opposite was true. Taking estrogen and progestin increased the risk of dementia.

ESSENTIAL

In light of the new finding about HRT, many women are not renewing their prescriptions and some are suffering with menopausal hot flashes and other symptoms of menopause. Studies on St. John's wort, dong quoi, vitamin E, magnesium, calcium, omega-3 fatty acids, evening primrose oil, and homeopathic medicines may all have a place in the management of menopausal symptoms. See a local naturopathic doctor for more information.

Some doctors choose to ignore the findings of the study and depend on their knowledge of the patient to determine risk of estrogen and progestin. The FDA, however, on February 11, 2004, announced that hormone replacement therapy products containing either estrogen or a combination of estrogen and progestin must attach a warning label to the packaging that states taking these products increases the risk of dementia. The box is already quite full with the warnings that combined estrogen-progestin therapy is associated with an increased risk of heart attacks, strokes, blood clots, and breast cancer.

Chapter 20

What the Future Holds

The Alzheimer's Association February 2004 baby boomer survey found that only 17 percent of Americans believe that nothing can be done to reduce the risk of getting Alzheimer's, and only 18 percent feel that nothing can be done once a person has the disease. As far as finding a cure, only 29 percent think that science is on the brink of more significant advances. And only 24 percent believe a cure will be found in their lifetime. What can be done to change those perceptions?

Current Treatments

In the past decade, only five medications have been approved by the FDA for the treatment of Alzheimer's:

- Tacrine (Cognex): approved in 1993
- Donepezil (Aricept): approved in 1996
- Rivastigmine (Exelon): approved in 2000
- Galantamine (Reminyl): approved in 2001
- Memantine (Namenda): approved in 2003

Only four of these medications are in common use because there are intolerable side effects with Tacrine, which causes liver damage. All but Namenda are cholinesterase inhibitors, which inhibit the breakdown of a major memory and thinking neurotransmitter, acetylcholine. Since these medications do not cure Alzheimer's but only help delay progression, there is a far-reaching search for more effective treatments.

The only other treatments for Alzheimer's are drugs to treat behavioral symptoms and moods. They play a significant role in Alzheimer's care, but they are symptomatic aids and do not affect the root cause of the disease.

An American Medical Association (AMA) Alzheimer's briefing on June 7, 2001, talked about a number of different research avenues that are being pursued in the battle against Alzheimer's. Such avenues include studies showing how the immune system can be trained to sweep up amyloid plaque, new drugs called neurotrophic factors that can prevent nerve cell death, and new drugs that prevent the formation of fibrillary tangles in the brain.

Sweeping Up Amyloid Plaque with Vaccines

An Alzheimer's vaccine is the most talked about way of training the immune system to digest and remove amyloid plaque. In July 2000 an encouraging bulletin from the United Kingdom reported that there was an Alzheimer's vaccine on the horizon and that it was "safe to use." Researchers conducted a clinical trial of 100 people and the results looked highly encouraging because there seemed to be no negative reactions to the first tests.

Alzheimer's Disease and Associated Disorders Journal, in their March 2004 issue, report on new experimental vaccine research. Dr. Sam Gandy at the Farber Institute for Neurosciences found that, "Vaccinating with amyloid brings an immune response that stimulates removal of amyloid from the body." Dr. Gandy is a professor of neurology, biochemistry, and molecular pharmacology and vice chairman of the Alzheimer's Association Scientific Advisory Council.

The vaccine is a synthetic form of naturally occurring beta amyloid protein, which is the main substance in plaques. When the vaccine is injected into mice, there is an immune response mounted by brain immune cells to attack the amyloid in the vaccine and that response spreads to nonvaccine amyloid plaques. The attack results in breakdown of amyloid, and then the debris is cleared from the brain by normal mechanisms in the brain.

Vaccine Trial Halted

In January 2002, however, the next stage of vaccine trials experienced a setback when a life-threatening side effect was exposed. About fifteen of the 360 test subjects suffered severe brain swelling. By March 2002, the research trial was stopped.

One subject who died in an unrelated fall was autopsied. When the subject's brain was examined, there were fewer plaques than in Alzheimer's patients who did not receive the vaccine. But, there was significant brain swelling and an unusual collection of immune-system cells, called T cells, which normally are not found in the brain. These immune cells could have caused the inflammation and brain damage found in the autopsied brain.

Vaccine Research Resumed

By October 2002, the company that makes the vaccine said they had sufficient evidence that the proper antibodies were formed to the amyloid vaccine and that a significant number of people who were in the clinical trial improved. Therefore, they decided to modify the vaccine to overcome the problem with inflammation and began more clinical trials. Critics of the vaccine say that there is no proof that clearing plaques will diminish the symptoms of Alzheimer's.

Neurotrophic Factors

Neurotrophic factors comprise a family of proteins that are considered responsible for the growth and survival of neurons during development, and for maintaining adult neurons throughout life. *Neuro* means "nerve" and *troph* means "nourish." For the last several decades, scientists believed that, unlike other cells of the body, brain cells of the central nervous system could not regrow. That meant that if nerve cells were damaged after a head injury or due to conditions like Alzheimer's, they would die and not be replaced. We thought we had a limited number of nerve cells to last our whole life.

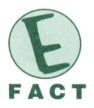

FACT

San Francisco biotech company Ceregene was issued a new patent that covers the delivery of neural growth factors to the brain, using both viral and nonviral gene methods of delivery. Ceregene plans to deliver neural growth factors to specific regions in the brain, where they could potentially block the destruction of certain cell populations. An Alzheimer's trial is planned for late 2004.

Research shows, however, that neurotrophic factors are capable of making damaged neurons regrow their dendrite processes in test tube and animal models. This breakthrough represents important research possibilities for all brain disorders, such as Alzheimer's disease, Parkinson's disease, and Lou Gehrig's disease. In development are ways to enhance the ability of neurotrophic factors to induce the regrowth of neurons damaged in Alzheimer's disease and improve their neurological symptoms. In the process, hundreds of questions have to be answered that will take years of research. While there may be answers in the future, there is nothing on the immediate horizon for the treatment of Alzheimer's.

Drugs That Prevent Neurofibrillary Tangles

A July 2002 issue of *European Journal of Biochemistry* stated that drugs to inhibit and disrupt tangles were being pulled from drugs already on the market for other diseases. One such drug, quinacrine, is an anti-malarial agent, and another, chlorpromazine, is used to treat schizophrenia. They are both being investigated as a possible treatment of Creutzfeldt-Jakob Disease and may hold promise for treating Alzheimer's. Other blockers of amyloid fibril formation cited in the journal include anti-cancer and antibiotic drugs, nicotine, and melatonin.

Medical Research

A more recent review article on the pharmacological treatment of Alzheimer's, in *Fundamental & Clinical Pharmacology* August 2003 by Dr. Allain and colleagues, cited the following "main entry pathways for drug discovery in Alzheimer's":

- Supplementation therapy
- Anti-apoptotic compounds
- Substances with a mitochondrial impact
- Anti-amyloid substances

- Anti-protein aggregation
- Lipid-lowering drugs

We've described the anti-amyloid vaccine and the anti-protein or anti-tangle drugs, which leaves four other avenues of drug research, according to Dr. Allain. Supplementation therapy is proceeding along the lines of nutrients explored in Chapter 9 and Chapter 19; however, it usually does not receive the same level of funding as patented drugs. Lipid-lowering drugs have, thus far, proven to be ineffective when given for the sole purpose of preventing Alzheimer's. We are left to review anti-apoptotic compounds and substances with mitochondrial impact.

Anti-Apoptotic Compounds

The November 1999 issue of *Mechanisms of Ageing and Development* reviewed the evidence that deprenyl is a neuroprotectant and suppresses apoptosis induced by particular free radicals. In animal studies, it was found that deprenyl protected the cells even after the medication was stopped, suggesting that it may be able to repress the apoptotic death program. These findings gave rise to the possibility that deprenyl may delay the deterioration of aging neurons as well as damaged neurons in neurodegenerative disorders such as Alzheimer's.

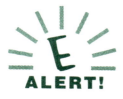

Researchers study substances called "cognitive enhancers" or "smart drugs" or "nootropics" that may improve mental abilities. (In Greek, *noos* means "mind" and *tropos* means "change.") Although there are many companies that make smart drinks, smart power bars, and diet supplements containing certain "smart" chemicals, we are still awaiting scientific proof.

A November 2001 paper in the *European Journal of Pharmacology* indicated that deprenyl protects neurons from oxidative damage while maintaining the mitochondrial membrane potential by having a positive effect on anti-apoptotic proteins. The authors concluded that deprenyl reduced the number of damaged nerve cells and made the nerve cells less susceptible to oxidative damage.

Human Studies and Deprenyl

A paper on deprenyl in the Cochrane Database of Systematic Reviews, 2000, found only fifteen clinical trials. Each trial measured cognitive effects of the drug, and twelve of the trials measured effects on behavior and mood. Eight trials indicated some benefits of deprenyl in the treatment of cognitive deficits, and three trials showed benefit in the treatment of mood and behavior.

The conclusion of the reviewer is that, in spite of some evidence of benefit, there is still not enough evidence to support its routine use. A second Cochrane Review of deprenyl in 2003 found that using the drug for Alzheimer's symptoms was still controversial, few doctors were prescribing it, and it was not being approved for use in Europe and elsewhere.

In this review, seventeen trials were included. The reviewer found that, whereas deprenyl initially showed promise as a neuroprotective agent, results in clinical trial were disappointing. It appears to be a relatively safe drug without significant adverse effects, but it also seems to have little clinical benefit. The rather strong conclusion reached by the reviewer is that "there would seem to be no justification, therefore, to use it in the treatment of people with Alzheimer's disease, nor for any further studies of its efficacy in Alzheimer's disease."

Mitochondria and Alzheimer's

In July 2000, researchers at the University of Virginia published their findings in the *Annals of Neurology* linking the hallmark signs of Alzheimer's, brain cell damage and death, to abnormalities in mitochondrial genes. Mitochondria are the site of energy production in the cells. They are descended from primitive bacteria and contain small pieces of circular DNA that are passed from mothers to children. Prior research had shown that abnormalities in mitochondrial genes are associated with rare brain diseases. This study extended mitochondrial gene abnormalities to Alzheimer's disease.

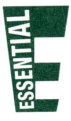

The mitochondria's main work is the Kreb's cycle, which tries to get the maximum number of electrons out of the food we eat. These electrons (in the form of hydrogen ions), with the help of vitamins B_2 and B_3, plus oxygen, are used to drive pumps that produce ATP, which is the body's source of energy that carries out movement, transport, entry and exit of products, cell division—basically everything.

Neurologist Dr. James Bennett, the principle investigator, believes defective genes are the cause of deposition of abnormal amyloid in Alzheimer's brains. His team found that defective mitochondrial genes caused increased oxidative stress, which led to activation of cell death pathways and oversecretion of amyloid and the formation of plaque.

Linking the possible cause of amyloid to mitochondrial gene defects opened the door to new research to find drugs to reduce oxidative stress in the mitochondria. However, several antioxidant supplements, such as vitamins C and E and beta carotene, already exist that should be tested in this regard.

The latest research on genes themselves is a study in the journal *Neurology*, February 10, 2004, that investigated 1,036 individuals from 266 families, living mostly in the Dominican Republic and Puerto Rico. These families were chosen because they had two or more members with Alzheimer's disease. They were tested to assess memory, attention, abstract reasoning, language, and visual-spatial function. And after accounting for age, education, and general intelligence, the researchers found that about half of memory ability of the participants was due to genetic factors.

The Latest Breakthrough Drug in Alzheimer's

We will continue to hear about the latest breakthrough research in the coming years. The following research is on a drug that is hailed as a breakthrough, but it is only in the early research stages. Often you see this type of headline only to learn that the drug is in the test tube research stage. And for the hundreds of drugs that are tested, only a modest few come to market. That's why funding of research is important, and that's also why doing all you can to improve your lifestyle and diet are important, too, because it may be very hard to find that magic pill.

A Cancer Drug for Alzheimer's

The laboratories of the Fisher Center for Alzheimer's Research at the Rockefeller University in New York City report that a fairly new cancer drug, called Gleevec, used successfully in leukemia and stomach cancer, may prove useful in the search for effective Alzheimer's treatments. A study published in the September 29, 2003, issue of the *Proceedings of the National Academy of Sciences* reports on their findings.

The drug was able to lower production of the toxic brain protein called beta-amyloid that is the cornerstone of Alzheimer's brain damage. Paul Greengard, Ph.D., 2000 Nobel Laureate in Physiology or Medicine and Director of the Fisher Center for Alzheimer's Research at the Rocke-feller University, along with other members of his laboratory at the Fisher Center, were the first to demonstrate that estrogen and testosterone are able to lower the levels of beta-amyloid.

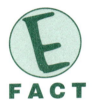

FACT

In chronic myeloid leukemia the body produces abnormal white blood cells because of damage to DNA that changes a chromo-some, which then creates an abnormal protein that tells the body to send out a constant signal to make abnormal cells. Gleevec seems to interfere with the abnormal protein and block it from telling the body to keep producing abnormal white blood cells.

The Early Stages of Testing

Presently, testing is on rat brain cell cultures and the drug has not yet been tested on human brains. And, Gleevec itself will probably not be used in pill form because it can't cross into the brain. The drug may be changed, however, to allow it to penetrate into the brain. Dr. Greengard feels that by unraveling the ways in which Gleevec targets beta-amyloid, it should be possible to develop medicines that safely enter the brain and have similar or better beta-amyloid lowering effects.

The Future of Diet and Supplements

"An apple a day may keep Alzheimer's away" is the message from a study by Dr. Thomas Shea published in the March 2004 issue of *Journal of Nutrition, Health and Aging*. Apple juice, because of its antioxidant effects, protects the brain against oxidative damage, which is the main contributor to age-related brain disorders. He found that in a group of mice, apples improve memory and learning.

Dr. Mark Mattson presented research at the 2004 annual meeting of the American Association for the Advancement of Science and published in the March 2004 *Proceedings of the National Academy of Sciences*. He and his research team found that fats in the neurons trigger the degenera-tion that leads to Alzheimer's. Cholesterol and other fats that build up in the brain are said to trigger a "neurodegenerative cascade." As the fats become rancid they destroy neurons in the vicinity and cause Alzheimer's. The reason for the buildup of fats in the brain is because of the amyloid plaques present in aging and present in larger amounts in Alzheimer's.

Dr. Mattson explained that "We had suspected that changes in fat metabolism in the membranes of nerve cells played a role in Alzheimer's but we had not been able to establish a direct link. With this study, we have been able to illustrate how alterations in membrane lipids can lead to neuronal dysfunction and death." The study also gives credence to the use of antioxidants like vitamin C, vitamin E, beta carotene, and selenium. Using vitamin E in a group of mice, Dr. Mattson's group was able to show that this antioxidant was able to reduce the level of cholesterol in neurons, which resulted in fewer killed neurons.

Dr. Mattson concluded that "Our work suggests that dietary modifications and drugs that inhibit the accumulation of . . . cholesterol may prove effective in suppressing the processes that lead to the disease."

Professor Elaine Perry, of the University of Newcastle upon Tyne in northern England, told members of a medical conference on the psychiatry of old age held in February 2004 that the plant extracts of sage and lemon balm produced promising results in studies to improve memory and behavior in Alzheimer's. Dr. Perry said that "In controlled trials in normal volunteers, both extracts improved memory, and lemon balm improved mood. Lemon balm reduced agitation and improved quality of life in people with Alzheimer's disease." She also said that "Extracts of both sage and lemon balm are clearly worth pursuing as potential treatments."

Chelation and Alzheimer's

The American Federation for Aging Research reported on how metals affect Alzheimer's. Apparently, amyloid that builds up in significant quantities in the Alzheimer's brain harbors atoms of zinc, copper, and iron inside its structure. Researchers theorize that the metal may hold the key to the brain damage in Alzheimer's and possibly its treatment.

How this might occur could be because metals like copper, zinc, and iron can all react with oxygen and create toxic free radicals that damage

DNA and protein and are implicated in the excess amyloid formation of Alzheimer's. Copper, especially, can promote the production of these free radicals; however, zinc has antioxidant properties, which protect against free radical damage. Unless zinc is present in high doses, it can act as a free radical.

Current research at Harvard Medical School, the University of Melbourne, and Prana Biotechnology Ltd. in Australia is directed at feeding mice that are prone to developing Alzheimer's copper chelating drugs that grab onto copper and flush it out of the body. These new metal-binding drugs effectively "melted" the amyloid plaques in living mice in as little as nine weeks.

WebMD medical news on Monday, December 15, 2003, reported on a novel treatment approach to severe cases of Alzheimer's that seems to show excellent promise. A December 2003 issue of *Archives of Neurology* reported that heavy metal chelation therapy, which chelates, or pulls metals out of the body also lowered the abnormal protein called amyloid found in Alzheimer's brains. Roger N. Rosenberg, M.D., editor of the *Archives of Neurology*, gave the opinion that chelation therapy may be a promising new Alzheimer's treatment.

Clioquinol

Clioquinol, besides being an antibacterial, antiparasitic, and antidiarrheal drug is also a metal chelator. Researchers found that it lowered levels of amyloid in people with moderately severe forms of Alzheimer's. Investigators feel that lower levels of this amyloid protein in the blood can be an indication of lower levels in the brain and possibly a slower progression of Alzheimer's. Since chelation treatment pulls out heavy metals, it may work by preventing zinc and copper from binding to amyloid and thereby dissolving it and preventing buildup.

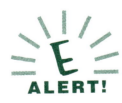
ALERT!

An epidemic of a disease associated with weakness, paralysis, and blindness, which was named SMON, occurred in Japan between 1957 and 1970. The disease was shown to be caused by clioquinol, which was used for diarrhea. But since that time there have only been neurotoxic effects reported with an overdose of the drug. Medical historians suspect there was an additional factor involved with the epidemic.

In this study, researchers compared the effects of clioquinol with a placebo in a group of thirty-six people with moderately severe Alzheimer's disease for thirty-six weeks. Half of the patients were given twice-daily doses of the drug and the other half were given a placebo. By study's end, not only was there a drop in blood levels of amyloid, but Alzheimer's patients that had taken clioquinol also had better scores on mental function tests and experienced few side effects.

The Other Side of Chelation

Researchers who think the underlying cause of Alzheimer's is the buildup of beta-amyloid protein feel this chelation study is proving their theory. By chelating out the protein, there is improvement in mental function. Dr. Boyd Haley, however, takes the other side of the argument and advises that it is copper, zinc, and mercury that are present in dental fillings and present in amyloid plaque that are being chelated out of the brain and causing the improvement in mental function.

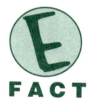

FACT

In 2003, the Alzheimer's Association awarded $150 million in research grants for Alzheimer's research. And federal research funding for Alzheimer's reached $520 million. However, there is need for more Alzheimer's research and more funding.

A Personal Journey

Tom Warren became his own expert in such things as chelation and dental fillings after being diagnosed with Alzheimer's. As part of his investigations, he had a CT scan that showed brain atrophy consistent with Alzheimer's. Mr. Warren did a lot of investigations of his own and tried a number of therapies including chelation therapy and having his mercury dental fillings removed. After four years, he was symptom free and his CT scan was normal. He wrote *Beating Alzheimer's: A Step Towards Unlocking the Mysteries of Brain Diseases* to help other people find their way.

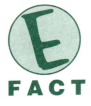

FACT

In the chelation process a water-soluble chelating molecule such as EDTA can wrap itself around a heavy metal molecule that is fat-soluble and is relatively trapped in fatty body tissues. The body needs about seventy friendly trace metals, but there are twelve poisonous heavy metals, such as lead, mercury, aluminum, arsenic, cadmium, nickel, etc., that interfere with enzyme systems and metabolism of the body.

The Future of Diagnosis

Presently, there are no inexpensive screening tools to diagnose a predisposition to Alzheimer's or even the very early stages. Researchers are investigating possible biological markers for Alzheimer's disease that could be identified in the blood, urine, or spinal fluid. Psychologists are also creating more sensitive cognitive tests to look for slight memory changes that could be associated with the development of Alzheimer's.

Diagnostic imaging techniques, the MRI and PET scans, are also being tested for their accuracy in diagnosing Alzheimer's. Their costs, however, may be prohibitive in using them as screening tools. Even now, PET scans can be used to diagnose very early Alzheimer's. They are used in clinical trials of various Alzheimer's drugs, anti-inflammatory drugs, vitamins C and E, and beta carotene to assess their effect on brain aging.

Every day there are new research papers, new press releases, and new hopes in the battle against Alzheimer's. Part of the disquiet about a disease like Alzheimer's is that it seems so hopeless. When you hear that there is no "cure" it's only natural to give up. While scientists search for "the cure," however, realize that there is enough information about the treatment and prevention of Alzheimer's that you can pursue for yourself or your loved one right now. The fact that there is something to be done can ignite purpose and hope. You will find that putting your mind to work on a solution instead of giving up is one of the best ways to stave off the disease. Ⓔ

Appendix A
Resources

Books

Bell, Virginia, and David Troxel. *The Best Friends Approach to Alzheimer's Care.* (Health Professions Pr, 2003).

Berman, Claire. *Caring for Yourself While Caring for Your Aging Parents: How to Help, How to Survive.* (Owl Books, 2001).

Brackey, Jolene. *Creating Moments of Joy for the Person with Alzheimer's or Dementia: A Journal for Caregivers.* (Purdue University Press, 2000).

Castleman, Michael, et al. *There's Still a Person in There: The Complete Guide to Treating and Coping with Alzheimer's.* (Perigee, 2000).

Coste, Joanne Koenig. *Learning to Speak Alzheimer's: A Groundbreaking Approach for Everyone Dealing with the Disease.* (Houghton Mifflin Company, 2003).

DeBaggio, Thomas. *Losing My Mind: An Intimate Look at Life with Alzheimer's.* (Free Press, 2002).

Dowling, James R. *Keeping Busy: A Handbook of Activities for Persons with Dementia.* (Johns Hopkins University Press, 1995).

Fitzray, B. J. *Alzheimer's Activities: Hundreds of Activities for Men and Women with Alzheimer's Disease and Related Disorders.* (Rayve Productions, 2001).

Kuhn, Daniel, and David A. Bennett. *Alzheimer's Early Stages: First Steps for Family, Friends, and Caregivers.* (Hunter House, 2003).

Loverde, Joy. *The Complete Eldercare Planner, Second Edition: Where to Start, Which Questions to Ask, and How to Find Help.* (Three Rivers Press, 2000).

Mace, Nancy L., and Peter V. Rabins. *The 36-Hour Day: A Family Guide to Caring for Persons with Alzheimer's Disease, Related Dementing Illnesses, and Memory Loss in Later Life.* (Warner Books, 2001).

Marcell, Jacqueline. *Elder Rage, or Take My Father . . . Please!: How to Survive Caring for Aging Parents.* (Impressive Press, 2001).

Petersen, Ronald C., M.D. (Editor) *Mayo Clinic on Alzheimer's Disease.* (Mayo Clinic, Kensington Pub Corp, 2002).

Shenk, David. *The Forgetting: Alzheimer's: Portrait of an Epidemic.* (Anchor, 2003).

Sheridan, Carmel. *Failure Free Activities for the Alzheimer's Patient.* (Elder Books, 1997).

Strauss, Claudia J. *Talking to Alzheimer's: Simple Ways to Connect When You Visit with a Family Member or Friend.* (New Harbinger Publications, 2001).

Associations

Alzheimer's Association: *www.alz.org*
Alzheimer's Disease Education and Referral Center (ADEAR): 1-800-438-4380; *www.alzheimers.org/adear*
Alzheimer's Society U.K.: *www.alzheimers.org*
American Association of Retired Persons (AARP): 202-434-2277
American Health Assistance Foundation (AHAF): 1-800-437-2423
American Health Care Association (AHCA): 1-800-555-9414; *www.ahca.org* or *www.ncal.org*
Area Agencies on Aging: Check your phone book under "Aging" in the State Government pages
Benefits CheckUp: The National Council on the Aging, *www.benefitscheckup.org*
Eldercare Locator: 1-800-677-1116; *www.aoa.dhhs.gov*
FamilyCareAmerica: *www.familycareamerica.com*
HealthFinder: *www.healthfinder.gov*
Medicare: 1-800-772-1213; *www.medicare.gov*
National Hospice Organization: 1-800-658-8898
Resource Directory for Older People: 1-800-222-2225
Social Security Information Hotline: 1-800-772-1213

Appendix B
Questions to Ask the Nursing Home

From ✑ *www.thirdage.com*

Does staff respond quickly to requests for assistance?

Are residents involved in a variety of activities?

What are the base costs? What are add-on costs (e.g., laundry, bandages, beauty salon)?

Is the facility Medicare or Medicaid certified?

How will the staff monitor your loved one's care?

Is there an adequate staff-to-resident ratio?

Is privacy respected?

Is there a qualified social worker on staff?

Does the home have contact with community groups such as pet therapy programs and Scouts?

Does the resident or family participate in developing the care plan?

Is there fresh water at bedside?

How many residents share a bathroom? Do bathrooms have hand grips or rails near all toilet and bathing areas? Is there a call button inside?

Who plans the meals? How are special dietary needs met?

What arrangements are made for honoring religious preferences?

Is there a family council for residents? When does it meet and who coordinates it?

Is there a physician available for emergencies?

What is the billing procedure? Will you be informed of any changes?

How is personal laundry handled? Will you need to do it yourself?

Is there a system to protect wanderers?

Index

THE EVERYTHING SERIES!

BUSINESS

Everything® **Business Planning Book**
Everything® **Coaching and Mentoring Book**
Everything® **Fundraising Book**
Everything® **Home-Based Business Book**
Everything® **Leadership Book**
Everything® **Managing People Book**
Everything® **Network Marketing Book**
Everything® **Online Business Book**
Everything® **Project Management Book**
Everything® **Selling Book**
Everything® **Start Your Own Business Book**
Everything® **Time Management Book**

COMPUTERS

Everything® **Build Your Own Home Page Book**
Everything® **Computer Book**

COOKBOOKS

Everything® **Barbecue Cookbook**
Everything® **Bartender's Book, $9.95**
Everything® **Chinese Cookbook**
Everything® **Chocolate Cookbook**
Everything® **Cookbook**
Everything® **Dessert Cookbook**
Everything® **Diabetes Cookbook**
Everything® **Indian Cookbook**
Everything® **Low-Carb Cookbook**
Everything® **Low-Fat High-Flavor Cookbook**
Everything® **Low-Salt Cookbook**
Everything® **Mediterranean Cookbook**

Everything® **Mexican Cookbook**
Everything® **One-Pot Cookbook**
Everything® **Pasta Book**
Everything® **Quick Meals Cookbook**
Everything® **Slow Cooker Cookbook**
Everything® **Soup Cookbook**
Everything® **Thai Cookbook**
Everything® **Vegetarian Cookbook**
Everything® **Wine Book**

HEALTH

Everything® **Alzheimer's Book**
Everything® **Anti-Aging Book**
Everything® **Diabetes Book**
Everything® **Dieting Book**
Everything® **Herbal Remedies Book**
Everything® **Hypnosis Book**
Everything® **Massage Book**
Everything® **Menopause Book**
Everything® **Nutrition Book**
Everything® **Reflexology Book**
Everything® **Reiki Book**
Everything® **Stress Management Book**
Everything® **Vitamins, Minerals, and Nutritional Supplements Book**

HISTORY

Everything® **American Government Book**
Everything® **American History Book**
Everything® **Civil War Book**
Everything® **Irish History & Heritage Book**
Everything® **Mafia Book**
Everything® **Middle East Book**
Everything® **World War II Book**

HOBBIES & GAMES

Everything® **Bridge Book**
Everything® **Candlemaking Book**
Everything® **Casino Gambling Book**
Everything® **Chess Basics Book**
Everything® **Collectibles Book**
Everything® **Crossword and Puzzle Book**
Everything® **Digital Photography Book**
Everything® **Easy Crosswords Book**
Everything® **Family Tree Book**
Everything® **Games Book**
Everything® **Knitting Book**
Everything® **Magic Book**
Everything® **Motorcycle Book**
Everything® **Online Genealogy Book**
Everything® **Photography Book**
Everything® **Pool & Billiards Book**
Everything® **Quilting Book**
Everything® **Scrapbooking Book**
Everything® **Sewing Book**
Everything® **Soapmaking Book**

HOME IMPROVEMENT

Everything® **Feng Shui Book**
Everything® **Feng Shui Decluttering Book, $9.95 ($15.95 CAN)**
Everything® **Fix-It Book**
Everything® **Gardening Book**
Everything® **Homebuilding Book**
Everything® **Home Decorating Book**
Everything® **Landscaping Book**
Everything® **Lawn Care Book**
Everything® **Organize Your Home Book**

All Everything® books are priced at $12.95 or $14.95, unless otherwise stated. Prices subject to change without notice.
Canadian prices range from $11.95–$31.95, and are subject to change without notice.

EVERYTHING® KIDS' BOOKS

All titles are $6.95

Everything® **Kids' Baseball Book, 3rd Ed.** ($10.95 CAN)
Everything® **Kids' Bible Trivia Book** ($10.95 CAN)
Everything® **Kids' Bugs Book** ($10.95 CAN)
Everything® **Kids' Christmas Puzzle & Activity Book** ($10.95 CAN)
Everything® **Kids' Cookbook** ($10.95 CAN)
Everything® **Kids' Halloween Puzzle & Activity Book** ($10.95 CAN)
Everything® **Kids' Joke Book** ($10.95 CAN)
Everything® **Kids' Math Puzzles Book** ($10.95 CAN)
Everything® **Kids' Mazes Book** ($10.95 CAN)
Everything® **Kids' Money Book** ($11.95 CAN)
Everything® **Kids' Monsters Book** ($10.95 CAN)
Everything® **Kids' Nature Book** ($11.95 CAN)
Everything® **Kids' Puzzle Book** ($10.95 CAN)
Everything® **Kids' Riddles & Brain Teasers Book** ($10.95 CAN)
Everything® **Kids' Science Experiments Book** ($10.95 CAN)
Everything® **Kids' Soccer Book** ($10.95 CAN)
Everything® **Kids' Travel Activity Book** ($10.95 CAN)

KIDS' STORY BOOKS

Everything® **Bedtime Story Book**
Everything® **Bible Stories Book**
Everything® **Fairy Tales Book**
Everything® **Mother Goose Book**

LANGUAGE

Everything® **Inglés Book**
Everything® **Learning French Book**
Everything® **Learning German Book**
Everything® **Learning Italian Book**
Everything® **Learning Latin Book**
Everything® **Learning Spanish Book**
Everything® **Sign Language Book**
Everything® **Spanish Phrase Book,** $9.95 ($15.95 CAN)

MUSIC

Everything® **Drums Book (with CD),** $19.95 ($31.95 CAN)
Everything® **Guitar Book**
Everything® **Playing Piano and Keyboards Book**
Everything® **Rock & Blues Guitar Book (with CD),** $19.95 ($31.95 CAN)
Everything® **Songwriting Book**

NEW AGE

Everything® **Astrology Book**
Everything® **Divining the Future Book**
Everything® **Dreams Book**
Everything® **Ghost Book**
Everything® **Love Signs Book,** $9.95 ($15.95 CAN)
Everything® **Meditation Book**
Everything® **Numerology Book**
Everything® **Palmistry Book**
Everything® **Psychic Book**
Everything® **Spells & Charms Book**
Everything® **Tarot Book**
Everything® **Wicca and Witchcraft Book**

PARENTING

Everything® **Baby Names Book**
Everything® **Baby Shower Book**
Everything® **Baby's First Food Book**
Everything® **Baby's First Year Book**
Everything® **Breastfeeding Book**
Everything® **Father-to-Be Book**
Everything® **Get Ready for Baby Book**
Everything® **Getting Pregnant Book**
Everything® **Homeschooling Book**
Everything® **Parent's Guide to Children with Autism**
Everything® **Parent's Guide to Positive Discipline**
Everything® **Parent's Guide to Raising a Successful Child**
Everything® **Parenting a Teenager Book**
Everything® **Potty Training Book,** $9.95 ($15.95 CAN)
Everything® **Pregnancy Book, 2nd Ed.**
Everything® **Pregnancy Fitness Book**
Everything® **Pregnancy Organizer,** $15.00 ($22.95 CAN)
Everything® **Toddler Book**
Everything® **Tween Book**

PERSONAL FINANCE

Everything® **Budgeting Book**
Everything® **Get Out of Debt Book**
Everything® **Get Rich Book**
Everything® **Homebuying Book, 2nd Ed.**
Everything® **Homeselling Book**
Everything® **Investing Book**
Everything® **Money Book**
Everything® **Mutual Funds Book**
Everything® **Online Investing Book**
Everything® **Personal Finance Book**
Everything® **Personal Finance in Your 20s & 30s Book**
Everything® **Wills & Estate Planning Book**

PETS

Everything® **Cat Book**
Everything® **Dog Book**
Everything® **Dog Training and Tricks Book**
Everything® **Golden Retriever Book**
Everything® **Horse Book**
Everything® **Labrador Retriever Book**
Everything® **Puppy Book**
Everything® **Tropical Fish Book**

REFERENCE

Everything® **Astronomy Book**
Everything® **Car Care Book**
Everything® **Christmas Book, $15.00**
    ($21.95 CAN)
Everything® **Classical Mythology Book**
Everything® **Einstein Book**
Everything® **Etiquette Book**
Everything® **Great Thinkers Book**
Everything® **Philosophy Book**
Everything® **Psychology Book**
Everything® **Shakespeare Book**
Everything® **Tall Tales, Legends, &**
    Other Outrageous
    Lies Book
Everything® **Toasts Book**
Everything® **Trivia Book**
Everything® **Weather Book**

RELIGION

Everything® **Angels Book**
Everything® **Bible Book**
Everything® **Buddhism Book**
Everything® **Catholicism Book**
Everything® **Christianity Book**
Everything® **Jewish History &**
    Heritage Book
Everything® **Judaism Book**
Everything® **Prayer Book**
Everything® **Saints Book**
Everything® **Understanding Islam**
    Book
Everything® **World's Religions Book**
Everything® **Zen Book**

SCHOOL & CAREERS

Everything® **After College Book**
Everything® **Alternative Careers Book**
Everything® **College Survival Book**
Everything® **Cover Letter Book**
Everything® **Get-a-Job Book**
Everything® **Hot Careers Book**

Everything® **Job Interview Book**
Everything® **New Teacher Book**
Everything® **Online Job Search Book**
Everything® **Resume Book, 2nd Ed.**
Everything® **Study Book**

SELF-HELP/ RELATIONSHIPS

Everything® **Dating Book**
Everything® **Divorce Book**
Everything® **Great Marriage Book**
Everything® **Great Sex Book**
Everything® **Kama Sutra Book**
Everything® **Romance Book**
Everything® **Self-Esteem Book**
Everything® **Success Book**

SPORTS & FITNESS

Everything® **Body Shaping Book**
Everything® **Fishing Book**
Everything® **Fly-Fishing Book**
Everything® **Golf Book**
Everything® **Golf Instruction Book**
Everything® **Knots Book**
Everything® **Pilates Book**
Everything® **Running Book**
Everything® **Sailing Book, 2nd Ed.**
Everything® **T'ai Chi and QiGong Book**
Everything® **Total Fitness Book**
Everything® **Weight Training Book**
Everything® **Yoga Book**

TRAVEL

Everything® **Family Guide to Hawaii**
Everything® **Guide to Las Vegas**
Everything® **Guide to New England**
Everything® **Guide to New York City**
Everything® **Guide to Washington D.C.**
Everything® **Travel Guide to The Dis-**
    neyland Resort®, Cali-
    fornia Adventure®,

Universal Studios®, and
the Anaheim Area
Everything® **Travel Guide to the Walt**
    Disney World Resort®, Uni-
    versal Studios®, and
    Greater Orlando, 3rd Ed.

WEDDINGS

Everything® **Bachelorette Party Book,**
    $9.95 ($15.95 CAN)
Everything® **Bridesmaid Book, $9.95**
    ($15.95 CAN)
Everything® **Creative Wedding Ideas**
    Book
Everything® **Elopement Book, $9.95**
    ($15.95 CAN)
Everything® **Groom Book**
Everything® **Jewish Wedding Book**
Everything® **Wedding Book, 2nd Ed.**
Everything® **Wedding Checklist,**
    $7.95 ($11.95 CAN)
Everything® **Wedding Etiquette Book,**
    $7.95 ($11.95 CAN)
Everything® **Wedding Organizer,**
    $15.00 ($22.95 CAN)
Everything® **Wedding Shower Book,**
    $7.95 ($12.95 CAN)
Everything® **Wedding Vows Book,**
    $7.95 ($11.95 CAN)
Everything® **Weddings on a Budget**
    Book, $9.95 ($15.95 CAN)

WRITING

Everything® **Creative Writing Book**
Everything® **Get Published Book**
Everything® **Grammar and Style Book**
Everything® **Grant Writing Book**
Everything® **Guide to Writing Chil-**
    dren's Books
Everything® **Screenwriting Book**
Everything® **Writing Well Book**

Available wherever books are sold!
To order, call 800-872-5627, or visit us at everything.com

Everything® and everything.com® are registered trademarks of F+W Publications, Inc.

The American
CRAFT BEER
COOKBOOK

155 Recipes from Your Favorite Brewpubs & Breweries

JOHN HOLL

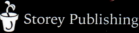

Storey Publishing

*For my father, John, who taught me the value of the written word,
the importance of good food and drink, and
the pleasure of great conversation with great company.*

*The mission of Storey Publishing is to serve our customers by
publishing practical information that encourages
personal independence in harmony with the environment.*

Edited by Margaret Sutherland
Art direction and book design by Alethea Morrison
Text production by Liseann Karandisecky

Cover photography by © Lara Ferroni
Author photo by Mars Vilaubi
Interior photography by © Lara Ferroni, except pages ii, iii, viii, 3, 13,
    43, 45, 53, 54, 63, 109, 131, 152, 153, 159, 171, 174, 175, 194, 231, 238,
    239, 273, and 286–288 by Mars Vilaubi

Indexed by Christine R. Lindemer, Boston Road Communications

© 2013 by John Holl

The information in this book is true and complete to the best of
our knowledge. All recommendations are made without guarantee on
the part of the author or Storey Publishing. The author and publisher
disclaim any liability in connection with the use of this information.

Storey books are available for special premium and promotional
uses and for customized editions. For further information, please call
1-800-793-9396.

Storey Publishing
210 MASS MoCA Way
North Adams, MA 01247
www.storey.com

Printed in China by Toppan Leefung Printing Ltd.
10 9 8 7 6 5 4 3 2 1

Library of Congress Cataloging-in-Publication Data

Holl, John.
  The American craft beer cookbook / by John Holl.
    pages cm
  Includes index.
  ISBN 978-1-61212-090-4 (pbk. : alk. paper)
  ISBN 978-1-60342-864-4 (ebook)
  1. Cooking (Beer) 2. Cooking, American.
  3. Microbreweries—United States.
  I. Title.
TX726.3.H65 2013
641.6'23—dc23

                2012047101

*Storey Publishing is committed to making environmentally responsible
manufacturing decisions. This book was printed on paper made from
sustainably harvested fiber.*

CONTENTS

FOREWORD

What beverage is the most popular and diverse in the world, a superior accompaniment to great food, a lubrication to good fellowship, an anchor to robust health, a source of deliciousness celebrated by royalty and common people alike for centuries, and is perhaps even the spark that started civilization itself? All this — and it often costs less than a fancy coffee at the corner shop?

If you're reading this, no doubt you know the answer. But beer has had a strange and twisting path into our collective glasses over the past hundred years. If you were in New York City in the year 1890, you would have seen the world's most diverse food culture side-by-side with the most interesting beer culture in the world. Does that assertion surprise you? Think about it. Great American cities teemed with all the peoples of the world, and from their home countries they brought dozens of languages, thousands of recipes, and often a love for their native beers. So our immigrant nation made dozens of types of beer, brewed by thousands of American breweries. We had breweries specializing in porter, breweries that made their names in pale ales and India Pale Ales, breweries making ranges of new lager beers, breweries that aged all their beer in oak, breweries that brewed only Bavarian-style weissbier. And we also imported many of the great beers of Europe. We had everything. And then, slowly and carelessly, we lost it all.

Over the twentieth century we turned cheese into plastic, bread into a chemical sponge, and beer back into water. They called it "progress," but something was missing: flavor. American food had become boring. Many people proudly said "I'm a meat and potatoes man," an intonation that was supposed to display a sort of all-American sturdiness blended with a distrust of fancy foreign pleasures. American beer became simple fizz, largely flavorless, another highly engineered modern food product, sparkling the most pallid yellow. By the 1980s, though, something began to stir. Our food started to become interesting again. Salsa overtook ketchup on American tables. Sushi went from the exotic restaurant to the airport, the supermarket, the campus, and the baseball stadium. And American beer came roaring back along with American food. Today, the United States can boast the most vibrant beer culture in the world. We have whole television channels dedicated to cooking. So the question is simple: we've got great beer and we've got great food — how do we put them together and have a good time doing it?

This may be my favorite cookbook sentence of the year: *"This flavorful recipe is also fun to make, thanks to the blowtorch."* John Holl is clearly a guy you want to hang out with. Our guide here is not only a knowledgeable beer enthusiast but also a reporter's reporter, and he has traveled the country's brewpubs and breweries to show you how much fun you can have with craft beer in your kitchen and at your dinner table. In a page or two per recipe, many of them sumptuously photographed, John lays out the preparation, a short story about the brewery and the people behind it, and a range of beers that will pair beautifully. With his book in your hands, you can go to the supermarket, the butcher, and the fishmonger and put together dozens of awesome beer dinners. Or you can make a quick and delicious dinner with a great beer pairing on an average Tuesday night. From Belgian Endive with Gruyère and Prosciutto, paired with a tripel, to Duck Chile Rellenos paired with a red IPA, this book leads you through a world of flavors both familiar and new. Even if you're already an avid cook and a craft beer fan, you're going to find a lot of things here to delight and surprise you.

Some people are puzzled when I tell them that brewing is much more like cooking than it is like winemaking. As a brewmaster, my nearest nonbrewing peers are chefs. Craft brewing, like cooking, is an act of expression and creation — the brewer has an idea and then gathers ingredients together to create the beer he or she has dreamed up. As a result, craft beer can taste like sea air, like bananas, like ginger, like chocolate or coffee, like cherries, like rum, like virtually anything at all. This versatility gives beer vast superiority over other beverages when it comes to compatibility at the table. I love wine and many other drinks, but frankly, when it comes to food pairing, nothing compares to the range of flavor in craft beer.

Ten years ago I wrote a book about beer and food pairing. The book was supposed to have contained recipes, many of which I'd gathered from some of the top chefs in the country. As the book stretched out to hundreds of pages, my editor told me that we'd need to cut the recipes; the book had simply become too big. Over these past ten years, many people have asked me when I would put out a revised version of the book with the recipes restored. So here I want to thank John Holl for saving me thousands of hours of hard work — now I don't need to go back to work on that book. John has gathered up even better recipes and done a splendid job, and I'm ready to follow his lead. I suggest you do the same. I have a fridge full of fun beers, several good knives, a whisk, and a blowtorch — it's party time!

— Garrett Oliver,
Brewmaster, The Brooklyn Brewery
Editor-in-Chief, *The Oxford Companion to Beer*
and author, *The Brewmaster's Table*

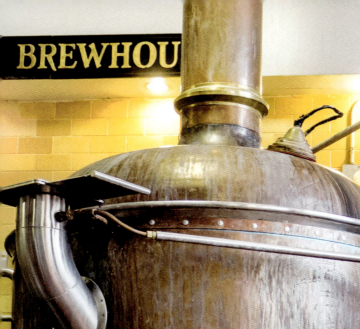

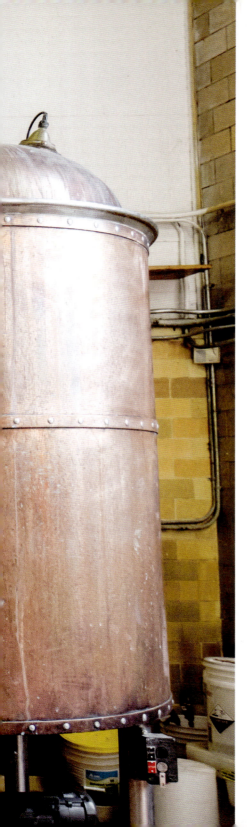

INTRODUCTION

Beer has long lived in the shadow of wine. It is treated as a second-class citizen at many dinner parties, fine restaurants, and even casual meals. In the general consciousness of American dining, vino has received all the glory: it's served in special glasses next to the dinner plate, writers devote countless pages to its characteristics, and it is the hostess gift of choice.

Fortunately that attitude has changed in recent years, thanks in part to the growth of the craft beer movement and increased educational writing about the beverage. Today, more than at any other time in the country's history, we have access to a dizzying array of beer styles from professionals who know how to wield their ingredients.

I firmly believe that beer pairs better than wine with food.

Beer is so varied, so complex, and offers such a cornucopia of flavors that it finds ways to complement, contrast with, and elevate all cuisine — from the lowly chip and dip to the most perfectly aged steak. There are so many different beer tastes that it's actually more flexible than wine when it comes to creating the perfect pairing.

Don't believe me? What about spicy Thai takeout? Try an IPA. Butternut squash soup? A brown ale. Beef carbonade? A Flemish red ale. Oysters? A stout (trust me).

All these brews are appealing, all are flavorful, and all are completely removed from the bland light lagers that permeated the beer scene from the 1950s to the late 1980s. That was a period of time that also saw an ideological shift in our general approach to food — we embraced a culture of convenience. Microwavable meals, McDonald's, Wonder Bread, and Velveeta became routine ingredients in our lives. They are cheap and tasty enough, and above all, they save time in our busy days.

For a long time, it seemed like there was not a lot of pride in producing the food we were consuming. Sure, there were restaurants and small community movements that savored local, flavorful, and fresh foods, but the availability of mass-produced sustenance caused many to lose their way.

Then the light switch flipped and people began to care about not only what they were eating, but where it came from. There were a lot of reasons for this shift: the rise of cooking shows and celebrity chefs and a general movement toward becoming more environmentally responsible and health conscious. Palates developed, better education about food and drink became widely available, and now more people are eating local.

Many chefs and brewers say people with more adventurous palates have also helped usher in a beer renaissance. It helps that chefs are drinking good beer, and restaurants run by the likes of Thomas Keller, Mario Batali, Gordon Ramsay, Todd English, and countless others now feature stellar beer menus right alongside their wine lists.

It's been a long road for beer to get the respect it deserves in the United States, but we are now in a frothy golden age, where the beers produced by the country's more than 2,100 breweries are not only technically perfect, but imaginative, eye-opening concoctions that have turned a millennia of brewing on its head. To that end it's no longer acceptable to refer to the beverage as "suds" or "brewski" or any other name that takes away from its stature.

It is also no longer valid for someone to say he or she just doesn't like beer. With more than 100 style variations and just about every possible ingredient under the sun finding its way at some point or another into a beer these days, there is a taste that can please anyone, so long as beer is approached with an open mind.

The soul of beer is just four ingredients: water, malt, hops, and yeast. However, each of these elements can be tinkered with, and given the varieties of hops, count-less yeast strains, and how the malt is prepared, an infinite number of combina-tions can be brewed and fermented.

Beer's ingredients enhance its relationship with food. Malts can impart fla-vors of caramel, chocolate, coffee, and biscuit, among many others. Hops can give aromas of tropical fruit, pine, spice, and herbs. Yeast can reveal a wide range of flavors, from clove to bubble gum. This is a simplified list, but the right combina-tion of flavors in a beer can transform a meal. Take some time to learn about the ingredients and you won't be sorry. Over time it will be easier to distinguish cer-tain flavors in beers that can pair well with a variety of cheeses, meats, dressings, and other foods.

This book is a collection of recipes gathered from breweries, brewpubs, chefs, and beer-centric restaurants around the country. They represent local flavors and sensibilities and create an overall sense of where we are today on the culinary road where beer and food meet. The recipes range from burgers and bites to choice cuts of meat and fresh seafood. There are salads that stand out and desserts that delight. With each one a suggested beer pairing is offered to round out the meal.

In some cases, the recipes are established menu items that have been served and enjoyed for years. Still others were created for this book. Some are very simple to make, and others require some kitchen skill, but each brings a wealth of flavor and depth and a chance to try a new beer.

There is such a wonderful choice of craft beer on the market these days (and more being added by the hour) that it would be nearly impossible to catalog each offering from each style. So, this book mostly sticks to styles. Many package stores offer wide selections of beer and have knowledgeable staff who can help you select the right Baltic porter, wheat wine, black IPA, or whatever beer your recipe calls for. If you can swing it, pick up a few bottles from different breweries. As with other beverages, each brewer puts his or her own stamp and spin on a recipe.

Also, it is worth seeking out your local brewery. It's believed that the majority of Americans now live no more than 10 miles from a brewery (although in some rural areas it's quite a few more). The breweries featured here are small businesses. They are parts of communities because the brewers chose to hang their shingles there. Keeping that in mind, I urge you to support them as well as your local food providers when sourcing ingredients.

Farmers' markets will sell many of the garden treasures called for in these pages (and often other great ingredients). Seek out butchers who can not only source excellent cuts of meat, but save you from doing much of the prep work. I always try to use the best ingredients possible. Some things are worth the extra few bucks for better taste.

When you have explored the recipes in this book at home, take your newfound knowledge into the world at large. Next time you're out to dinner and thinking about ordering that glass of wine, take a minute to scan the beer menu. Having a steak? Ditch the cabernet in favor of a robust porter. Grilled fish? Perhaps a Kölsch, rather than a chardonnay.

Consider the malt, hops, and yeast flavors in a beer and how they will complement or positively contrast with what is being served on the plate. Chances are you'll bring your dinner to a whole new level.

Host a beer party. Many of the recipes in this book can be served family style. Call together friends and task them with making a dish and bringing the corresponding beer. This is a great way to try quite a few styles (in moderation) without anyone breaking the bank or slaving too long in the kitchen. Discuss the flavors, and challenge each other on tastes and to explore the pairing. Not everyone will agree, and that's part of the beauty of beer.

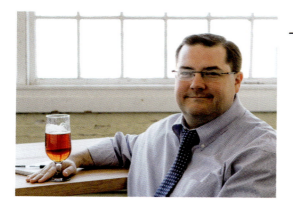

— *John Holl*

Halcyon Chicken Breakfast
Enchilada. see page 16

Beer and Brunch

A Great Way to Start the Day

Super Ultra Free-Range Pancakes

1 cup unbleached pastry flour

½ cup whole wheat pastry flour

½ cup quick-cooking rolled oats, such as Bob's Red Mill

¼ cup ground flaxseed meal

¼ cup garbanzo bean flour

1½ teaspoons baking powder

½ teaspoon fine sea salt

2 eggs

1 cup whole milk or unsweetened almond, coconut, or soy milk

1 cup water, plus more as needed

2 tablespoons unsalted butter, melted, plus more for serving

1 teaspoon vanilla extract

2 cups hulled and chopped strawberries or whole blueberries

½ cup ground walnuts or cashews (optional)

2 tablespoons honey
Flaxseed oil, for the skillet
Maple syrup, for serving

This take on traditional pancakes benefits from using organic or local ingredients (as available), while walnuts or cashews add a nice bit of crunch. Use this recipe to make waffles too. You can make several batches in advance and freeze them; when you're ready to eat them, microwave the pancakes for a few seconds to quickly thaw, and then pop them in the toaster oven for a minute or so to finish warming. Pair the pancakes (or the waffles) with a coffee stout or porter for that extra breakfast boost. Southern Tier Jahva is a great fit.

1 Combine the unbleached flour, whole wheat flour, oats, flaxseed meal, garbanzo bean flour, baking powder, and salt in a medium bowl and blend together with a whisk until combined.

2 Beat the eggs in a separate bowl until foamy, and then whisk in the milk, water, melted butter, and vanilla until combined. Add the egg mixture to the flour mixture, and whisk until smooth. Add the berries, nuts, if using, and honey, and mix until combined.

3 Coat the surface of a large skillet or griddle with flaxseed oil and warm over medium heat. Working in batches, pour 1/2-cup portions of the batter into the skillet and cook until the surface of the pancake becomes bubbly, about 5 minutes. Flip the pancake and cook until golden brown, about 2 1/2 minutes longer. Serve immediately with maple syrup and butter.

Makes 4–5 servings

PROFILE ★ **Southern Tier has quickly grown** from a local brewery to a regional brand with beers available in multiple states and several foreign countries. With offerings like the oak-aged Unearthly Imperial IPA, Crème Brûlée milk stout, Pumking Ale, refreshing Hop Sun, and more, after you've sampled a few bottles, it's easy to see why fans continually line up.

Breakfast Pigs in a Blanket

The basis of this dish is a playful riff on traditional pigs in a blanket, but this version lives in breakfast land. After making the sausage, simply wrap it in a pancake and drizzle with maple syrup before serving. This dish goes really well with a smoked beer, such as Jackie O's Hog Wash, which adds depth to the savory and sweet meal. Use your favorite pancake recipe with this dish or try the Super Ultra Free-Range Pancakes on the facing page.

1 pound ground beef tenderloin
1 pound ground pork
6 ounces ground veal
1 tablespoon chopped fresh rosemary
1 tablespoon chopped fresh thyme
1 tablespoon minced fresh Italian parsley
1 tablespoon chopped fresh sage
Salt and freshly ground black pepper
2 ounces cheddar cheese, shredded (½ cup)
6–8 thin pancakes (add additional milk to the batter to keep the pancakes thin)
Maple syrup, for serving

1 Preheat the oven to 350°F. Blend the beef, pork, and veal in the bowl of a food processor until combined.

2 Add the rosemary, thyme, parsley, and sage to the meat mixture and process until incorporated. Transfer the meat mixture to a large bowl, season with salt and pepper to taste, and then fold in the cheddar.

3 Form the sausage mixture into small, 1-ounce hot dogs, place them in a baking dish, and bake for 15 minutes, or until a thermometer inserted into the center of the sausages reads 165°F.

4 Prepare your preferred style of pancakes or the Super Ultra Free-Range Pancakes on page 6.

5 Wrap a pancake around each sausage and serve immediately with maple syrup.

Makes 6–8 servings

A Few Beers to Try with This Recipe

- *Dark Horse Fore Smoked Stout*
- *New Holland Charkoota Rye*
- *Victory Otto*

PROFILE ★ **There is something instantly familiar** and comfortable about *Jackie O's*. Maybe it's the old-world feeling radiated by the warm wood accents or the welcoming attitude conveyed by many Irish pubs. In an age where prefab bars go up quickly and feel a little too plastic, it's a relief to visit a bar where everything has been around for a few generations. Brewmaster Brad Clark has carefully created beers that are at once familiar but intriguing, brews that deserve closer attention as they swirl in your glass.

Shrimp and Grits

4 slices bacon

1 cup instant grits

½ pound medium shrimp, peeled and deveined

½ white onion, finely diced

2 teaspoons blackened seasoning, preferably Chef Paul Prudhomme's Blackened Redfish Magic spice

1 teaspoon freshly ground black pepper

1 teaspoon granulated garlic

¼ cup Chablis, or any dry white wine

1½ cups heavy cream

¼ cup freshly grated Parmesan cheese Chopped scallions, for garnish

A Few Beers to Try with This Recipe

- *Alaskan Summer Ale*
- *Flying Dog Tire Bite Golden Ale*
- *Front Street Coastal Kölsch*
- *Harpoon Summer Beer*
- *New Holland Full Circle*
- *Saint Arnold Fancy Lawnmower*
- *Samuel Adams East-West Kölsch*
- *Schlafly Kölsch*

A staple of Southern cuisine, shrimp and grits can be served any time of day. However, this particular variation makes for a bold breakfast, and it's a great way to start off any day on the right foot. This recipe gets its depth and rich flavor from the cream and the bacon and its reserved grease. It is a relatively simple recipe thanks to instant grits, which absorb the other flavors and lay down a good base. A bright Kölsch with a nice hop bite and some dryness, such as Front Street Brewery's Coastal Kölsch, is the perfect pairing.

1 Cook the bacon in a medium skillet over medium heat until brown and crisp, about 4 minutes. Transfer the bacon to a paper towel–lined plate to cool, reserving any bacon grease in the skillet. Roughly chop the bacon and set aside.

2 Prepare the grits in a small saucepan according to the package instructions. (For a richer version, use chicken broth and milk in place of water.) Remove the saucepan from the heat and cover to keep warm.

3 Toss the shrimp, onion, spice mixture, black pepper, and garlic with the bacon grease in the skillet and cook over high heat, stirring occasionally, until the shrimp are evenly coated and cooked through, 2 to 3 minutes.

Transfer the shrimp mixture to a medium bowl, cover, and set aside.

4 Add the wine to the skillet, stirring and scraping up the flavorful bits from the bottom of the pan. Let the wine reduce for 1 minute. Add the cream and Parmesan; bring to a boil, and then simmer, stirring occasionally, until the sauce starts to thicken, 5 to 6 minutes. Put the shrimp back in the sauce and warm through.

5 Spoon the reserved grits into two serving bowls and pour the shrimp and sauce over the grits. Sprinkle the bacon on top and garnish with chopped scallions.

Makes 2 servings

PROFILE ★ **Established in 1995, Front Street Brewery** has that comfortable neighborhood atmosphere that makes even first-time visitors feel like regulars. With its expansive menu and brewer Kevin Kozak's expertly made beers, this brewpub is one to visit time and time again. If you're feeling brave, ask your server about the ghost that lives on the upper level and occasionally roams among the brewing tanks.

8 eggs
4 cups sunflower oil, for
    frying
2 pounds pork sausage,
    casings removed
1 cup all-purpose flour
    Spices such as cayenne
    pepper, mace, sage, or
    dry mustard powder
4 cups plain dried
    breadcrumbs

Scotch Egg

Praise the inventor of this delectable treat: part breakfast, part snack, all goodness. The Scotch egg begins with a hard-boiled egg and adds a protective layer of sausage before giving the whole thing the deep-fried treatment. Served warm with a side of spicy mustard for some kick (try the spicy Two Hearted Mustard on page 71), it's not your average morning meal. It also makes a good appetizer. Pair with a dry Irish stout (commonly seen on tap through a Guinness-style nitro pour); the roastiness of dark malts is a pleasing complement to the egg.

1 Preheat the oven to 350°F.

2 Place four of the eggs in a medium saucepan, cover with water, and bring to a boil. Remove the pan from the heat, cover, and let the eggs sit in the hot water for 10 to 12 minutes. Remove the eggs from the hot water, cool, and peel.

3 Heat the oil in a deep fryer (or deep pot) to 375°F.

4 Flatten the sausage into four thin patties and wrap one patty around each egg. (This step is easier if the patties are made on plastic wrap. The plastic can be used as a guide when wrapping the sausage around the egg.)

5 In a small bowl, whisk together the flour and a pinch of the spices. Lightly coat the eggs with the seasoned flour.

6 Beat the remaining four eggs in a small bowl and place the breadcrumbs in another bowl. Coat the floured eggs with the beaten eggs, and then roll each egg in the breadcrumbs to cover evenly.

7 Deep-fry the eggs until golden brown, 3 to 5 minutes. Remove from the oil, transfer to a baking dish, and bake for 10 minutes. Cut the eggs in half and serve immediately.

Makes 2–4 servings

A glass filled to the middle gives the holder two different ways to consider the situation. Pessimistic? Half empty. Optimistic? Half full. The folks behind this relatively new Connecticut brewery are the hopeful, forward-thinking sort who believe the best is yet to come. *Half Full Brewery* is the dream of Conor Horrigan, who quit his full-time job to travel Europe and advance his beer education. Upon returning to the States, he learned the craft of brewing from the venerable New England Brewing Company and finally hung his own shingle. With the help of brewer Jennifer Muckerman, Half Full Brewery is giving residents of the Nutmeg State reason to drain their glasses and order another.

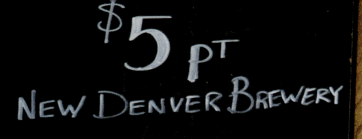

$5 PT

NEW DENVER BREWERY

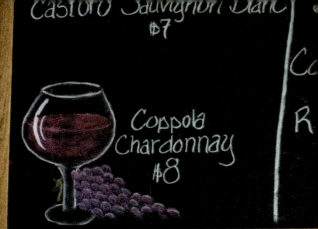

Castoro Sauvignon Blanc
$7

Coppola
Chardonnay
$8

Beer-mosa

Why should champagne get all the fun at brunch? A typical mimosa recipe calls for the sparkling wine to be mixed with orange juice, but the right beer paired with citrus leads to a tasty, eye-opening experience. For the best results use a wheat beer.

Combine the juice, beer, and triple sec, if using, in a champagne flute and stir gently. Garnish with a strawberry and serve immediately.

Makes 1 cocktail

5 ounces orange juice or grapefruit juice
3 ounces beer (see suggestions at right)
½ ounce triple sec (optional)
Fresh strawberries

Suggested Beer-mosa Beers

- *Breckenridge Agave Wheat*
- *Clownshoes Clementine*
- *Dogfish Head Namaste*
- *(512) Wit*
- *Grand Teton Tail Waggin' Double White Ale*
- *Samuel Adams Imperial White*
- *Sierra Nevada Kellerweis*
- *Southampton Double White Ale*

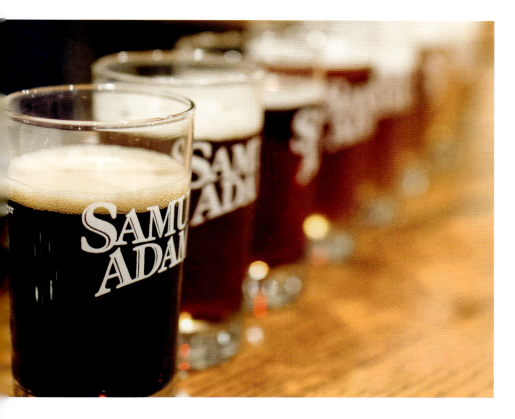

Ugly Pug Sweet Potato Pancakes

1 cup all-purpose flour, sifted
2 tablespoons sugar
1 teaspoon baking powder
½ teaspoon ground cinnamon
Ground cloves
1 medium sweet potato, cooked and mashed (about ⅔ cup)
2 tablespoons unsalted butter, melted
1 egg, beaten
1¼ cups Schwarzbier, at room temperature
Cooking spray

A Few Beers to Try with This Recipe

- *The Bruery Saison Rue*
- *Full Sail Session Black*
- *Ommegang Hennepin*
- *Pretty Things Jack D'or*
- *Rahr & Sons Ugly Pug*
- *Shiner Black Lager*
- *Sprecher Black Bavarian*

Too often sweet potatoes are eaten only for dinner. But with their natural sugars and agreeable disposition toward spices, they are perfect for breakfast. Pair this recipe with a Schwarzbier, like Rahr's Ugly Pug, or a spicy saison, which will add depth to the sweetness of the dish.

1 Whisk the flour, sugar, baking powder, cinnamon, and a pinch of cloves together in a small bowl until combined.

2 Mix the sweet potato, butter, egg, and beer together with a spatula in a large bowl until the ingredients are combined and the beer foam subsides. Mix the dry ingredients into the sweet potato mixture and stir until thoroughly blended.

3 Coat a griddle with cooking spray and warm it over medium-high heat. Working in batches, scoop 2 large tablespoons of the batter onto the hot griddle and cook until the bottom of the pancake is nicely browned and tiny bubbles form along the top edges, 3 to 5 minutes. Flip the pancake and cook until evenly browned, 3 to 5 minutes longer. Repeat the process with the remaining batter. Serve hot.

Makes 15 pancakes

PROFILE ★ **The Rahr family** has been in the beer business since 1847, when William and Natalie Rahr emigrated from Germany to Wisconsin and opened a brewery. They later opened a malting facility that supplied their venture, as well as many other local breweries. The original brewery eventually closed, but the malting business continued to thrive and remains a well-known name among brewers.

William's great-great-grandson and namesake, Frederick William "Fritz" Rahr, Jr., opened *Rahr & Sons Brewing Company* 165 years later in Fort Worth, Texas. Since 2004, the brewery has served traditional ales and lagers, along with some specialty offerings that pay homage to the family history as well as its Texas roots.

Roasted Root Vegetable Hash

Corned beef usually gets the hash treatment in the early morning hours, but the earthiness of root vegetables brings a new dimension to breakfast. The beauty of this recipe is its versatility. Use root vegetables that are in season, and mix and match them to create a colorful and hearty dish. You can serve this as an accompaniment or you can poach or fry eggs and put them on top of the hash to create a meal in itself. You can also add smoked salmon or pork belly for a protein boost. Pair the hash with a hoppy red ale to round out the flavors.

1 large onion
1 pound fingerling or Yukon Gold potatoes, finely diced
1 pound yams or sweet potatoes, finely diced
1 pound rutabagas or carrots, finely diced
1 pound turnips or parsnips, finely diced
3 garlic cloves, minced
1 teaspoon chopped fresh thyme leaves
1 teaspoon chopped fresh oregano or rosemary leaves
3 tablespoons extra-virgin olive oil
Salt and freshly ground black pepper

1 Preheat the oven to 400°F.

2 Finely dice half of the onion and thinly slice the other half. Combine the onion, potatoes, yams, rutabagas, turnips, garlic, thyme, oregano, and olive oil in a large mixing bowl; toss to coat the vegetables with the oil. Season with salt and pepper to taste.

3 Transfer the vegetable mixture to a baking sheet or a large glass baking dish. Roast for 30 to 40 minutes, stirring the vegetables every 5 to 10 minutes, until lightly browned around the edges and tender. Serve hot.

Makes 8 servings

PROFILE ★ **Ninkasi is the Sumerian goddess of beer,** and the brewery that now bears her name is blessed. Jamie Floyd and Nikos Ridge launched the brewery in 2006 in a German restaurant already outfitted with brewing equipment. The reception was swift and positive, and they soon found themselves in a building of their own, operating a 50-barrel brewhouse. Ninkasi has embraced hop-forward beers as well as some delightful malty brews that are always flavorful and sought after. Active in their community, and respected by their fellow brewers, the Ninkasi team is continuing good work in the goddess's name.

TALLGRASS BREWING COMPANY

MANHATTAN, KANSAS

Halcyon Chicken Breakfast Enchilada

This breakfast sticks to your ribs and sets you up right for the rest of the day. Creamy, spicy, and hearty, this recipe requires at least 1 hour of marinating time before cooking and serving. It pairs well with the beer used to marinate the chicken — an American wheat — because of its slightly sweet flavor that offsets the spicy pepper and tangy cheese.

CHICKEN AND MARINADE

- 1 cup Tallgrass Halcyon Wheat, or similar witbier
- ¼ cup extra-virgin olive oil
- 2 garlic cloves, minced
- 2 tablespoons chopped yellow onion
- 2 tablespoons chopped fresh chives
- 2 (5-ounce) boneless, skinless chicken breasts

SCRAMBLED EGGS

- 1 teaspoon butter
- 8 large eggs, whisked

SAUCE

- 2 tablespoons unsalted butter
- 2 tablespoons all-purpose flour
- 2 cups heavy cream
- 1 cup vegetable broth
- 6 ounces Swiss cheese, shredded (1½ cups)
- 4 ounces cream cheese, softened
- 1 teaspoon granulated garlic
- ¼ teaspoon salt
- ¼ teaspoon white pepper
- ½ teaspoon diced habañero pepper
- ½ cup Tallgrass Halcyon Wheat, or similar witbier

ENCHILADAS

- 4 large flour tortillas
- 8 ounces cheddar cheese, shredded (2 cups)
- 2 tablespoons chopped fresh chives

1 MARINATE THE CHICKEN: Combine the beer, olive oil, garlic, onion, and chives in a ziplock bag or airtight container. Add the chicken and refrigerate for at least 1 hour or as long as overnight.

2 Prepare a medium fire in a gas or charcoal grill. Remove the chicken from the marinade and discard the marinade. Grill the chicken until cooked through, about 12 minutes per side. The chicken can be cooked a day ahead and reserved in the refrigerator until you're ready to assemble the enchiladas.

3 SCRAMBLE THE EGGS: Melt the butter in a skillet over medium heat. Pour in the eggs and use a heatproof spatula to constantly scramble the eggs as they cook. The eggs are done when they are firm and lose their gloss, about 5 minutes.

4 MAKE THE SAUCE: Melt the butter in a medium saucepan over medium heat. Whisk in the flour to form a smooth paste and then cook for 2 minutes, whisking constantly. Add the cream and broth and whisk until incorporated, about 3 minutes, taking care not to let the sauce boil. Slowly add the Swiss cheese and cream cheese and whisk until blended. Add the garlic, salt, pepper, and habañero, and mix. Add the beer and stir until the foam subsides. Reduce the heat and simmer the sauce, stirring occasionally, while assembling the enchiladas.

5 ASSEMBLE THE ENCHILADAS: Warm the tortillas on a grill or in a microwave. Slice the chicken breast and place a few slices inside a tortilla. Top with one-quarter of the eggs and ½ cup of the cheddar. Roll up the tortilla and smother with the warm cheese sauce. Repeat with the remaining tortillas and filling. Top with the chives and serve immediately.

Makes 4 servings

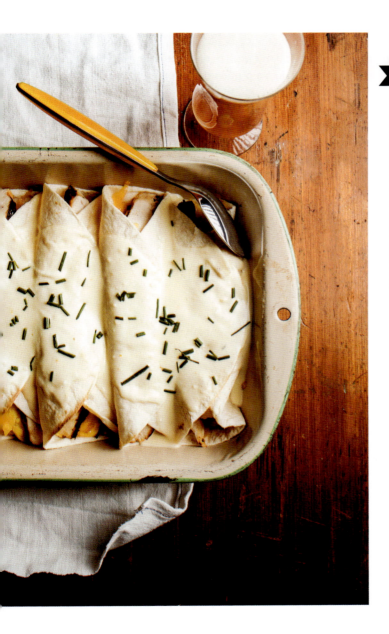

Before he was a brewer, Jeff Gill was a geologist, so it makes sense that he would have a good idea of how to locate ideal water sources for the beers made by his *Tallgrass Brewing Company*. Jeff and his wife, Tricia, chose Manhattan, Kansas, for the venture, not only for the water, but because it's a fine place to raise a family.

Using quality ingredients along with inventiveness, Tallgrass is a growing brewery, and one that has embraced canning as the preferred method for getting fresh beer to the people.

Corned Beef Hash

3 tablespoons unsalted butter

1 cup finely chopped yellow onion

3 cups finely chopped, cooked corned beef

3 cups finely chopped, cooked russet potatoes

Fresh Italian parsley, minced

Salt and freshly ground black pepper

The difference between good hash and bad hash is vast. There is rarely a middle ground. One way to ensure all the ingredients come together properly is to take your time. This is not a weekday preparation, but a weekend one; make it when minutes don't matter and the aromas can waft throughout the house, giving slowpokes a pleasant reason to wake. Another necessity for excellent hash is uniformly and finely chopped ingredients, which ensures proper mixing and thorough cooking. This is a simple recipe that doesn't weigh down the hash with a lot of ingredients, giving the salty, tender beef a chance to shine. Serve the hash with eggs prepared however you like them (poached or over-easy are classics) and a side of hot buttered toast. And skip the orange juice; this brunch dish goes well with an amber ale or dry Irish stout.

A Few Beers to Try with This Recipe

- *Bear Republic Red Rocket Ale*
- *Duck-Rabbit Amber Ale*
- *Flying Fish ESB Ale*
- *Fort Collins 1900 Amber*
- *Odell Red*
- *Rogue Ales American Amber Ale*
- *Ruth McGowan's Cloverdale Ale*
- *Widmer Brothers Drop Top Amber Ale*

1 Melt the butter on a griddle or in a large skillet over medium heat. Add the onion and cook, stirring occasionally, until soft and fragrant, 2 to 3 minutes.

2 Combine the corned beef and potatoes in a medium bowl, and then stir in the sautéed onions. Spread the mixture evenly on the hot griddle. Increase the heat to high and press down on the mixture with a spatula or kitchen weight. Do not stir the mixture; you want a nice brown crust to form. Cook for 3 to 5 minutes, taking care not to burn.

3 When the hash has browned, flip it over and brown it on the other side, again pressing down with the spatula or weight. Cook until the potatoes and corned beef are evenly browned, about 2 minutes longer.

4 Remove the hash from the heat and sprinkle with parsley. Season with salt and pepper to taste and serve immediately.

Makes 4–6 servings

PROFILE ★ **There is something soothing** about a comfortable pub, a place where friendships are formed with fellow customers and staff, where happy occasions are celebrated and losses mourned. *Ruth McGowan's* is that kind of place. Plus, it features a quality brewery, a solid kitchen, and a staff dedicated to the cause.

Mary Ann and Mike Brigham opened the brewpub on St. Patrick's Day 2002, naming it in honor of Mike's grandma, the feisty and stout-hearted Ruth McGowan. Looking around at the pub, you see couples catching up after a long workweek or students matching talents and wits at shuffleboard or darts. You see many pints of the brewery's Cloverdale Ale (with labels that cleverly highlight LOVE ALE) and other brews, and plates of good-looking (and good-tasting) food. One other thing that makes Ruth's special is the Irish music session nights, a gathering of musicians who collectively play tunes from the old country as well as more contemporary fare. Fiddle, mandolin, guitar, banjo, pipes, accordion, concertina, flute, and whistle players gather in the dining hall to perform, drink, and enjoy. Yes, this is a comfortable pub, and the folks of Sonoma County are lucky to have it.

Smoked Bologna Mousse on Chicken
Skin Crostini. see page 36

Appetizers

The Very Best of the Beginning

Gouda Fondue

While fondue was most popular in the 1960s and '70s, it is enjoying a resurgence as chefs and party hosts embrace the communal appeal of people standing around a bubbling pot of melted cheese. This two-cheese fondue blend gets its kick from the mustard powder and cayenne, while the addition of a lager soothes some of the heat. Have skewers and dipping options like bite-size pieces of apples, a grilled baguette, or fresh vegetables on hand. Drink a premium American lager with this rich dish.

10 ounces Full Sail Session Premium Lager, or similar American pale lager
½ garlic clove, minced
12 ounces smoked Gouda, rind removed and shredded (about 3 cups)
8 ounces Monterey Jack cheese, shredded (2 cups)
1 teaspoon Worcestershire sauce
⅛ teaspoon cayenne pepper
1½ teaspoons cornstarch
½ teaspoon dry mustard powder
1 tablespoon water
⅛ teaspoon freshly ground black pepper
Sliced apples, fresh vegetables, and crusty artisanal bread, for dipping

A Few Beers to Try with This Recipe

- *Avery Joe's Premium American Pilsner*
- *Bell's Lager of the Lakes*
- *Full Sail Session Premium Lager*
- *Pretty Things American Darling*
- *Shmaltz Coney Island Sword Swallower*

1 In a fondue or similar pot, combine the beer and garlic and bring to a simmer. Gradually add the Gouda and Monterey Jack cheese, stirring constantly to evenly distribute. Bring the mixture to a gentle simmer, stirring until all the cheese is melted and the fondue is smooth. Stir in the Worcestershire and cayenne.

2 Whisk the cornstarch, mustard powder, and water together in a small bowl to make a slurry. Stir the slurry into the cheese mixture and continue to cook at a low simmer, uncovered, for 20 minutes to let the flavors develop.

3 Stir in the pepper, taste, and season with additional black pepper and cayenne as needed. Transfer to a fondue pot or serving bowl and serve with a platter of accoutrements.

Makes 4–6 servings

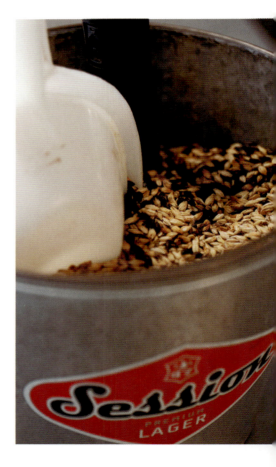

Nestled inside the scenic town of Hood River, *Full Sail Brewing Company* does craft beer the right way. That is to say, it releases beers that use quality ingredients and are full of flavor, and its staff has some fun doing it. The brewery, which opened in 1987, stands in what was once a cannery and is employee owned. The 47 employees each have a financial stake in the business and keep things running smoothly to ensure that their beer gets into customers' eager hands.

Full Sail releases a bevy of brews that include award-winning beers like Session Premium Lager, Session Black Lager, and the holiday Session Fest, and a full range of styles, from the heavenly, sinful Black Gold (an imperial stout aged in bourbon barrels) to the hearty Wassail, a winter warmer. The location in Oregon gives the brewery team access to a variety of locally grown hops, and they use them well. Proponents of local and independently owned businesses, they regularly host events that showcase the best of what they love.

Slow-Cooked Doppelbock BBQ Meatballs

- 2 cups Sprecher Doppel Bock, or similar doppelbock
- 1 cup ketchup
- ½ cup Sprecher Root Beer BBQ Sauce
- ¼ cup brown sugar
- 2 tablespoons red wine vinegar
- ¼ teaspoon garlic powder
- ¼ teaspoon salt
- ¼ teaspoon freshly ground black pepper
- 3 pounds frozen cocktail meatballs

Just like the old saying "set it and forget it," this is an easy recipe that lets a slow cooker do all the work for you. Combine the ingredients and return to the slow cooker a few hours later to a wonderful aroma and ready-to-serve bites. The recipe calls for Sprecher Root Beer BBQ sauce (available through the brewery's website, or feel free to substitute another pop-inspired sauce), and it does make all the difference in flavor. The recipe yields a lot of meatballs, so it's a great choice for a large gathering.

1 Combine the beer, ketchup, barbecue sauce, brown sugar, vinegar, garlic powder, salt, and pepper in a slow cooker. Add the meatballs and stir gently to make sure they are covered with the sauce (add more beer if necessary).

2 Cover the slow cooker and cook on low heat for 6 to 8 hours. Halfway through the cooking time, check to see if you need to add more beer.

3 Serve the meatballs on a large platter with toothpicks for picking them up. Place the extra sauce in a small bowl for dipping.

Makes about 20 cocktail servings

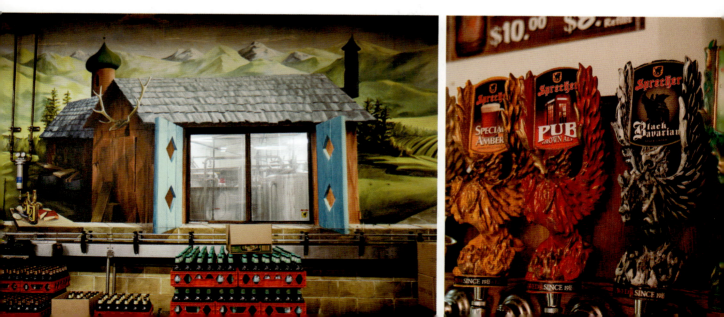

Randal (Randy) Sprecher worked as a brewing supervisor for the once-proud Pabst Brewing Company — a staple of Milwaukee's storied brewing past. In 1985, he struck out on his own, opening a brewery and soda company in his own name, and helped usher in a new generation of microbreweries. Visit **Sprecher** today and you'll see decades of hard work and great skill in action. Relax in the brewery's comfortable tasting room, try the full lineup of beers and sodas, and then pick up some cheese and sausage from the fridge in the gift shop to round out the full Wisconsin experience. In addition to its well-crafted beers, Sprecher also produces a line of gourmet sodas packed with real flavor, interesting combinations, and just the right amount of sweetness. Early on, Randy saw the need to have locally owned breweries in the city he loves, and today, Sprecher Brewing is among the top attractions for beer lovers. It has continued the proud tradition Milwaukee has enjoyed for generations.

Bourbon Sweet Potato Tarts
with Imperial Stout Sauce

TARTS
- 3 large sweet potatoes
- 4 tablespoons unsalted butter
- 3 tablespoons dark brown sugar
- 1 teaspoon orange zest
- 2 tablespoons fresh orange juice
- 1 egg
- ¼ cup heavy cream
- ½ teaspoon ground cinnamon
- ½ teaspoon ground allspice
- ¼ teaspoon ground nutmeg
- 1 teaspoon bourbon (optional)
- 30 small phyllo cups or tartlet shells

TOPPING
- ½ cup chopped pecans
- 2 tablespoons dark brown sugar
- 1 tablespoon all-purpose flour
- 2 tablespoons unsalted butter, melted

SAUCE
- ¼ cup maple syrup
- ¼ cup dark brown sugar
- ¼ cup Oakshire Hellshire II, or similar imperial stout aged in bourbon barrels

These tarts could almost be a dessert, but why should you wait to get through several courses to taste this multiflavored treat? Perfect as an appetizer, this recipe can also be used as a side dish to pork loin dishes, ham, or turkey. The sauce calls for a generous pour of a Russian imperial stout aged in bourbon barrels. In recent years, American brewers have taken to aging beer in barrels no longer needed by distilleries. (Charred oak barrels can be used only once for bourbon, according to tradition.) Strong stouts are a popular choice for this treatment because their higher alcohol content stands up to the wood and bourbon flavors absorbed by the beer. There are not many reasons to use a quality bourbon stout for anything other than drinking, but this recipe is one of them.

1 Preheat the oven to 400°F.

2 Place the sweet potatoes in a 9- by 13-inch glass baking dish and bake for 45 minutes to 1 hour, or until soft when pricked with a fork. Remove the potatoes from the oven to cool slightly and reduce the temperature to 300°F.

3 MAKE THE TOPPING: When the potatoes are nearly done, mix the pecans, brown sugar, and flour in a small bowl, and then drizzle with the melted butter. Stir to combine and set aside.

4 MAKE THE SAUCE: Bring the maple syrup, brown sugar, and beer to a simmer in a small saucepan, and then continue to simmer the sauce, uncovered, until reduced by half.

5 ASSEMBLE THE TARTS: Peel the potatoes while hot and mash the flesh in a bowl with the butter, brown sugar, orange zest, orange juice, egg, cream, cinnamon, allspice, nutmeg, and bourbon, if using. Stir to combine well.

6 Arrange the empty phyllo cups on a baking sheet and fill each with a few tablespoons of potato mixture. Sprinkle each tart with the topping. Bake the tarts for 15 minutes.

7 Drizzle the tarts with the sauce and serve immediately.

Makes 30 small tarts

Hard against the train yard in Eugene is *Oakshire Brewing*. It's a production facility that even without a restaurant has embraced pairing its beers with excellent food. This recipe came from brewmaster Matt Van Wyk, who perfected it with practice. The brewery's three year-round beers are found only in the Pacific Northwest and Alaska — a lucky break for residents, but bad news for the rest of us.

Founded by brothers Jeff and Chris Althouse in 2006, the brewery enjoys a reputation for releasing flavorful beers, and those who make the beer are not afraid to speak their minds. Van Wyk, for example, has been leading the charge in recent years against the term "India black ale" or "black IPA" in favor of "Cascadian dark ale." His passionate arguments have won over a lot of people who enjoy this new style and want to call it by a deserving name. Stop by Oakshire's tasting room at the brewery to try their beers for yourself. There's also a newly opened public house for full pints, and you can grab some great meals from the food trucks that set up shop outside.

A Few Beers to Try with This Recipe

- *Deschutes Abyss*
- *FiftyFifty Eclipse*
- *Firestone Walker Barrel Aged Velvet Merkin*
- *Full Sail Bourbon Barrel Aged Imperrial Stout*
- *Goose Island Bourbon County Stout*
- *Great Crescent Bourbon's Barrel Stout*

Pork Belly Corn Dogs with Truffle Mustard

The creative geniuses at Dogfish have helped to turn the beer world on its head, so it should come as no surprise that they take carnival fare as humble, tired, and ubiquitous as the corn dog and turn it into a culinary wonder. This is a recipe done in stages and one that requires overnight preparation; I suggest reading all the way through before starting. The corn dogs are well worth the effort, though; put them out and you'll attract a line of hungry fans as long as the line for the best Ferris wheel.

CORN DOGS

- 5 pounds pork belly, skin removed
  Wooden skewers
- 2 cups all-purpose flour
- ⅔ cup yellow cornmeal
- ¼ cup sugar
- 1½ teaspoons baking powder
- ½ teaspoon baking soda
  Pinch of salt
- 1 egg, beaten
- 1¼ cups buttermilk
- 2 tablespoons clover honey
  Vegetable oil, for frying (1 gallon if using a large heavy pot or to recommended fat level if using a deep fryer)
  Truffle mustard, for serving (recipe follows)

TRUFFLE MUSTARD

- 1 yellow onion, roughly chopped
- ½ cup red wine vinegar
- 1½ cups Dijon mustard
- 1 cup soybean or vegetable oil
- 2 tablespoons truffle oil
  Salt and freshly ground black pepper

1 Preheat the oven to 300°F.

2 Cut the pork belly into pieces about 5 inches long by 2 inches wide (corn dog size). Place the belly in a roasting pan, cover with aluminum foil, and bake for 4 hours, or until most of the fat is rendered. Remove the pan from the oven carefully as it will be full of melted fat.

3 Carefully remove the pork belly from the pan, place flat on a plate, cover with plastic wrap, and refrigerate overnight. Reserve 2 tablespoons of the rendered fat, covered, at room temperature.

4 **MAKE THE MUSTARD:** Combine the onion, vinegar, and mustard in a blender and blend until smooth.

5 Slowly add the soybean oil to emulsify, and then add the truffle oil. Season with salt and pepper to taste. Serve immediately or store in a sealed container for up to 4 days.

6 **MAKE THE CORN DOGS:** Skewer each piece of chilled pork belly.

7 To make the batter, combine 1 cup of the flour with the cornmeal, sugar, baking powder, baking soda, and salt in a mixing bowl. Combine the egg, buttermilk, honey, and reserved pork belly fat in a separate bowl and blend well. (If the fat has congealed, heat it in the microwave in short bursts to liquefy before adding it to the bowl.) Make a well in the middle of the dry ingredients and add the wet ingredients; whisk to incorporate.

8 Heat the oil to 350°F in a deep fryer or large pot. Put the remaining 1 cup flour in a shallow dish.

9 Dredge each piece of pork belly first in flour and then in corn batter. Deep-fry until golden brown, 4 to 5 minutes. Drain the corn dogs on a paper towel–lined plate to absorb excess grease. Serve the corn dogs immediately with truffle mustard for dipping.

Makes 10 corn dogs and 1 quart of mustard

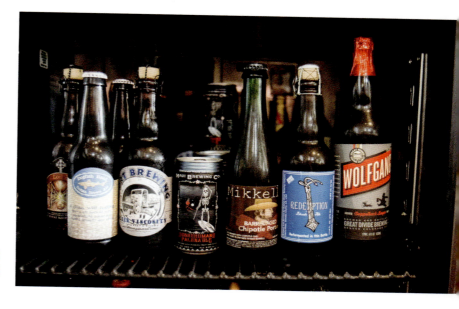

PROFILE ★ **The wizards of wonder,** the brave brewers of ***Dogfish Head***, have changed the way many people think about beer and taught their fans that no ingredient is too obscure, strange, or rare to put into a brew. Led by founder Sam Calagione, the inspired team of free-thinking brewers, chefs, and other employees has gained a loyal — even rabid — following from all areas of beer geekdom. Thanks to their beers like India Brown Ale and 90 Minute IPA (and sister beers 60 Minute and 120 Minute), they have introduced many people to aggressively hoppy beer. They have also given a much-needed boost to the East Coast, which gets trounced by the West Coast when it comes to hop usage.

Dogfish Head releases a dizzying array of beers with clever and quirky labels. Recently the brewery has partnered with musicians and record labels to pay homage to musical greats like Miles Davis and Pearl Jam. Many of their exploits and methods were featured on a Discovery Channel show called *Brew Masters*, but to get the true feeling of what this "off-centered" brewery is all about, head to the company headquarters in Delaware. They are the brewery with the tree house in the front yard.

Fried Green Tomatoes with Sun-Dried Tomato Ale Mustard

A staple of Southern cuisine, fried green tomatoes get a new twist from some spice and a generous beer bath. Prepare the mustard the day before you make the tomatoes; the overnight storage is important to help the flavors blend. Enjoy with a red ale; the malty sweetness will combat some of the spice.

MUSTARD

- ½ cup sun-dried tomatoes, thinly sliced
- 1 cup red ale
- 1 tablespoon puréed chipotle in adobo
- 3 cloves roasted garlic (see recipe on page 234 for roasting instructions)
- 1 cup grainy mustard
- ⅓ cup Dijon mustard
- 1 teaspoon cider vinegar

TOMATOES

- Vegetable oil, for frying
- 1 cup cornstarch
- ½ cup yellow cornmeal
- ½ cup all-purpose flour
- 1½ teaspoons baking powder
- 1 teaspoon kosher salt
- ½ teaspoon cayenne pepper
- 2 cups triple ale
- 4 green tomatoes, cut into ¼-inch slices

1 MAKE THE MUSTARD: The day before you want to serve the tomatoes, soak the sun-dried tomatoes in an airtight container with the red ale and chipotle pepper for at least 3 hours or up to overnight. Drain the liquid and place the tomatoes in the bowl of a food processor; add the garlic, grainy mustard, Dijon, and cider vinegar. Process until just combined. Do not blend until smooth; you want to see solid flecks of tomato. Transfer to a serving dish.

2 MAKE THE TOMATOES: Heat the oil in a deep fryer or large pot to 350°F. Mix the cornstarch, cornmeal, flour, baking powder, salt, and cayenne in a shallow bowl; whisk to combine. Slowly add the ale to the dry mixture, whisking until smooth.

3 Dredge each tomato slice in the batter until well coated. Deep-fry the tomato slices until golden brown, 2 to 4 minutes. Drain on a paper towel–lined plate and serve hot with the mustard.

Makes 4 servings

PROFILE ★ **Craft beer has struggled to take root** in the South, where other beverages and offerings from larger breweries traditionally dominated the scene. That is now changing, as seen, in part, by brewers like *Below the Radar*, a brewpub in Huntsville that is focusing on hearty, stick-to-your-ribs fare with a modern flair and small-batch beers (many aged in oak barrels that once held wine, rum, or whiskey). It also boasts an impressive 32-tap lineup of guest beers, offering some of the best the country and the world have to offer.

Hopocalypse Ceviche

DRAKE'S BREWING

SAN LEANDRO, CALIFORNIA

The spiciness of the habañero marries beautifully with the hops of Hopocalypse, a big chewy double IPA. The bright citrus hop notes in the ale also play very well with the lime juice and blood orange in the ceviche.

½ cup Drake's Hopocalypse, or similar double IPA
1 cup freshly squeezed lime juice
2 garlic cloves, minced
Salt
2 pounds whitefish (snapper, bass, cod are favorites), diced into ½-inch cubes
2 avocados, peeled, pitted, and diced
1 small red onion, diced and rinsed
1 medium habañero pepper, ribs removed and minced (optional but recommended)
½ cup cilantro leaves, chopped
1 tablespoon ground coriander
½ cup blood orange segments
Tortilla chips, for serving

1 Whisk together the Hopocalypse, lime juice, garlic, and salt to taste in a small bowl. Put the fish in a shallow dish and pour in the marinade. Cover and let marinate for 2 hours.

2 Fold the avocado, onion, habañero, cilantro, and coriander into the fish mixture. Mix gently until combined. Season with additional salt to taste.

3 Garnish the ceviche with orange segments, and serve with crispy tortilla chips.

Makes 4–6 servings

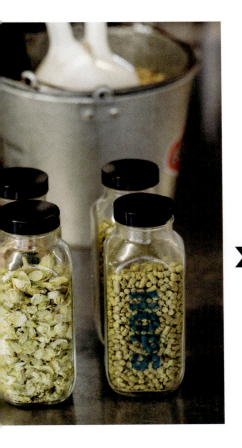

PROFILE ★ **Perfectly at home** in what was once a powerhouse for a construction equipment facility, *Drake's* is a California institution. They have been making and serving beers since 1989 and set an early tone for what is taken for granted today: extreme beers. They don't do anything small, as demonstrated by their high-ABV brews, strong use of hops, and delightfully deep barrel-aging program. The original owner and brewer, Roger Lind, used to deliver beer himself and is credited with bringing good beer to the market and inspiring others to do the same. Today, the Drake's tasting room is a place to fill up on favorites and try experimental brews. One of the great taprooms, it's worth a special visit.

Loose Cannon Wings

This is a great take on a traditional pub favorite. The citrus hop presence from the Loose Cannon (or similar India pale ale) blends nicely with the fruit juice in the marinade, giving great flavor to the wings without the mess associated with a sticky sauce. Grilling the wings is also healthier than deep-frying, meaning you can have a few more than usual without any guilt.

- ¼ cup kosher salt
- ¼ cup packed light brown sugar
- 1 tablespoon Southwest seasoning or cayenne pepper
- 1 teaspoon red pepper flakes
- 1 cup water
- ⅓ cup orange juice
- ¼ cup lemon juice
- 1 tablespoon lime juice
- ½ cup chopped yellow onion
- 1 lime, thinly sliced
- ¼ cup roughly chopped fresh cilantro leaves
- 1 tablespoon minced garlic
- 1 (12-ounce) bottle Heavy Seas Loose Cannon IPA, or similar beer
- 2½ pounds chicken wings
  Olive oil
  Ranch dressing, for serving (optional)

1 Combine the salt, brown sugar, Southwest seasoning, pepper flakes, water, orange juice, lemon juice, and lime juice in a large ziplock bag; close the bag and shake until the salt and sugar are completely dissolved. Add the onion, lime slices, cilantro, garlic, and beer and shake to combine and degas the beer.

2 Add the chicken wings to the bag and shake the bag so that the wings are submerged. Refrigerate for at least 8 hours and up to 12 hours.

3 Remove the wings from the refrigerator and discard the brining solution. Pat the wings dry with paper towels and set aside to come to room temperature, about 30 minutes.

4 Prepare a low fire in a gas or charcoal grill. Brush the wings with olive oil to prevent sticking. Grill until golden brown, 3 to 5 minutes per side. Serve the wings hot with a side of ranch dressing, if using.

Makes 6–8 servings

It was a circumnavigated route that led to *Heavy Seas*, a brewery based in Maryland but with a reach well beyond the state's borders. Captained by Hugh Sisson, a man who has been part of the beer business for most of his career, Heavy Seas Beer is brewed by Clipper City Brewing Company. Sisson first came to prominence as a brewer in the late 1980s, when he founded Maryland's first brewpub, Sisson's. It was an immediate hit, and a few years later, Hugh moved to the production end of things with Clipper City.

Heavy Seas reflects a commitment to modern brewing methods combined with tradition and history. The brewery bottle-conditions its beers, meaning yeast lives in bottles or casks, naturally fermenting the beers while they are waiting to be consumed. Bottle conditioning also adds depth of flavor to beers. A brewery committed to the importance of food and beer, Heavy Seas hosts several events throughout the year that promote worthy pairings.

Saison Vos Mussels

Mussels love beer, and these mollusks that play an important role in Belgian cuisine especially love Belgian-style beer — in this case a saison. Pair with a side of fries or crusty bread and a tall glass of saison for a quick and easy meal.

SLY FOX BREWING COMPANY

PHOENIXVILLE, PENNSYLVANIA

1 pound fresh mussels, cleaned
1 tablespoon extra-virgin olive oil
3 small shallots, diced
2 garlic cloves, chopped
1 cup Sly Fox Saison Vos, or similar saison
2 tablespoons unsalted butter
2 tablespoons minced fresh parsley
Salt and freshly ground black pepper

1 Rinse the mussels well in cold water, making sure they are still alive: tap the shells of any open mussels; if they don't close, they are dead and should be discarded.

2 Heat the olive oil in a large skillet over medium-high heat. Add the shallots and garlic and sauté until translucent; do not let the mixture brown. Reduce the heat to medium, pour in the beer, and bring to a simmer. Add the mussels, cover, and simmer for 5 to 7 minutes, or until all the mussels have opened. Take care not to overcook. Discard mussels that do not open.

3 Turn off the heat, add the butter and parsley, and stir thoroughly. Season to taste with salt and pepper. Transfer the mussels and all the juices to a serving dish and enjoy hot.

Makes 1–2 servings

PROFILE ★ **Having one packaging line** is difficult for many, but the folks at *Sly Fox* package their beers in traditional 12-ounce cans — including a line with removable lids — kegs for draft accounts, and even special 750 ml cage-and-cork bottles. This is par for the course for this Pennsylvania-based beer institution. The company was founded in December 1995 by the Giannopoulos family. Things were going along just fine until Brian O'Reilly arrived in the spring of 2002. He quickly developed an off-premises sales program to gain Sly Fox beers a place on the taps at some of Philadelphia's best bars and taverns. Things exploded from there, and they show no signs of slowing down. One event not to miss is the annual Bock Fest & Goat Race on the first Sunday of May, which draws crowds of 4,000 or more every year.

American Wheat Beer Steamed Clams

2 pounds clams
4 tablespoons unsalted butter
1 small white onion, chopped
1 garlic clove, minced
1 sprig fresh thyme
2 cups American wheat beer
1 tablespoon chopped fresh parsley

Clam Tips: Fresh clams can be found at your local seafood store or grocer. Look for those packed on ice. I prefer littleneck clams, as they are ridiculously easy to prepare. The beauty of the jet age is that fresh seafood is available in practically every part of the country, meaning you do not have to be near saltwater to enjoy this great summer treat.

IMPORTANT: Clams that do not open after being steamed for a few minutes should be thrown away.

A Few Beers to Try with This Recipe

- *Harpoon UFO*
- *Pyramid Haywire Hefeweizen*
- *Southern Tier Hop Sun*
- *Three Floyds Gumballhead*

The beauty of this recipe is the simplicity. To steam clams, you need a liquid, so why not beer? With this preparation, I considered several styles but ultimately settled on unfiltered American wheat beer with a nice balance between the yeast and malt. Unlike German hefeweizens, American wheat beers do not have banana and clove notes, but they do tend to have a bit more citrus behind them. For me, that worked better with the flavor and seasoning of the clams.

1 Scrub the clams under cold running water to remove any sand or dirt.

2 Melt 2 tablespoons of the butter in a large pot over medium heat. Add the onion and sauté, stirring occasionally, until it turns translucent, about 3 minutes. Add the garlic and sauté 1 minute longer. Add the thyme and beer and bring to a simmer.

3 Add the clams, cover, and steam until the clams open, 5 to 10 minutes. Transfer the clams to a serving bowl with a slotted spoon.

4 Add the remaining 2 tablespoons butter to the broth and add the parsley. Stir until the butter is melted. Transfer the sauce to a smaller bowl and serve as a dipping sauce with the clams.

Makes 2–4 servings

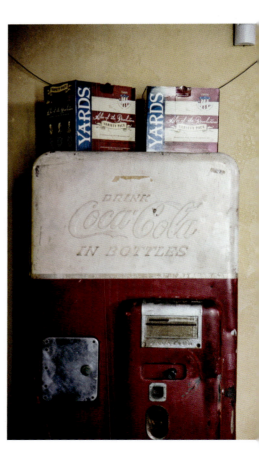

Hummus

Hummus is incredibly easy to make at home. The creamy and protein-rich snack is also something of a blank canvas; it's fine on its own but feel free to improve it with any number of ingredients such as chopped olives, minced garlic, roasted red peppers, pesto, pine nuts, or anything else that suits your taste buds. Enjoy with toasted pita chips or julienned vegetables, or use it as a sandwich spread. A malty maibock makes a wonderful companion.

OTTER CREEK BREWING

MIDDLEBURY, VERMONT

1 (15.5-ounce) can chickpeas, drained
¼ cup extra-virgin olive oil, plus more for seasoning
¼ cup freshly squeezed lemon juice
¼ cup tahini (sesame paste)
Garlic salt

1 Combine the chickpeas, olive oil, lemon juice, and tahini in the bowl of a food processor and blend until smooth. Season with garlic salt and additional oil as needed to achieve the desired flavor and consistency.

2 Transfer the hummus to a bowl, and serve immediately with desired accompaniments or refrigerate in an airtight container for up to 4 days.

Makes 2 cups

A Few Beers to Try with This Recipe

- *Capital Maibock*
- *Narragansett Bock*
- *Otter Creek Spring Bock*
- *Ramstein Maibock*
- *Rogue Deadguy*
- *Sierra Nevada Glissade*

PROFILE ★ **In March 1991, Otter Creek** brewed its first Copper Ale. Based on strong sales, the brewery moved to a larger facility with a 60,000-barrel capacity a few years later. Known for its solid and easy-drinking beers, Otter Creek now ships beers to 15 states. The brewery works with local farmers to source as many local brewing ingredients as possible and in return makes spent grain available to farms as a valuable feed supplement for dairy cattle. It also donates spent hops and yeast to local farmers to use as fertilizer.

TRÖEGS BREWING COMPANY

HERSHEY, PENNSYLVANIA

Smoked Bologna Mousse on Chicken Skin Crostini

2 pounds chicken skin
Vegetable oil, for deep frying
Salt and freshly ground black pepper
1 pound thickly sliced smoked bologna, rind removed, roughly chopped
¾ cup mayonnaise
½ cup coarse mustard
½ cup sour cream
1 shallot, minced
¼ cup cold water
10 sweet pickles, thinly sliced

A Few Beers to Try with This Recipe

- *Capital Autumnal Fire*
- *Fort Collins Doppelbock*
- *Schlafly Doppelbock*
- *Sprecher Doppel Bock*
- *Tröegs Troegenator Double Bock*

Chicken skin as a cracker? Yes! The crispy skin adds flavor and texture to an already tasty mousse. Sure, it might not be the healthiest thing, but everything in moderation. Chicken skins are easy to obtain — save skin from another recipe or just ask your butcher. This requires some advance preparation, so plan ahead. Everything comes together quickly when you're ready to serve. Consider pairing this dish with a doppelbock (like Tröegs' Troegenator), as the malt character complements the strength of the mousse.

1 Lay the chicken skin on a baking sheet, stretching it as far as possible so it stays flat. Refrigerate overnight, uncovered.

2 Cut the chicken skin into 4-inch squares with a paring knife. Pour 4 inches of oil into a deep skillet or chef's pan and heat to 350°F. Working in batches, fry the chicken skin until crispy, 20 to 30 seconds. Transfer the chicken skin to a paper towel–lined plate, season with salt and pepper to taste, and allow to cool slightly.

3 Combine the bologna, mayonnaise, mustard, sour cream, shallot, and water in the bowl of a food processor. Process until fully incorporated into a mousse. Season with salt and pepper to taste.

4 Pipe or spoon the mousse onto the crispy chicken skin pieces. Garnish with a sliver of sweet pickle and serve.

Makes about 2 dozen crostini

Grown brothers John and Chris Trogner were living apart but found common inspiration in beer, and that led them to open a brewery that has thrived, grown, and earned a loyal following. John Trogner was working in real estate in Philadelphia and found himself frequenting the nearby Dock Street brewpub to escape the realities of the job. Younger brother Chris had moved to Colorado to experience the skiing scene and soon found himself enamored with the state's rich beer culture. For years, the siblings talked about launching a business together and then found their calling in the fermenting sciences.

John headed to Colorado and worked at a brewery washing kegs and doing the things one must do to learn every aspect of the trade. Chris focused on marketing and business development. Soon, they were back in Pennsylvania, and in 1997 they opened *Tröegs*. First located in Harrisburg, they recently moved to a larger, modern, and thoroughly impressive location in Hershey. Their well-executed beers such as Nugget Nectar, Java Head Stout, and Sunshine Pils have earned them dedicated customers and numerous awards. With its offerings now available in the mid-Atlantic states, the brewery is expanding its footprint and is no doubt inspiring new generations of brewers to take up the cause.

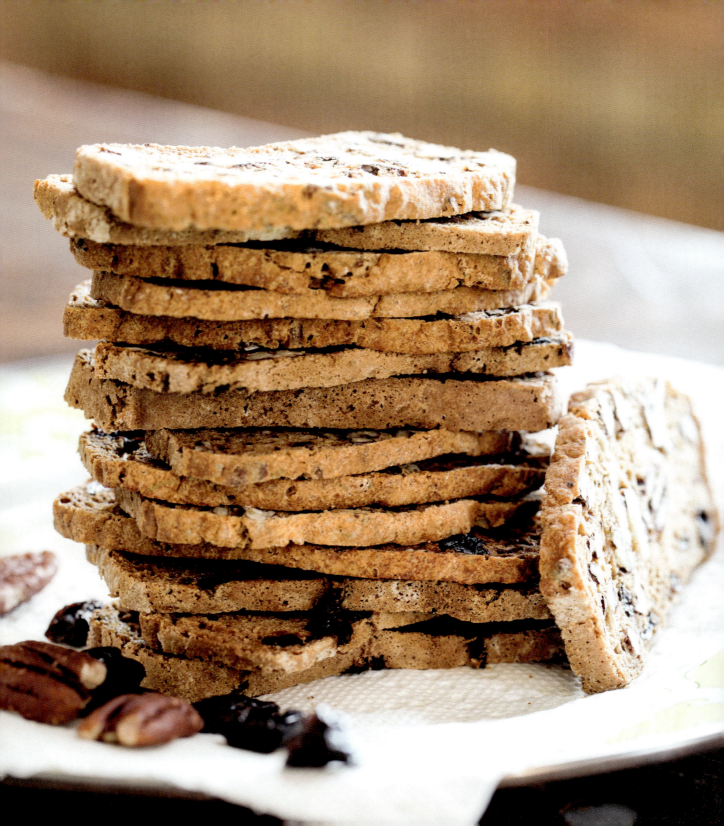

Gluten-Free Fruit and Nut Crisps

For those with a gluten sensitivity, crunchy game-day snacks can be hard to come by. This recipe, paired with a gluten-free beer to wash it down, has you covered. Lakefront makes a gluten-free beer called New Grist that is widely available. More gluten-free beer options are coming onto the market each month. Check with your local store for selections.

Gluten-free flour, for dusting pans

2 cups gluten-free all-purpose baking mix (brands such as Bisquick, King Arthur, and Arrowhead Mills all offer gluten-free options)

⅓ cup dark brown sugar

1½ teaspoons baking soda

1¼ teaspoons salt

2 cups buttermilk

1½ cups chopped walnuts and/or pecans

1 cup dried cranberries or dried cherries

1 tablespoon chopped fresh rosemary leaves

2 teaspoons xanthan gum

1 Preheat the oven to 350°F. Grease two 4- by 8-inch loaf pans, dust them with gluten-free flour, and line them with parchment paper. Now grease and flour the parchment paper, removing any excess flour by inverting the pans and patting them gently over the sink.

2 In a medium mixing bowl, combine the baking mix, sugar, baking soda, and salt, and stir well. Add the buttermilk and mix well. Add the nuts, dried cranberries, and rosemary. Add the xanthan gum and stir briskly.

3 Divide the batter evenly between the prepared baking pans and bake for about 45 minutes, or until golden brown. Cool the pans on a rack for 10 to 15 minutes, then invert the loaves onto the rack and let cool to room temperature.

4 Wrap the loaves in plastic wrap and freeze until firm, about 30 minutes.

5 Preheat the oven to 300°F and remove the loaves from the freezer. Slice the loaves into ¼-inch (or thinner) slices. Lay the slices on baking sheets and bake for 15 to 20 minutes, flipping once, until the crisps are a honey brown color.

6 Let the crisps cool completely on a rack before serving. Store in an airtight container for up to a week.

Makes about 48 crisps

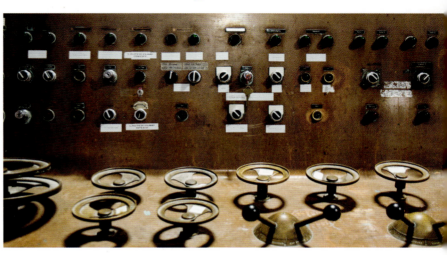

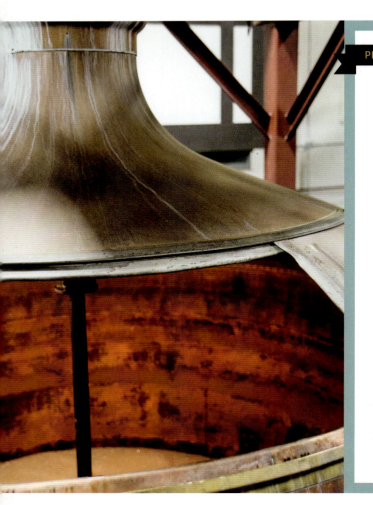

Milwaukee is a city with a proud brewing tradition. Giant brands like Schlitz, Miller, and Pabst built empires and raised generations on their beers. Today, with the landscape changing and many large breweries now memories, Milwaukee is home to a number of craft breweries that have raised the beer bar, perhaps none more than *Lakefront*, a brewery founded by the Klisch brothers in 1987.

Lakefront has grown considerably since it opened and continues to produce a solid line of beers that run the gamut of flavors and styles. It distributes to multiple states, but a visit to the brewery proves the commitment that Lakefront has to its city, heritage, and environment. Housed in what was once the Milwaukee Electric Railway and Light Co. coal-fired power plant, the brewery is forward-thinking on environmental issues — as highlighted on the tour — and with its hospitality. The tour is only one of a handful in the country that has a bar midway through to let thirsty visitors fill up (it's also where Bernie Brewer's Chalet is housed, a treat for baseball fans). The tour ends with crowds singing the theme from *Laverne and Shirley*, a nice kitschy touch and a nod toward local pop culture. Visit on a Friday for the traditional fish fry in the large Palm Garden. It's one of the great experiences in today's craft beer world.

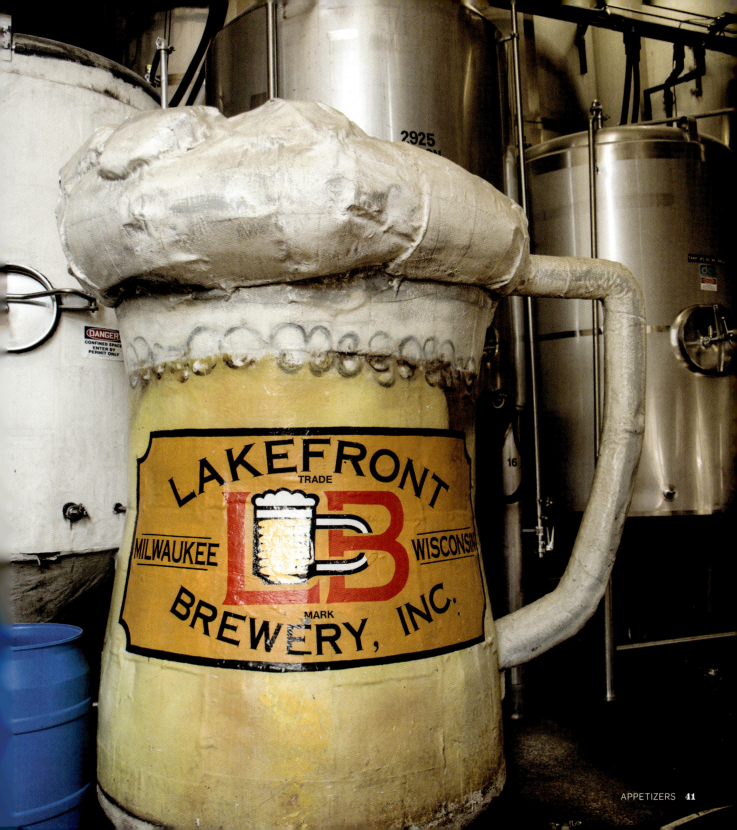

Chicken Wings with Bacon Barbecue Sauce

1 cup roughly chopped
   applewood-smoked bacon
12 large chicken wings
2 tablespoons extra-virgin
   olive oil
¼ cup diced yellow onion
¼ cup dark brown sugar
1 cup New Albanian Bob's Old
   15-B Porter, or similar
   robust porter
1 tablespoon unsalted butter
2 cups veal or beef broth
½ cup Worcestershire sauce
1 tablespoon puréed chipotle
   in adobo
1 teaspoon dried oregano
1 teaspoon dried thyme
¼ teaspoon garlic powder

Note: This recipe yields a bit of extra sauce. Leftover sauce is great on burgers, with other grilled meats, or as a dip for bread. Or simply make a double batch of wings!

This recipe combines two wonderful things — bacon jam and barbecue sauce — and liberally spreads the mixture on that trusty pub standby, the chicken wing. This is a versatile recipe that can be used on a variety of smoked or barbecued meats; it even works well with escargots. Chef Matt Weirich also suggests replacing the chicken wings with duck wings. Lager is the common accompaniment, but try pairing these wings with a robust porter; the slightly burnt, smoky notes from the malts bring an extra level of flavor to the bacon and chipotle.

1 Preheat the oven to 400°F. Put the bacon in a heavy skillet and cook it in the oven until crispy. Transfer the bacon to a paper towel–lined plate, reserving the fat in the skillet. Reduce the oven temperature to 350°F and move the skillet to the stovetop.

2 Toss the chicken wings in the olive oil, arrange them on a baking sheet, and bake for 1 hour, or until crisp and cooked through.

3 Add the onion to the bacon fat in the skillet and cook over medium-high heat, stirring occasionally, until golden brown, 5 to 7 minutes. Be careful handling the skillet; it will still be hot from the oven.

4 Add the brown sugar to the skillet and cook over medium heat, stirring occasionally, until it dissolves. Add the beer, scraping the bottom of the skillet with a spatula to loosen any brown bits. Stir in the butter and simmer until the liquid is reduced by half, stirring occasionally.

5 After the beer has reduced, add the broth to the skillet and reduce until the jam is thick, stirring occasionally and being careful not to burn it, 10 to 20 minutes.

6 Add the Worcestershire, chipotle, oregano, thyme, and garlic powder to the skillet and stir to fully incorporate.

7 Transfer the sauce and bacon to a blender, let cool for 8 to 10 minutes, and then purée until smooth. Remove the chicken wings from the oven, place them in a large bowl, and pour in enough sauce to liberally coat the chicken. Serve immediately.

Makes 12 wings and plenty of leftover sauce

A Few Beers to Try with This Recipe

- *Avery New World Porter*
- *Bell's Porter*
- *Deschutes Black Butte Porter*
- *Great Lakes Edmund Fitzgerald Porter*
- *New Albanian Bob's Old 15-B Porter*
- *Sierra Nevada Porter*
- *Smuttynose Robust Porter*

PROFILE ★

With two locations in a renaissance city across the Ohio River from Louisville, the ***New Albanian Brewing Company*** has become a beacon of great beer in what is firmly whiskey country. Over the years, they have been blessed with talented brewers who create beer concoctions that keep people coming back for more. Spearheaded by the uncompromising and passionate Roger A. Baylor, New Albanian Brewing Company is a brewery that encourages conversations on all the taboo topics — sex, politics, and religion included. At times, tables can seem more like *The McLaughlin Group* than a local pub, but that's all part of the charm. There is simply not enough space to say all that is good about NABC. It is best experienced in person.

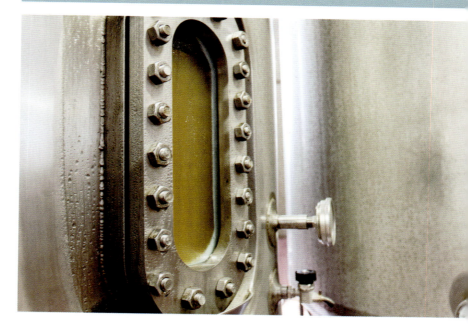

Spent-Grain Beer Bread

Finding spent grain is not terribly hard. All breweries (and many homebrewers) have it in spades, and most are willing to either give it away or sell it for a nominal fee. Nutrient-rich and flavorful, spent grain is hearty and adds weight to this bread, making it perfect for light toasting and eating with a slather of rich butter.

¾ cup warm water
2 tablespoons active dry yeast
¾ cup whole milk
¼ cup unsalted butter
4½ tablespoons sugar
1 tablespoon salt
1 cup sweet apple juice
¼ cup molasses
1½ cups spent grain
1 cup whole wheat flour
4–5 cups all-purpose flour
Vegetable oil, to coat bowl
Cornmeal
1 egg, lightly beaten

1 Pour the warm water into a small mixing bowl, sprinkle the yeast on top, and let dissolve. Set aside.

2 Combine the milk and butter in a medium saucepan over medium-low heat and cook until the butter melts. Remove the saucepan from the heat and whisk in the sugar, salt, apple juice, and molasses. Pour the mixture into a large bowl.

3 When the yeast mixture is foamy, combine it with the milk mixture. Add the spent grain, reserving 2 tablespoons, and the whole wheat flour to the bowl.

4 Start to mix the dough, gradually adding the all-purpose flour until the dough is workable and does not stick to your hands. Knead for several minutes.

5 When the dough is no longer sticking to your hands, transfer it to a large bowl coated with oil and let it rise until doubled in size, 30 to 60 minutes.

6 Line a baking sheet with parchment paper and sprinkle it with cornmeal.

7 Punch the dough back down to its original size. Separate the dough into 2 loaves and transfer the loaves to the prepared baking sheet. Use a pastry brush to brush the loaves with egg wash and then sprinkle with the reserved spent grain. Let the bread rise until almost doubled in size.

8 Meanwhile, preheat the oven to 325°F. Bake the loaves for 45 minutes, or until golden brown and a toothpick inserted in the middle comes out clean. Cool slightly, then slice and serve.

Makes 2 loaves

A sanctuary in the mountains of northern New Hampshire, ***Woodstock Inn Station & Brewery*** welcomes visitors and locals to its attached restaurant and hotel with perfect hospitality and charm. The train depot from a neighboring town was moved and incorporated onto the inn building, and other rooms at the lodge once served as cabins for hikers passing through. Recent renovations have left the brewery better than ever. Thanks to area skiing, great views for leaf peeping, hiking, and swimming, Woodstock is a year-round destination. Several times a year, the brewery hosts weekends where guests can get the full brewing experience and work with the brewer on a seven-barrel system. It's a fun vacation that any beer lover will appreciate.

Belgian Endive with Gruyère and Prosciutto

3½ cups water
¾ cup Weyerbacher Merry Monks, or similar golden Belgian ale
2 tablespoons apple cider vinegar
1 teaspoon salt, plus more for seasoning
6 heads Belgian white endive
Freshly ground black pepper
4 ounces sliced Gruyère, cut into 12 strips
6 slices prosciutto or similar dry ham, cut in half lengthwise

This relatively simple recipe will impress your guests with its harder-than-it-looks presentation. For this recipe, a Belgian-style abbey tripel comes in handy and keeps a theme of national unity. Belgian endive is called "white gold" by natives, who use the tangy, leafy vegetable in just about everything from soup to entrées. In this recipe, it provides a fresh, crisp base for the rich ham and cheese.

1 Preheat the oven to 400°F.

2 Bring the water, beer, vinegar, and salt to a simmer in a medium pot. Add the whole endive and simmer until just tender, 4 to 6 minutes. Drain the endive, allow to cool slightly, and then cut each head in half lengthwise. Season with salt and pepper to taste.

3 Lay a strip of cheese over the cut side of each endive half, and then wrap a slice of prosciutto around the endive and place it in a medium baking dish. You will have 12 wrapped endive bundles.

4 Bake the wrapped endive for about 10 minutes, or until the cheese melts and the ham is crispy on top. Serve warm.

Makes 6 servings

A Few Beers to Try with This Recipe

- *Boulevard Long Strange Tripel*
- *Captain Lawrence Xtra Gold*
- *Flying Fish Exit 4*
- *New Belgium Trippel Belgian Style Ale*
- *Victory Golden Monkey*
- *Weyerbacher Merry Monks*

PROFILE ★ **When Dan and Sue Weirback** opened their brewery in 1997, they decided to go back to the traditional spelling of the family name: *Weyerbacher* (pronounced why-er-bock-er). After first brewing mainstream recipes, Dan found his stride making big beers. Customers looking for something different in the local market responded enthusiastically and more beers followed; each new addition was flavorful, strong, and well made. Consider their oak-barrel-aged barley wine, imperial pumpkin ale, or robust stouts, each worth your time and attention. Now closing in on 20 years in the business, Weyerbacher is available in many states on the East Coast, and the brewery has grown in size and reputation. That's welcome news for those who appreciate big beers.

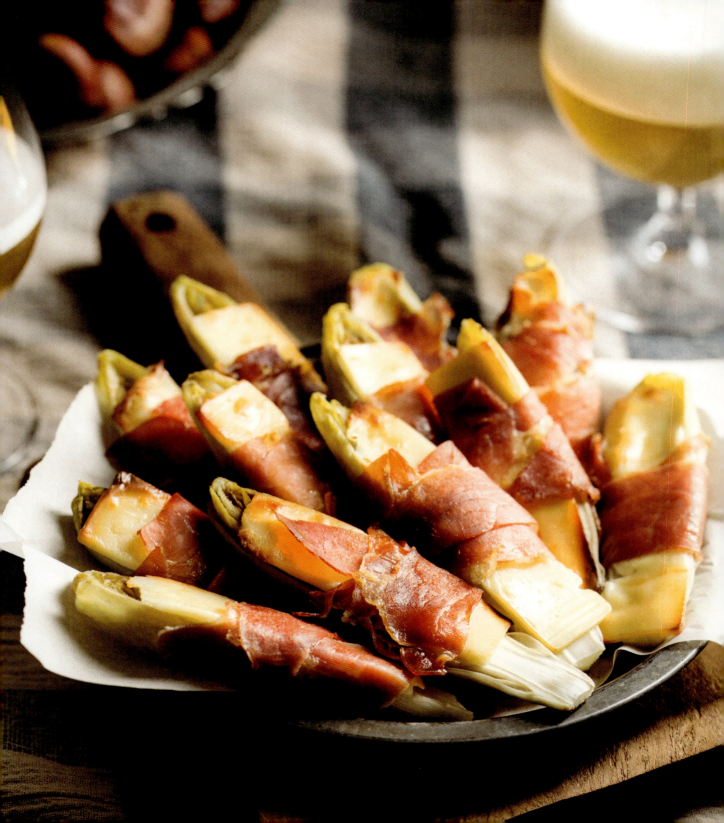

1½ cups sour cream
1 cup marinated artichoke hearts, drained and roughly chopped
3 tablespoons shredded Asiago cheese, plus additional for serving
1 garlic clove, minced
½ teaspoon ground celery seed
½ teaspoon ground white pepper
2 cups mayonnaise
½ teaspoon dried thyme
½ teaspoon cayenne pepper
Chopped scallions, for serving

Artichoke Dip

Creamy and satisfying, this dip is popular at restaurants all over the country, but it's also simple to make at home and is great with toasted pita chips, tortilla chips, or vegetables for dipping. A red lager makes a wonderful accompaniment.

1 Preheat the oven to 350°F.

2 Combine the sour cream, artichokes, cheese, garlic, celery seed, and white pepper in a medium bowl and stir to combine. Add the mayonnaise, thyme, and cayenne, and blend well. Continue to stir the mixture until all ingredients are incorporated.

3 Transfer the dip to a small oven-proof dish suitable for serving and bake for 20 to 25 minutes, or until an instant-read thermometer inserted into the center of the dish reads 140°F. Garnish with shredded Asiago and scallions, and serve warm.

Makes 4½ cups

PROFILE ★ **With the right combination of upscale and comfort,** *Upstream Brewing Company* has focused on giving guests the best possible experience since opening in 1996. With two locations in the Omaha area, the focus is on local food (like the beef Nebraska is known for) and quality pints. As an after-dinner bonus, both locations have rooms with pool tables to get the muscles moving and keep the good times going.

Roasted Bone Marrow

GALENA BREWING COMPANY

GALENA, ILLINOIS

Nutrient-rich bone marrow is too often overlooked, but after a short time in a hot oven, it emerges as a savory, buttery beef spread. Go easy on the seasoning, and make sure you have good crusty bread or crostini on hand for serving. This simple recipe is big on flavor, and after just one taste, it's sure to become a favorite. Pair with a slightly spicy rye-infused ale or lager that sports bready characteristics.

8–12 center-cut beef or veal
  marrow bones, cut into
  2½- to 3-inch pieces
Kosher salt and freshly
  ground black pepper
French baguette, thinly
  sliced and lightly toasted
Extra-virgin olive oil, for
  drizzling (optional)

1 Preheat the oven to 400°F.

2 Place the bones, cut side up, in an oven-proof skillet and season with salt and pepper to taste. Bake for 20 to 25 minutes, or until the centers are soft and the marrow begins to separate from the bone.

3 Remove the bones from the oven. Use a small spoon to remove the marrow from the center of the bones and spread it on crostini. Sprinkle with additional salt or a drizzle of olive oil, if desired.

Makes 4 servings

PROFILE ★ **On the far end of the main drag in Galena,** the brewery sits inside a comfortable but cavernous space. It is a wonderful addition to this artisan-friendly tourist town a short drive from the banks of the Mississippi River. With strong offerings from the kitchen and quaffable pints, this brewery is helping to educate beer drinkers on the versatility and approachability of craft beer. On any given day, there are busloads of visitors who have never experienced a craft beer. With the pub's open layout, they can see firsthand how the beer is made (the brewing system is fully visible behind the bar) while tasting whatever is on offer. For history buffs, *Galena Brewing* has a wall of brewery memorabilia, from old bottles and labels to other interesting items. Warren and Kathy Bell have created a beer destination in this quaint town, and visitors are wealthier because of it.

Soft Rye Pretzels

see photo, **page 66**

1½ cups warm water, 85–90°F
15 grams sugar
20 grams active dry yeast
420 grams bread flour
115 grams rye flour
85 grams barley flour
20 grams kosher salt
65 grams unsalted butter, melted
    Vegetable oil, for oiling bowl
12 cups plus 1 tablespoon water
⅔ cup baking soda
1 egg yolk
    Sea salt

A Few Beers to Try with This Recipe

BRITISH IPAS

- *Berkshire Lost Sailor IPA*
- *Brooklyn East India Pale Ale*
- *Left Hand 400 Pound Monkey*
- *Middle Ages ImPaled Ale*

VIENNA LAGERS

- *Blue Point Toasted Lager*
- *Devils Backbone Vienna Lager*
- *Great Lakes Eliot Ness*
- *Trapp Vienna Lager*

This style of pretzel is soft, dense, and chewy. Best enjoyed fresh and warm right out of the oven, these treats are better than any ballpark variety, and the touch of rye gives the dough a pleasant spice kick. Serve with mustard, the Gouda Fondue on page 22, or the Bavarian Cheese Spread on page 74. Pair these beauties with either a British IPA or a Vienna lager.

1 Combine the water, sugar, and yeast in a small bowl. Mix gently and let rest until the yeast begins to foam.

2 Combine the bread flour, rye flour, barley flour, and salt in the bowl of a stand mixer fitted with a dough hook. When the yeast mixture is foamy, slowly add it and the butter to the flour mixture with the mixer on slow speed, and mix until just combined, about 20 seconds. Turn off the mixer and let the dough rest for 20 minutes.

3 Mix the dough on slow speed for 1 minute, and then increase the speed to medium and mix for 2 minutes longer, or until the dough forms a ball and pulls cleanly away from the sides of the bowl.

4 Remove the dough from the bowl and knead it on a lightly floured work surface for 2 minutes. Put the dough into an oiled bowl, cover with a moist towel, and let rise in a warm place until doubled in size, 60 to 90 minutes.

5 Preheat the oven to 450°F. Portion the dough into 12 equal pieces. Roll each piece into a 20-inch-long rope of even diameter. Fold the rope into the pretzel knot shape and press the dough together firmly where it intersects at the twist and the ends.

6 Bring 12 cups water and the baking soda to a boil in a large pot. Working in batches of 3 or 4, depending on the size of your pot, slowly lower each pretzel into the boiling water and cook for 30 to 45 seconds, pushing down and re-submerging the pretzels with a slotted spoon as needed. Transfer the pretzels to a wire rack to dry.

7 When all the pretzels are boiled, arrange them on large baking sheets lined with parchment paper and bake for 6 minutes.

8 Meanwhile, whisk the 1 tablespoon water and the egg yolk together in a small bowl. Remove the pretzels from the oven and brush with the egg wash. Sprinkle with salt and bake for 8 to 10 minutes longer, or until dark brown. Serve warm. The pretzels will keep for about a day unwrapped, but not overnight. Wrapping in plastic will melt the salt and distort the crust.

Makes 12 pretzels

So strong is its commitment to serving locally made food that ***Bull City Burger and Brewery*** lists on its menu the items not made on-site: soda and ketchup. Everything else is made in-house, from the burgers to the sauerkraut. The brewery works with local farmers, cares about the environment (and proves it through green initiatives), and makes some of the best pints in a town already known for good beer. In short, Bull City Burger and Brewery is everything a hamburger joint should be.

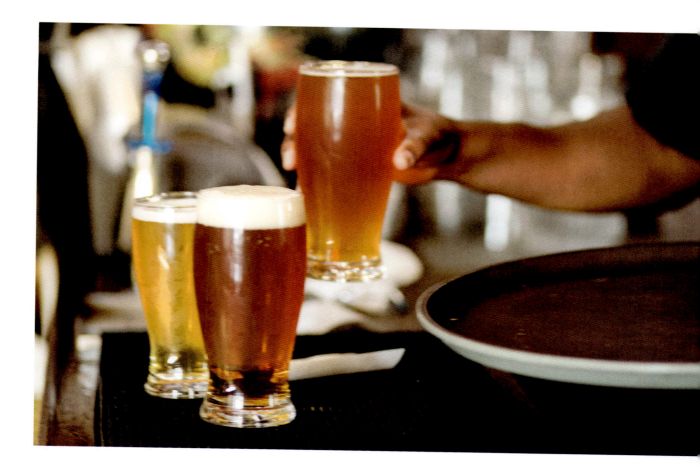

Sardines on Toast with Romesco Sauce and Pickled Onions

Forget those little fish that come in cans or on a pizza. Real sardines are larger and more flavorful than their oil-soaked counterparts. This recipe brings the fish, a punch of spice from the sauce, and a pucker from the pickled onions together into a joyous mosaic of flavor that will make you forget the tinned-variety sardine forever. While this recipe requires a bit of advance preparation, the wide-eyed look of wonder from your guests will be thanks enough.

PICKLED ONIONS
- 1 medium red onion, sliced into ⅛-inch rings on a mandolin or with a sharp knife
- 1 tablespoon salt
- ½ teaspoon black peppercorns
- 2 cups red wine vinegar
- ¾ cup sugar
- ¾ cup water

CROSTINI
- 1 baguette, cut on a bias into 12 ¼-inch slices (process the remainder of the baguette into breadcrumbs for the romesco sauce)
  Extra-virgin olive oil

ROMESCO SAUCE
- 1 ancho chile
- 1 plum tomato, chopped
- ¼ cup diced yellow onion
- 1 garlic clove
- 4 tablespoons extra-virgin olive oil
- ¼ cup breadcrumbs
- ¼ cup peeled almonds
- 1 tablespoon sherry vinegar
- ½ teaspoon chili powder
- ½ teaspoon paprika
  Salt and freshly ground black pepper

SARDINES
- 6 fresh sardines
- ¼ cup extra-virgin olive oil
- 1 tablespoon sea salt
  Freshly ground black pepper

1 MAKE THE PICKLED ONIONS: Place the red onion in a heatproof bowl. Combine the salt, peppercorns, vinegar, sugar, and water in a small saucepan and bring to a boil. Boil until the sugar has dissolved, and then pour the hot pickling liquid over the raw onion. Cover and refrigerate for at least 3 hours before serving.

2 MAKE THE CROSTINI: Preheat the oven to 350°F. Brush each baguette slice with olive oil and arrange the slices on a baking sheet. Bake for 6 minutes, or until toasted and crispy.

3 MAKE THE ROMESCO: Raise the oven temperature to 400°F. Place the ancho chile in a medium heatproof bowl. Bring 1 quart of water to a boil and pour over the chile. Let stand for 10 minutes, and then drain and set the chile aside.

4 Toss the tomato, yellow onion, and garlic with 2 tablespoons of the olive oil in a small bowl. Transfer the mixture to a baking sheet and roast for 10 minutes, or until the vegetables develop a slight char. Leave the oven on.

5 Heat the remaining 2 tablespoons olive oil in a medium skillet over medium heat. Add the breadcrumbs and almonds and sauté until lightly toasted.

6 Combine the ancho chile, the tomato mixture, the almond mixture, and the sherry vinegar, chili powder, and paprika in a blender and purée until smooth. Season to taste with salt and pepper.

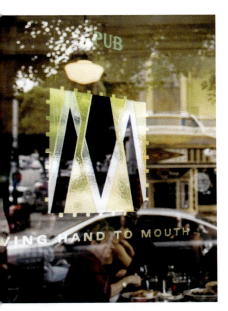

7 **MAKE THE SARDINES:** Using the back of a boning knife, scrape the skin of the sardines to remove the scales. To filet each fish, use your boning knife to cut against the bones of the fish, removing the flesh from the spine. After removing the filets from the carcasses, clean off any remaining blood and bones from the filets and cut each one down the middle, creating 12 pieces.

8 Place the sardines on a baking sheet, drizzle with the olive oil, and lightly season with salt and pepper. Roast for 3 minutes.

9 **ASSEMBLE THE TOASTS:** Spoon about 1 tablespoon of romesco onto each crostini, making sure the crostini are completely covered with sauce.

10 As soon as the sardines come out of the oven, place one piece on top of each sauced crostini and sprinkle with a pinch of sea salt. Garnish each toast with a few slices of picked onion and serve.

Makes 12 crostini

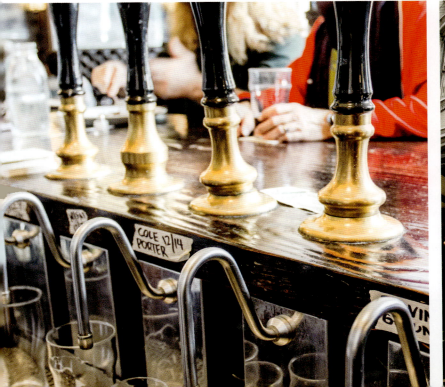

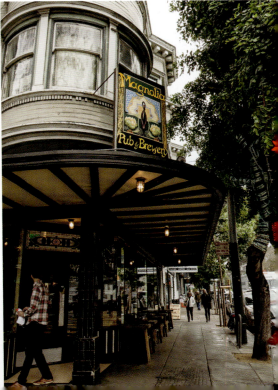

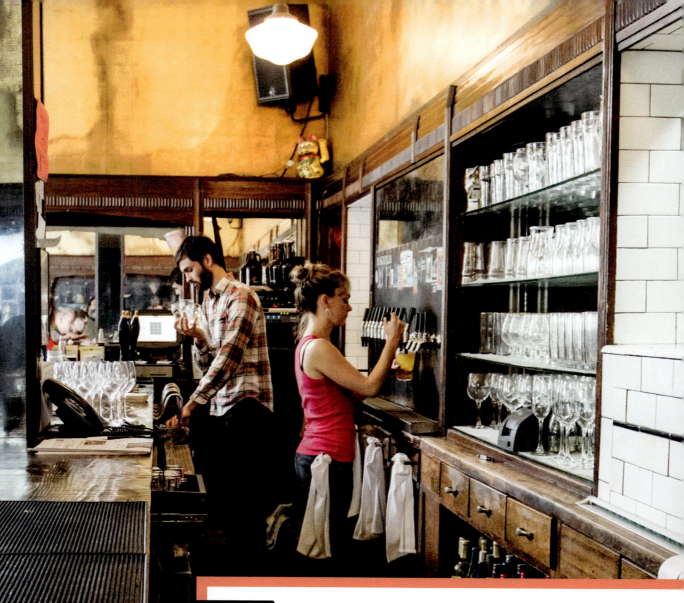

Steak and Blue Cheese Tartare

There is something carnal about eating raw meat and experiencing its natural flavors. Bison, with its tender texture and meaty taste, takes on new dimensions when served tartare. Combine it with the bold flavors of truffles, blue cheese, and hot sauce in just the right proportions and they collaborate to create a great dish. The crunch of a kettle chip seals the deal. Pair this appetizer with a Belgian pale ale, a beer that marries the sensibilities and tradition of Belgian brewing with the ingenuity of American hop usage.

5 ounces bison sirloin, finely diced

¼ teaspoon finely chopped black truffle

1 egg yolk

4 drops Worcestershire sauce

1 teaspoon lemon juice

1 teaspoon Dijon mustard

1 teaspoon finely chopped parsley

½ ounce blue cheese, crumbled

Salt and freshly ground black pepper

4 handfuls kettle-cooked potato chips

½ teaspoon hot sauce

1 Mix the bison, black truffle, egg yolk, Worcestershire, lemon juice, mustard, and parsley together in a large mixing bowl until well combined. Fold in the blue cheese until incorporated. Season to taste with salt and pepper.

2 Arrange the chips in a single layer on a plate and place bite-size spoonfuls of the tartare on each chip. Drizzle with the hot sauce and serve immediately.

Makes 4–6 servings

A Few Beers to Try with This Recipe

- *Bayou Teche LA-31 Bière Pâle*
- *Brewery Ommegang BPA*
- *Captain Lawrence Liquid Gold*
- *Coast The Belafonte*
- *The Lost Abbey Devotion Ale*

PROFILE ★ **For those who appreciate good beer,** Belgium is a special and sacred place. So too is a Belgian brewery that opened in the late 1990s in upstate New York near the Baseball Hall of Fame. **Brewery Ommegang** was founded by Wendy Littlefield and Don Fernberg in 1997 and is now owned by Duvel Moortgat, a company that specializes in Belgian beers. (They also own the Duvel and Brasserie d'Achouffe brands.) As such, the company has access to the traditions and know-how of some of the world's best brewers. Ommegang's solid lineup of beers is released in cage- and cork-finished bottles and runs the gamut of flavors and styles. The brewery is also home to a must-attend festival each summer: Belgium Comes to Cooperstown, a celebration of great beer, live music, and camaraderie.

Barcade's Pickled Hop Shoots

2 pounds hop shoots
2 cups water
2 cups rice wine vinegar
⅔ cup sugar
⅓ cup coarse salt
4 garlic cloves
2 bay leaves
2½ teaspoons black peppercorns
2 teaspoons coriander seeds
1 teaspoon mustard seeds
1 teaspoon red pepper flakes
4 allspice seeds
¼ star anise

If you can get hop shoots — the season generally falls near the end of March — please be sure they have not been treated with herbicides or other chemicals. Hop shoots resemble young asparagus; they should be firm and about half the width of a pencil, with the leaves of the head bundled tightly together. Since their season is so short, pickling is a popular means of preserving hops. You can also eat them fresh with acidic or light creamy sauces, freshwater fish, and poultry. Be careful not to overcook them, as long cooking times will destroy their tender flavor. A quick poach in salted and sugared water or a light sauté works best. These hops make great finger food right out of the jar, or add a small pile to a cheese or charcuterie tasting.

1 Wash and sterilize two pint-size canning jars. Wash the hop shoots, dry them with a paper towel, and trim to fit inside the jars.

2 Bring the water, vinegar, sugar, and salt to a simmer over medium-high heat in a medium saucepan. Continue to simmer, stirring occasionally, until the sugar and salt are completely dissolved.

3 Meanwhile, fill a large pot with enough water to cover your canning jars by at least 2 inches and bring to a boil. Divide the garlic cloves, bay leaves, peppercorns, coriander seeds, mustard seeds, pepper flakes, allspice seeds, and star anise between the jars. Add the hop shoots to the jars, positioning them upright for appearances' sake.

4 Divide the brine between the jars, leaving ¼ inch of head-space between the top of the liquid and the top of the jars. Tap the jars to remove any air bubbles. Wipe the rims with a clean moist cloth, and put two-piece canning lids on the jars. Using canning tongs, place the jars in the boiling water, making sure that they are covered by at least 2 inches of water, return to a boil, and process for 10 minutes.

5 Transfer the jars to racks and allow to cool completely. When they have cooled, check to be sure that the lids are firmly in place. Sealed jars will keep for up to 1 year.

Makes 2 pint-size jars

Beer and video games? Yes please. *Barcade* is a bar for adults who love craft beer but are still kids at heart. Jersey City, New Jersey, is the second location for co-owners Paul Kermizian and Kevin Beard, following a successful (and continuing) run in Brooklyn. A Philadelphia location is also in the mix with plans for a Manhattan outpost in the works. Featuring nearly 25 taps of nothing but American craft brews and old-school video games like Tapper, Ms. Pac-Man, Double Dragon, Mappy, Burger Time, and about 35 others (for just 25 cents per play), the bar has become a popular neighborhood hangout and destination for many in the nearby suburbs.

Pork and Porter Hand Pie

Not long ago the *Washington Post* called hand pies "the next big thing in treats." Whereas cupcakes are smaller versions of cakes, hand pies are smaller versions of pies. They can be sweet or savory, as this recipe from Fullsteam Brewery's spin-off bakery, Bullytown, demonstrates. Hand pies are perfect for parties, for snacks, or simply as an original centerpiece for a light meal. Drink with a porter or brown ale to complement the dark beer used in the filling, or contrast it with a hoppy India pale ale.

CRUST

- 2 cups all-purpose flour
- ½ cup fine-ground cornmeal
- 1 teaspoon coarse salt
- 1 cup (2 sticks) cold unsalted butter, cut into ½-inch pieces
- ¼ cup ice water

FILLING

- ½ tablespoon extra-virgin olive oil
- 1 cup finely chopped yellow onion
- 2 medium garlic cloves, finely chopped
- ½ pound ground pork
- ½ pound ground pork sausage
- 3 Granny Smith apples, peeled, cored, and cut into 1-inch cubes
- 2 medium sweet potatoes, peeled and cut into 1-inch cubes
- ½ cup porter or smoked porter
- 1 teaspoon finely chopped fresh sage leaves
- 1 teaspoon finely chopped fresh thyme leaves
- Coarse salt and freshly ground black pepper
- 1 egg, lightly beaten

1 **MAKE THE CRUST:** Sift the flour, cornmeal, and salt into a medium bowl. Using two knives, cut in the butter until the mixture forms pea-size coarse crumbs. Slowly add the ice water and combine the ingredients with your hands until the dough forms a ball. Avoid overkneading the dough. Shape the dough into a 1-inch-thick disk, wrap tightly in plastic wrap, and refrigerate until firm, at least 1 hour or up to 2 days.

2 **MAKE THE FILLING:** Heat the olive oil in a large skillet over medium-high heat. Add the onion and cook, stirring occasionally, until soft, 3 to 4 minutes. Add the garlic and cook for 1 minute longer. Add the ground pork and pork sausage and cook, breaking the meat up with a wooden spoon, until the pork is no longer pink, 3 to 5 minutes.

3 Add the apples, sweet potatoes, porter, sage, and thyme to the skillet. Cover and cook until the sweet potatoes and apples are nearly tender, about 15 minutes. Season with salt and pepper to taste. Transfer the pork filling into a medium bowl, and place in the refrigerator to cool slightly until you're ready to fill the dough.

4 **ASSEMBLE THE PIE:** Divide the dough in half. On a lightly floured work surface, roll out one half of the dough to ⅛-inch thickness. With a knife or biscuit cutter, cut out eight 5-inch circles (rerolling the dough if necessary). Transfer the circles to a baking sheet lined with parchment paper. Repeat the process with the remaining dough, this time cutting out eight slightly larger 5¼-inch rounds. Chill the rounds on baking sheets for 1 hour, or until ready to use.

5 Preheat the oven to 450°F. Place a heaping ¹/₃ cup of the filling in the center of each smaller round of dough, leaving a ¹/₂-inch border around the edges. Brush the edges with the beaten egg and press a larger round of dough over the top of each pie, using your fingers to firmly seal the edges.

6 Crimp the edges of the dough with the tines of a fork and cut three small air vents in the top of each hand pie. Brush the hand pie tops with the beaten egg. Bake the hand pies, rotating the baking sheet halfway through, for 20 to 25 minutes, or until golden brown and bubbling. Serve warm.

Makes 8 pies

Chicken Satay with Peanut Sauce

There is a certain joy in eating meat on a stick. Maybe it's evolutionary instinct from our cave-dwelling ancestors or nostalgia for childhood foods. This recipe is simple to make, tasty, and most of all fun to eat. Pair with a fruit beer that complements the peanut and the sweet and salty spices. Note that the sauce is best served at room temperature.

CHICKEN

- 6 skinless, boneless chicken breasts
- ½ cup soy sauce
- ½ cup vegetable oil
- 6 tablespoons curry powder
- ¼ cup sugar

SAUCE

- 2 cups plain yogurt
- 1¾ cups creamy peanut butter
- 3 tablespoons ground ginger
- 3½ tablespoons soy sauce
- 3½ tablespoons lemon juice

A Few Beers to Try with This Recipe

- *Brown's Cherry Raspberry Ale*
- *Kuhnhenn Tenacious Cassis*
- *New Glarus Raspberry Tart*
- *Samuel Adams Cherry Wheat*
- *Short's The Soft Parade*
- *21st Amendment Hell or High Watermelon*
- *Vermont Forbidden Fruit*

1 **MAKE THE CHICKEN:** Slice each chicken breast into 4 strips. Thread the strips onto 10-inch skewers, using 2 strips per skewer and "pleating" the strips over and under the skewer.

2 Combine the soy sauce, vegetable oil, curry powder, and sugar in a shallow dish, and whisk to incorporate. Place the chicken skewers in the marinade, cover, and refrigerate for 4 to 5 hours.

3 **MAKE THE SAUCE:** Whisk the yogurt, peanut butter, ginger, soy sauce, and lemon juice together in a medium mixing bowl until incorporated. Refrigerate until 1 hour before serving.

4 Prepare a medium fire on a gas or charcoal grill. Remove the chicken from the marinade, discard the marinade, and grill the chicken skewers for 5 to 7 minutes. Cut into one to check for doneness. Do not overcook the chicken; the thin strips of meat will dry out quickly.

5 Serve hot with the dipping sauce on the side.

Makes 12 skewers

PROFILE ★ **There are many reasons** the *Vermont Pub & Brewery* sits at the top of so many best-of lists. There is the beer and food, of course, and the comfortable, welcoming atmosphere, and the inventiveness of the brewers and chefs. There is also a certain passion and pride that comes from the brewery, and that can be traced to Greg Noonan. He founded the brewery in 1988 after lobbying the state to grant pubs the right to brew for the first time since Prohibition. His dedication was firm, and although he has since passed away, he lives on in the memories of the brewers he inspired and in the ideas he promoted.

Frickles

MAD FOX BREWING COMPANY

FALLS CHURCH, VIRGINIA

Spicy and crunchy, yet still juicy, fried pickle slices are easy to make and the result is an irresistible nibble that disappears quickly at parties. If you do not have a deep fryer at home, you can use a Dutch oven or deep pot and an instant-read thermometer to heat the oil. If you start with whole pickles, you can achieve perfect slices by using a mandoline. While great by themselves, frickles are also delicious dipped in ranch or Thousand Island dressing, a spicy Thai sauce, or a tangy barbecue sauce. Pair with a crisp Kölsch (Mad Fox makes a world-class version) to round out the experience.

Vegetable oil, for frying
3 cups all-purpose flour
1 tablespoon garlic powder
1 tablespoon onion powder
1 tablespoon paprika
1 tablespoon freshly ground black pepper
1½ teaspoons dried oregano
1 teaspoon cayenne pepper
2 cups buttermilk
1 pound dill pickles, sliced into ¼-inch rounds

1 Heat the frying oil to 350°F in a deep fryer or large pot.

2 Combine the flour, garlic powder, onion powder, paprika, black pepper, oregano, and cayenne in a large mixing bowl. Pour the buttermilk into a separate bowl.

3 Coat the pickles with the flour, then dip them into the buttermilk, and then back into the flour mixture. (Use one hand for the flour and the other hand for the buttermilk to keep the flour from "caking" on your hand.)

4 Shake off any excess flour from the pickles and fry them in small batches until golden, 1 minute. Transfer the pickles to a paper towel–lined plate using a slotted spoon and drain any excess oil on the paper towels before serving. Repeat with the remaining pickles.

PROFILE ★ **There are beer and food experiences** and then there are *beer food experiences*. **Mad Fox** falls into the second category, the one where you want to exclaim out loud about how nearly flawless everything is, from the soup to the pints. The brewery's seasonal menu is a locavore's delight, and the beers — crafted by the respected and talented Bill Madden — are a pleasure to drink. Sitting down to a meal at Mad Fox leaves just one question: what to order. Here's a hint: there are no wrong answers.

Grebble with Sunflower Seed Pesto

Fried dough has different names in different cultures. In Germany, it's called grebble, and it is delicious. Gella's Diner and Lb. Brewing Co. offers pesto for dipping grebble (it's also great as a pasta sauce). In fact, this pesto is so popular that customers at the brewery order it to go by the quart. Luckily you only have to travel as far as your kitchen. Pair this snack with an IPA; the hop punch stands up well to the basil's herbaceous bite.

PESTO

- 2 cups fresh basil leaves
- 1 cup sunflower seeds
- ½ cup fresh parsley leaves
- ½ cup fresh spinach leaves
- 4 garlic cloves
- 1 tablespoon salt
- ½ teaspoon white pepper
- 2 cups extra-virgin olive oil

GREBBLE

- 1½ cups warm water, between 85 and 95°F
- 1½ teaspoons active dry yeast
- 4 cups all-purpose flour
- 1 teaspoon salt
  Vegetable oil, for frying

Note: Leftover pesto is great on pasta and vegetables or as a sandwich spread.

A Few Beers to Try with This Recipe

- *Bell's Two Hearted Ale*
- *Coast HopArt IPA*
- *Dogfish Head 60 Minute IPA*
- *Firestone Walker Union Jack IPA*
- *Foothills Hoppyum IPA*
- *Lagunitas IPA*
- *Odell IPA*
- *Sierra Nevada Torpedo*
- *Wynkoop Mile HIPA*

1 MAKE THE PESTO: Combine the basil, sunflower seeds, parsley, spinach, garlic, salt, and pepper in a blender, and pulse 10 times to chop and combine the ingredients. Slowly add the olive oil with the motor running, and blend until fully incorporated. Cover and refrigerate the pesto.

2 MAKE THE DOUGH: Pour the warm water into the bowl of a stand mixer, sprinkle with the yeast, and let rest for 10 minutes to proof.

3 Add the flour and salt to the bowl and mix for 3 minutes on medium speed with the dough hook. Alternatively, mix and knead the dough by hand. Cover the bowl with plastic wrap and let rest for 20 minutes.

4 Mix or knead the dough by hand again on a lightly floured work surface. Let ferment for 2 hours in a clean oiled bowl covered with plastic or a damp cloth.

5 Roll the dough out to ¼-inch thickness and cut into 10 equal-size pieces in any desired shape. Heat the oil to 340°F in a deep fryer or large pot and fry the pieces of dough until golden brown, about 2 minutes per side. Transfer the breads to a paper towel–lined baking sheet and serve immediately with the pesto sauce.

Makes 5 cups pesto and 10 pieces grebble

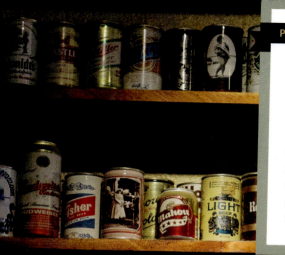

In the rural plains of Kansas, there is award-winning beer flowing from the taps of *Gella's Diner and Lb. Brewing Co.* Behind four renovated storefronts in downtown Hays, homebrewer-turned-pro Gerald Wyman is serving up tasty pints, and people are taking notice.

It was a winding route that led Gerald and his wife, Janet, to open the brewery. They had tried careers in oil and cattle but ultimately they settled on doing what they love. They met Chuck Comeau, an established businessman who shared a similar philosophy, and together they lined up investors and transformed long-forgotten buildings into a wonderful restaurant and brewery. There, innovative dishes are paired with great beers, and since 2005, business has been strong and the awards keep appearing on the wall.

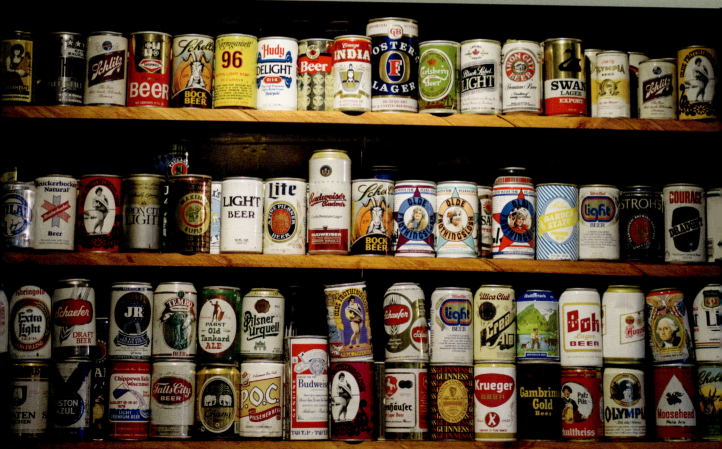

Amber Ale Cheese Bread

Packed with flavor and gooey cheese, this bread won't last long on the table. The amber ale brings a malty sweetness and a deeper texture to the bread. Dark Horse Amber uses a Belgian-like yeast strain that gives spice and fruitiness to the bread, so use that if you can. If not, a regular amber is fine.

Cooking spray
3¼ cups all-purpose flour, plus more for the pans
5 ounces aged white cheddar cheese, shredded (1¼ cups)
4 ounces Gruyère, shredded (1 cup)
¼ cup finely chopped parsley
1 tablespoon baking powder
1 garlic clove, minced
1 teaspoon dry mustard powder
1 teaspoon kosher salt
¼ teaspoon cayenne pepper
¼ teaspoon white pepper
1¼ cups Dark Horse Amber Ale, or similar amber beer
¾ cup sour cream
1 tablespoon Worcestershire sauce
1 egg
¼ cup shredded Parmigiano-Reggiano

1 Preheat the oven to 350°F. Grease and flour two 9-inch round cake pans and set aside.

2 Combine the flour, cheddar, ¾ cup of the Gruyère, and the parsley, baking powder, garlic, mustard powder, salt, cayenne, and white pepper in a large bowl. Stir until combined.

3 Whisk the beer, sour cream, Worcestershire, and egg together in a separate bowl. Pour the mixture into the dry ingredients and mix until just combined. Divide the dough between the prepared baking pans and push down with a spatula to evenly spread the dough across the pans.

4 Sprinkle the Parmigiano-Reggiano and the remaining ¼ cup Gruyère over the top of the dough, dividing it equally between the pans. Bake for 35 to 40 minutes, or until a knife inserted into the center of the loaves comes out clean. Remove the loaves from the oven and let cool for 10 minutes.

5 Run a knife along the edges of each pan and, when the bottom of the pan is cool to the touch, flip the bread out onto a wire rack to cool completely. Slice and serve immediately. Leftovers may be stored overnight in plastic wrap after the bread has completely cooled.

Makes 2 loaves

There is a lot to like about Dark Horse. Skilled in the fermented sciences, the company produces an inspired line of beers and does so with fun, bravado, and tongue-in-cheekness. Its artistically designed taproom is the place to be in Marshall, and the locals mix well with the steady stream of visitors. After all, they are all brought together for good beer. The brewery also has an expansive outdoor space that hosts a number of events such as a February chili cook-off, a summer crawfish boil, and a large anniversary party every September.

As proof that it is serious about its products and uncompromising when it comes to ideals, when the band Nickelback asked to display Dark Horse beer in a music video, the brewery, not being a fan of the band, turned them down.

Bavarian Cheese Spread and
Soft Rye Pretzels, see pages 74 and 50

Sauces and Spreads

**A Little Extra Oomph
Is All You Need**

Cherry Wee Mac Syrup

This syrup is an excellent topping for pancakes or waffles (try it with the Super Ultra Free-Range Pancakes on page 6), and equally good on ice cream. The Wee Mac ale adds notes of toffee and hazelnut and blends nicely with the other aromatic ingredients in the syrup. Sun King calls the beer a Scottish-style brown ale; it draws most of its flavor from roasted malts.

1 cup fresh or frozen tart or sour cherries, pitted
1 (16-ounce) can Sun King Wee Mac Scottish Ale, or similar brown ale
1½ cups granulated sugar
½ cup dark brown sugar
3 cinnamon sticks
1 (1-inch) piece fresh ginger, peeled
Kosher salt

1 Combine the cherries, ale, sugar, brown sugar, cinnamon sticks, ginger, and a pinch of salt in a large saucepan over medium-high heat and bring to a boil. Reduce the heat and simmer until the syrup is thick and can coat a spoon, 20 to 30 minutes.

2 Remove the cinnamon sticks and ginger from the saucepan.

Allow the syrup to cool slightly before serving with your desired accompaniments. (The syrup will thicken as it cools.) Transfer any leftover syrup to an airtight container and refrigerate for up to 1 week.

Makes 2 cups

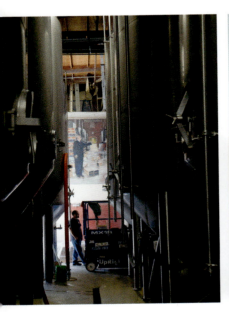

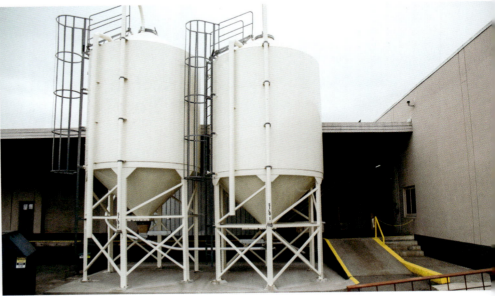

Before they started the ***Sun King Brewing Company*** in downtown Indianapolis, Dave Colt and Clay Robinson paid their dues by working at other brewpubs in the city. One of their duties was to polish the copper covering on the brew kettles. That time spent moving their arms in circular motions, rags in hand, was also used to develop recipe ideas, and it fueled their dream to get a business plan down and funding secured.

When they opened in 2009, they burst onto the state's brewing scene with authority. Just months after they brewed their first batches, several of their beers won medals at the World Beer Cup competition. More medals followed in subsequent contests. Demand for Sun King's beers was so strong early on that, for a while, it seemed they were placing orders for more new equipment as soon as previously ordered equipment was installed.

As the brewery continues to expand and entice people with its canned-beer offerings, Sun King has stayed true to its commitment to all things local. The brewery regularly partners with local businesses and charities, uses locally grown ingredients when possible, and has gained a loyal following for those efforts. It also helps that the brewing team is frequently breaking boundaries and coming up with unique recipes (a popcorn pilsner for example). A visit to the brewery's taproom reveals an eclectic scene of artists, musicians, folks in suits fresh from work, a mix of the old and the young, and every other demographic under the sun. All come for the beer; the line that snakes out the door on any given day is a testament to the quality being poured.

BELL'S BREWERY

KALAMAZOO, MICHIGAN

2 (12-ounce) bottles Bell's Double Cream Stout, or similar cream stout

4 cups dry mustard, preferably Colman's

2 cups dark brown sugar

4 teaspoons salt

2 teaspoons Indian saffron or turmeric

¼ cup plus 2 tablespoons apple cider

2 teaspoons Worcestershire sauce

Horseradish, grated (optional)

Note: You could also use in this recipe an American stout or Bell's Expedition Stout for a more strongly flavored mustard, or a porter for a "dark" beer mustard.

Double Cream Stout Mustard

Mustard is the workhorse of the condiment world. It lifts up an otherwise ordinary sandwich, adds heft to gravies, enhances dips, and is perfectly nice on its own, if you're into that kind of thing. There are many ways to manipulate this versatile condiment, and when you make it from scratch, the list of potential collaborating ingredients is nearly endless. To that end, the chefs at Bell's Brewery have shared two of their favorite scratch-made mustard variations. They're easy to make at home, so you won't need to go the store-bought route again. Like many good things, these mustards require some advance preparation and an overnight rest. Additionally, the recipes make A LOT of mustard, but you can store your homemade condiment for a long time — a month or two in a cool dark cupboard or up to 6 months in the refrigerator. Hermetic clamp storage jars are great looking and practical for storage.

1 Pour the stout into a large bowl, cover it with a kitchen towel or cheesecloth, and let it sit at room temperature overnight. (This lets some of the carbonation release.) Alternatively, pour the beer into a bowl and whisk until it begins to degas, 20 to 30 minutes.

2 Combine the mustard powder, brown sugar, salt, and saffron in a separate large bowl and slowly whisk in the stout, then the cider, and then the Worcestershire until the ingredients are smooth and fully incorporated.

3 Transfer the mustard mixture to a saucepan and slowly bring to a boil over medium heat to prevent foaming. Simmer, uncovered, stirring occasionally, until the sauce begins to thicken, about 20 minutes, and then remove the mustard from the heat.

4 Allow the mustard to cool, add the horseradish, if using, and transfer to a holding jar or container. Adjust the consistency to taste with water or a combination of beer and water. (When left at room temperature, the spiciness of mustard will increase. Refrigerate to stop the mustard from "aging" or from getting too spicy.)

Spicy Two-Hearted Mustard

1 Combine the mustard powder, brown sugar, chili powder, curry powder, and salt in a mixing bowl and whisk to incorporate.

2 Slowly whisk in the horseradish, beer, cider vinegar, olive oil, and lemon juice until smooth and fully incorporated.

3 Transfer the mustard mixture to a saucepan and slowly bring to a boil over medium heat to prevent foaming. Simmer the mustard, stirring occasionally, until slightly thickened, 20 to 30 minutes. Cool the mustard at room temperature for about 3 hours.

4 Transfer the mustard to a holding jar or container. Adjust the consistency if needed with water or a combination of beer and water.

5 cups dry mustard powder, preferably Colman's
2 cups light brown sugar
2 teaspoons chili powder
2 teaspoons curry powder
2 teaspoons salt
½ cup prepared horseradish
3 (12-ounce) bottles Bell's Two Hearted Ale, or similar American IPA
1 cup cider vinegar
1 cup extra-virgin olive oil
2 teaspoons lemon juice

PROFILE ★ **Bell's, one of the first-generation craft breweries,** has been around since 1985 and has grown steadily since then. A source of pride for Michigan residents, it carries a bit of a mythological aura for drinkers in states where Bell's does not distribute. As the oldest craft brewery east of the Rocky Mountains, it has made a name for itself from beers like Hopslam and Two Hearted Ale. Its beers are solid, pleasing, and wonderful representations of their styles, with a dash of creativity thrown in. Founded by Larry Bell, the original brewhouse (like others from its time) used whatever it could to brew and ferment. Today, Bell's employs more than 200 people and has a state-of-the-art facility. Its Eccentric Café is a great place to catch the latest beer release, enjoy a snack, and hang with like-minded beer fans.

½ cup extra-virgin olive oil
¼ cup Caldera IPA, or similar IPA
½ cup hulled and mashed strawberries
⅓ cup mashed grapefruit segments
1 tablespoon sugar
Salt and freshly ground white pepper

A Few Beers to Try with This Recipe

- Bear Republic Racer 5 IPA
- Caldera IPA
- Heavy Seas Loose Cannon American Hop3 Ale
- Napa Smith Organic IPA
- Oskar Blues Gubna
- Peak Organic Citra IPA
- Peak Organic Fall Summit Ale
- Weyerbacher Double Simcoe IPA
- Wolavers IPA

Caldera IPA, Strawberry, and Grapefruit Dressing

Tangy, sweet, and a little spicy, this dressing is perfect for summer salads that combine the best fruits and vegetables of the season. The Caldera IPA uses three hops in its recipe, including Amarillo, which has a citrus-like flavor that accentuates the grapefruit in the dressing.

1 Whisk the olive oil, IPA, strawberries, grapefruit, and sugar together in a medium bowl until the beer degasses and the sugar dissolves.

2 Strain the dressing through a fine-mesh strainer to remove any particles, and transfer to a lidded jar. Season to taste with salt and pepper. Use the dressing immediately or refrigerate for up to 3 days.

PROFILE ★ **Caldera was the first craft brewery in Oregon** to put its beers in cans. While some might view the can as a lesser vessel, it is actually an environmentally responsible way to transport beer. Cans are lighter than bottles and reduce shipping weight; they are easy to crush after consumption, which reduces recycling space; and they keep out light — beer's worst enemy. Caldera brews all its beers in small batches and uses whole-flower hops (rather than pelletized versions) to contribute a fuller flavor to the beers.

Shiner Beer Barbecue Sauce

K. SPOETZL BREWERY

SHINER, TEXAS

This classic recipe has been in the Shiner beer family for quite a while. Simple to whip up, it works well with chicken, fajitas, ribs, sausage, or hamburgers. The creator of this recipe, Brook Watts, also came up with a unique application method. Using a Shiner screw-top bottle, he pokes holes in the cap (from the inside out) with an ice pick or paring knife. He then pours the sauce into the bottle, reattaches the cap, and shakes the desired amount of sauce onto the meat. No basting brush required!

7 ounces Spoetzl Shiner
    Bock, or similar beer
Juice from 2 limes
2 tablespoons apple cider
    vinegar
1 tablespoon extra-virgin
    olive oil
1 tablespoon hot sauce
1½ teaspoons freshly ground
    black pepper
1 teaspoon salt
1 teaspoon chili powder
1 garlic clove, minced

1 Whisk the beer, lime juice, vinegar, olive oil, hot sauce, pepper, salt, chili powder, and garlic together in a large mixing cup to degas the beer and incorporate all the ingredients.

2 Transfer the sauce to an empty bottle, poke holes in the cap, and reattach. This bottle is perfect for sprinkling the sauce on your favorite grilled foods. The sauce will keep for 2 days in the refrigerator.

> **PROFILE ★** **Beer is universal,** but it is not always available. Witness what happened in 1909 when German immigrants arrived in the newly formed town of Shiner, Texas. Unable to find brews similar to the ones they enjoyed at home, they began their own venture, nicknamed "the little brewery." Several years later Kosmos Spoetzl came aboard as the first brewmaster, and eventually he assumed ownership. The **K. Spoetzl Brewery** would survive Prohibition and grow over the years, solidly serving southwestern Texas. Eventually it would expand beyond the Lone Star State and is known today for its traditional German brews as well as specialty batches that incorporate locally grown ingredients.

Bavarian Cheese Spread

Primarily used as a dip, this creamy delight is particularly wonderful with hot soft pretzels or as a topping for burgers and sandwiches. With its spicy hop flavor and balance of malt, a Helles lager is a quaffable complement. This recipe yields a lot of dip and is sure to be a hit at your next party.

6 small shallots, diced

3 (8-ounce) packages cream cheese, softened

¾ cup whole milk

2 cups (4 sticks) salted butter, cut into small pieces

2 pounds Brie, rind removed, cut into small cubes

3 tablespoons paprika

1 tablespoon cayenne pepper

1 tablespoon ground caraway seed

1 Pulse the shallots in the bowl of a food processor fitted with the steel blade attachment until finely ground. With the motor running, slowly add the cream cheese and milk and process until blended.

2 With the motor running, slowly add the butter and Brie to the food processor and blend until the mixture is smooth. Add the paprika, cayenne, and caraway seeds, and blend until fully incorporated.

3 Transfer the dip to a serving bowl, cover with plastic wrap, and chill for at least 1 hour or overnight to thicken. Serve cold. The dip keeps for up to 5 days covered and refrigerated.

Makes 1½ quarts

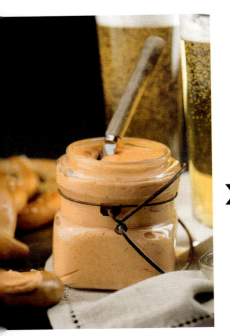

PROFILE ★ **Tony Simmons operates** the comfortable and hospitable *Pagosa Brewing Company and Grill* brewpub in a ski town in the southern part of Colorado near the New Mexico and Utah borders. During the winter months, Pagosa serves up award-winning pints and hearty dishes to skiers who have finished their last runs of the day, and skiers and non-skiers alike enjoy the beer and food year-round. The brewpub's tree-shaded 10,000-square-foot beer garden is a great place to sit and enjoy views of the nearby peaks.

Mole Poblano

This mole is a savory and spicy affair that pairs wonderfully with classic Mexican dishes such as enchiladas, burritos, and tacos. The mole brings forth the roasted character of stouts, porters, Schwarzbiers, and other beers that are brewed with dark malts. If your beer has strong bitterness, the sweetness of the mole will balance it, plus the dark malt flavors will live happily alongside the chocolate in the sauce. This tastes especially wonderful with grilled or smoked chicken thighs, and the mole yields enough for eight servings.

6 plum tomatoes, cut into wedges
¼ cup sesame seeds
4 garlic cloves, minced
10 guajillo chiles
5 ancho chiles
5 mulato chiles
1 cinnamon stick
½ cup breadcrumbs
1 cup chicken broth
½ cup raw sugar
2 tablespoons lard or vegetable oil
3 ounces Mexican chocolate, shaved

1 Preheat the oven to 375°F. Toss the tomatoes, sesame seeds, garlic, chiles, cinnamon stick, and breadcrumbs in a medium mixing bowl until combined. Spread the mixture onto a large baking dish and toast for 10 to 15 minutes, or until the chiles begin to smoke and the sesame seeds and breadcrumbs are golden brown.

2 Remove the cinnamon stick and transfer the chile mixture to a blender. Add the chicken broth and sugar and purée into a thick paste. Set aside.

3 Melt the lard (or warm the vegetable oil) in a large skillet over medium heat. Add the puréed paste, bring to a simmer, and add the chocolate a few shavings at a time until melted and incorporated.

4 Simmer the sauce until the mole has the consistency of a thick gravy and drips off a spoon, about 15 minutes.

Makes enough sauce for 8 servings

PROFILE ★ **Standing Stone is a welcoming place.** The family-owned brewpub has a feeling of comfortable familiarity. Maybe it's the staff, or the great food and exceptional beer, or how everyone there (customers too) just seems to be in a good mood. The wide windows that face the street offer a glimpse of the brewery where Larry Chase, the talented and affable brewer, works up the fermented magic that appears in your glass. Standing Stone also has an established commitment to sustainability (and the awards to prove it), giving you one more reason to love it.

Crawfish Bordelaise

The flavors of the Cajun tradition are comforting and jarring, pleasant and surprising, and liven up every meal. In this recipe, a Bordelaise sauce takes on a bayou flavor with crawfish and spice; it is perfect over a petit filet and solves the dilemma when you can't decide between surf and turf. Serve it with a Vienna lager.

1 teaspoon extra-virgin olive oil
6 tablespoons minced shallots
3 garlic cloves, minced
1 pound peeled crawfish tails
½ cup chopped plum tomatoes
Creole seasoning
½ cup dry red wine
1 cup demi-glace, homemade or purchased
2 tablespoons cold unsalted butter
¼ cup minced scallions
2 teaspoons finely chopped fresh parsley

1 Warm the olive oil in a skillet over medium heat. When it begins to shimmer, add the shallots and garlic, and sauté until tender and translucent, about 1 minute. Add the crawfish tails, tomatoes, and creole seasoning, and cook, stirring frequently, until the tails are well coated, about 2 minutes.

2 Add the wine and bring to a boil, and then reduce the heat to low and simmer for about 5 minutes. Add the demi-glace, and increase the heat to medium to return the sauce to a simmer. Continue to simmer until the sauce thickens slightly, about 5 minutes. Whisk in the butter 1 tablespoon at a time. When the butter has melted, remove the skillet from the heat and stir in the scallions and parsley.

Makes 2¼ cups

PROFILE ★ **The Devils Backbone Basecamp Brewpub** is a "big dark green building with a rust colored roof" according to the directions they hand out to people looking to visit the rural Virginia brewery. And why wouldn't you want to visit? Owner Steve Crandall and head brewer Jason Oliver have carved out a brewtopia. It's a comfortable place with stone and wood accents that give it a country charm conducive to relaxation and fun times. Locals have responded so favorably that Devils Backbone opened a production brewery with a taproom just a short drive away from the Shenandoah Valley. Making the most of its rural location, the brewery also hosts a large number of outdoor events — from festivals to competitions — and regularly draws crowds from around the country.

90 Shilling Rib Eye Marinade

This quick and easy marinade accentuates the flavors of grilled red meat and draws much of its flavor from the nutty, gently sweet beer. When the sugars from the beer hit the grill, they give the meat a nice caramelized char. This recipe makes enough marinade for up to 1½ pounds of beef, lamb, or pork.

¾ cup Odell 90 Shilling Ale, or similar Scottish ale
2 tablespoons soy sauce
2 tablespoons light brown sugar
½ tablespoon minced garlic
½ tablespoon kosher salt
1½ teaspoons freshly ground black pepper

1 Whisk the beer, soy sauce, brown sugar, garlic, salt, and pepper together in a small bowl until the beer degasses and the sugar dissolves.

2 Place the meat in an airtight container and pour the marinade over the meat. Refrigerate for at least 2 hours or up to 1 day before cooking. (The longer the meat and marinade spend together, the more robust the flavor.)

Makes ¾ cup

PROFILE ★ **Credited as the second craft brewery** to open in Colorado (long before the term "craft beer" was coined), *Odell Brewing Co.* started making beer inside a converted grain elevator that dated back to 1915. A dream shared by Doug, Wynne, and Corkie Odell, the brewery opened in 1989 and faced the challenge of educating neighbors who were deep in and loyal to Coors country. The response, say the Odells, was immediate and enthusiastic. The above-mentioned 90 Shilling and the Easy Street Wheat were the first two offerings from the brewery, and their rich and distinct flavors gained the infant business respect in the brewing world.

Now operating out of an updated brewery in Fort Collins, Colorado (a city that boasts nearly half a dozen craft breweries), the once-tiny operation covers more than 45,000 square feet and has a workforce of more than 80.

In addition to its flagship beers, Odell has wowed customers with wood- and barrel-aged beers that rival complex wines and are sometimes intentionally sour.

Watermelon Salad,
see page 84

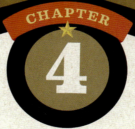

CHAPTER 4

Salads

**Not Just Leafy Greens
and Veggies**

Northern Michigan Salad
with Fruit Beer Vinaigrette

Relatively simple, this classic northern Michigan salad is a staple of a region where cherries are abundant and goat cheese is accessible from local farms. The dressing is a delightful blend of tart, bold, and sweet flavors that come from a fruit-infused beer, like Short's Soft Parade; it makes the whole salad pop with flavor. This bright dish is a perfect way to start a meal, or can become a light dinner when topped with grilled chicken.

VINAIGRETTE
- 2 tablespoons sugar
- 1 teaspoon garlic powder
- 1 teaspoon dry mustard powder
- 1 teaspoon onion powder
- ¼ teaspoon white pepper
- 6 tablespoons Short's Soft Parade, or similar fruit-infused rye ale
- 3 tablespoons apple cider vinegar
- 3 tablespoons white vinegar
- 1½ tablespoons all-purpose cherry juice concentrate
- 1 cup extra-virgin olive oil

SALAD
- 8 cups loosely packed mixed greens
- 4 ounces fresh goat cheese, crumbled
- ½ cup coarsely chopped dried cherries
- ¼ cup roughly chopped pecans

Note: It is fine to substitute other fruit ales, krieks, and lambics for the Short's Soft Parade ale.

1 **MAKE THE VINAIGRETTE:** Combine the sugar, garlic powder, mustard powder, onion powder, and white pepper in a mixing bowl. Whisk in the ale, cider vinegar, white vinegar, and cherry juice concentrate until blended. Slowly whisk in the olive oil to emulsify the vinaigrette.

2 **MAKE THE SALAD:** Place the greens, goat cheese, dried cherries, and pecans in a large salad bowl. Toss to combine.

3 Pour the vinaigrette over the salad, toss again, and serve immediately. Leftover dressing will keep for up to 3 days in an airtight container in the refrigerator.

Makes 4 first-course salads and about 1 cup dressing

In order to enjoy the flavorful, inventive, and downright delicious beers produced by the ***Short's Brewing Company***, you must live in Michigan, the only state where Short's beer is sold. This relatively small brewery has gained a big reputation in recent years thanks to its business and brewing philosophies as well as beers like Strawberry Short's Cake and Key Lime Pie.

At the Great American Beer festival a few years ago, beer legend Charlie Papazian used Twitter to compare Short's to the famed Dogfish Head. Within minutes the line at the Short's booth was 40 people deep, and it never let up. It's a similar situation at beer festivals in Michigan, where revelers line up for a taste of something new and guaranteed to shock their taste buds.

The brewery and pub sit in what was a century-old hardware store, and despite wide windows that open to the street, it has a bit of a speakeasy feel combined with an offbeat art gallery and a home basement pub (thanks to some vinyl bus seats that found new life as bar chairs). The menu is varied and there is plenty of live music, too. Short's is a great reason to visit northern Michigan.

Rocket Salad with Camembert Croquettes

There is no shortage of bars in Denver, but among beer people and foodies, Euclid Hall has emerged as a force to be reckoned with. Their scratch kitchen continually turns out a bevy of delights, including this unique salad. It requires a little more work than simply tossing vegetables together, but the result is a flavorful start to any dinner. The croquettes alone are a delight: combined with the bite of rocket, and the citrus and onion flavors, they're guaranteed to impress dinner guests. Pair with a doppelbock that stands up to the flavors of the salad.

CAMEMBERT CROQUETTES

- 12 (½-ounce) cubes Camembert
- 1 cup all-purpose flour
- 2 eggs
- ¼ cup water
- Panko breadcrumbs
- Peanut oil, for frying

CANDIED LEMON VINAIGRETTE

- 2 cups freshly squeezed lemon juice
- 2 cups sugar
- 2 cups water
- Zest of two lemons, julienned
- 1 tablespoon chopped shallots
- 1½ tablespoons chopped chives
- ½ cup canola oil
- Salt and freshly ground black pepper
- 3 cups organic baby arugula (rocket)

1 **BEGIN THE CROQUETTES:** Chill the Camembert cubes in the refrigerator for 1 hour to set before breading.

2 **MAKE THE VINAIGRETTE:** Boil the lemon juice in a small saucepan over medium heat until reduced by half, about 10 minutes.

3 Combine the sugar and water in a separate saucepan and simmer until the sugar is dissolved. Add the lemon zest and cook over medium heat until very tender, about 15 minutes.

4 Add the zest and syrup to the lemon juice reduction and reduce together over medium heat until the mixture is the consistency of maple syrup, about 10 minutes. Remove from the heat and set aside to cool slightly.

5 Whisk in the shallots and chives, and then slowly whisk in the canola oil to emulsify the dressing. Season to taste with salt and pepper. If the dressing seems too thick, add additional water.

6 **MAKE THE CROQUETTES:** Put the flour in a shallow dish; beat the eggs and water in another shallow dish; put the panko in a third shallow dish. Dip the cheese cubes in the flour, then twice in the eggwash, and finally in the panko. Refrigerate until ready to fry.

7 Pour 2 inches of peanut oil into a deep skillet and heat to 350°F. Fry the Camembert croquettes until crisp and golden brown, 2 to 3 minutes. Remove and set aside on a paper towel–lined plate.

8 Toss the arugula with a generous amount of vinaigrette and season with salt and pepper. Drizzle a small amount of vinaigrette on individual salad plates and then place a handful of dressed greens on each plate. Place two hot, crisp Camembert pieces next to the greens on each plate and serve.

Makes 6 servings

With its always inventive scratch kitchen, uncompromising beer list, and dedicated staff, *Euclid Hall* quickly established itself as a Denver destination for the craft beer faithful. Try the house-made sausages and schnitzels. Soak in the atmosphere of the building, which dates back to the late 1800s, and if possible, don't miss the opportunity to attend one of the special events or dinners. You're guaranteed to leave sated.

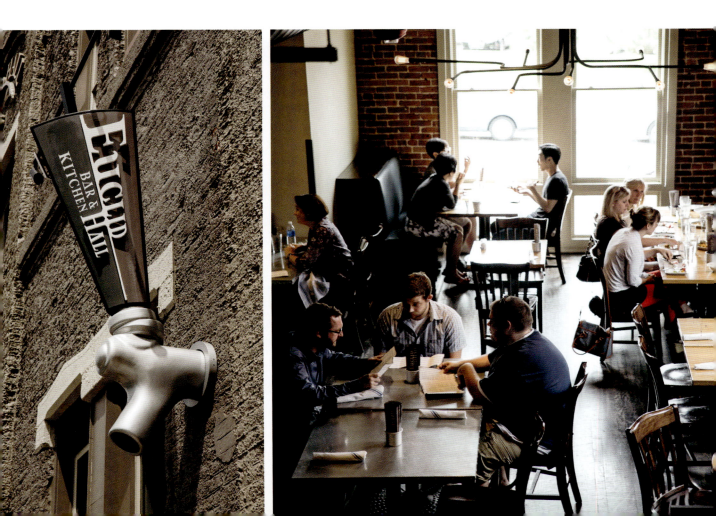

Watermelon Salad with Endive

see photo, page 78

1 small ripe watermelon, rind removed, diced into ¼-inch cubes

2 medium heirloom tomatoes, diced into ¼-inch chunks

8 large fresh basil leaves, thinly sliced

1 tablespoon extra-virgin olive oil

½ teaspoon sea salt

2 heads Belgian endive

4 ounces blue cheese, crumbled

Simple but flavorful, this salad combines sweet, bold, and tangy flavors and is a good start for just about any summer meal, when watermelon is at its seasonal best. Pair the salad with an oak-aged or sour ale such as Trinity's Old Growth Wild Brown Ale. Other breweries like Russian River, New Belgium, Jolly Pumpkin, Lost Abbey, and Allagash also routinely release sour ales, but they are subject to availability. The sour flavor offers a bold contrast to the fresh fruit.

1 Combine the watermelon, tomatoes, basil, olive oil, and salt in a large bowl. Allow the mixture to marinate in the refrigerator for up to 30 minutes.

2 Take the fresh endive and carefully peel off each leaf one by one until you reach the small leaves at the core. Rinse and trim the endive leaves and arrange on a platter or individual plates. (The endive will be the serving vessel for the salad.)

3 Divide the watermelon salad among the endive leaves. Sprinkle with the cheese and serve immediately.

Makes 4–6 servings

PROFILE ★ **There is a distinct pleasure** that comes from visiting a unique location. Visit enough bars and restaurants and, after a while, there are certain predictable elements that are unavoidable. However, *Trinity* happily breaks the mold with a custom-built pub made from nearly 100 percent recycled materials. Giving new life to discarded items has made Trinity unique, but that's not the only reason to visit. Their environmental commitments are firm, and they practice what they preach by using sustainable materials and sourcing local food for their kitchen. They even offer discounts to customers who arrive at the brewery by "human power."

Bavarian Sausage Salad

This is a dinner salad that will satisfy even the heartiest eater. It's simple to make and great for parties; serve this dish with hard pretzels and pair with a spicy IPA such as Urban Chestnut's Hopfen.

1 cup water
½ cup white wine vinegar
½ cup extra-virgin olive oil
6 large frankfurters or knockwurst, cooked and thinly sliced
8 ounces Swiss cheese, cubed
1 medium white onion, chopped
Salt and freshly ground black pepper
1 cup chopped fresh parsley

1 Whisk the water, vinegar, and olive oil together in a large bowl. Add the sausage, cheese, and onion, and season with salt and pepper to taste. Cover and chill the salad for at least 1 hour or up to overnight in the refrigerator.

2 When ready to serve, add the parsley to the salad, toss to combine, and serve cold.

Makes 4 servings

A Few Beers to Try with This Recipe

- *Bell's Two Hearted Ale*
- *Dogfish Head 60 Minute IPA*
- *Firestone Walker Union Jack IPA*
- *Foothills Hoppyum IPA*
- *Lagunitas IPA*
- *Odell IPA*
- *Sierra Nevada Torpedo*
- *Urban Chestnut's Hopfen*
- *Wynkoop Mile HIPA*

PROFILE ★ **By the time he was ready to open his own brewery,** Urban Chestnut's Florian Kuplent had logged countless hours perfecting recipes, learning established styles, and inventing some beer combinations of his own. **Urban Chestnut** produces a number of German beer styles. That's nothing new to St. Louis, but Kuplent does so with the kind of American flair that excites today's beer drinkers.

Curly Endive and Spring Dandelion Salad with Belgian White Apricot Vinaigrette and Pork Rillettes

Salads don't always have to be healthy and virtuous. Take for example this ambitious salad featuring carefully constructed elements and delicious ingredients that come together like a symphony on the plate. Rillettes are basically a meat paste, similar to pâté; stored in airtight sterilized jars, they can keep for upward of six months. A floral Belgian white accentuates the flavors of the endive, apricot, and pork.

ONIONS
- 1 tablespoon extra-virgin olive oil
- 1 large Vidalia, or similarly sweet, onion, thinly sliced
- Salt and freshly ground black pepper

RILLETTES
- 1 pound lard
- 3 yellow onions, finely chopped
- 1 (4- to 5-pound) boneless Boston butt pork roast
- Salt and freshly ground black pepper
- 5 garlic cloves, minced
- 1 celery stalk, trimmed, halved, and finely chopped
- 2 fresh thyme sprigs
- 2 bay leaves
- 1 teaspoon red pepper flakes
- 4 cups chicken broth
- 1 cup dry white wine

1 CARMELIZE THE ONIONS: Warm the olive oil over medium heat in a medium skillet. Add the Vidalia onions and 1/2 teaspoon salt, and cook, stirring occasionally, until the onions are caramelized and soft, about 8 minutes. Add additional salt and freshly ground black pepper to taste, and set aside.

2 MAKE THE RILLETTES: Melt the lard in a large enameled cast-iron lidded pot over medium heat. Add the yellow onions and cook, stirring occasionally, until they are very soft and translucent, about 10 minutes.

3 While the onions are cooking, cut the pork into 1-inch cubes and season with salt and pepper to taste. Add the pork, garlic, celery, thyme, bay leaves, pepper flakes, chicken broth, and wine to the pot. Increase the heat to medium-high and bring to a gentle boil. Reduce the heat to low, cover, and slowly simmer, stirring occasionally, for 3 hours, or until fork-tender.

4 Transfer the pork to the bowl of a standing mixer fitted with the paddle attachment, and mix on low speed until the pork is shredded. Remove and discard the celery, thyme sprigs, and bay leaves from the pot. Slowly add the remaining broth from the pot to the meat in the stand mixer and continue mixing on low speed until all the broth has been incorporated back into the pork. Season with salt and pepper to taste. Place the mixture in 2-ounce ramekins or molds and chill.

DRESSING

- ½ cup sugar
- ½ cup dried apricots
- ¼ cup roasted unsalted pistachios
- 1½ teaspoons salt
- 1 teaspoon dry mustard powder
- ½ cup champagne vinegar
- ½ cup Belgian white ale
- 2 cups olive oil
- Salt and freshly ground black pepper

SALAD

- 2 cups loosely packed curly endive
- 2 cups loosely packed young dandelion greens
- 2 cups cored and sliced radicchio, soaked in ice water to reduce bitterness
- Salt
- ½ cup Marcona almonds, toasted
- 8 paper-thin slices Serrano ham
- 4 ripe apricots, pitted and quartered

5 **MAKE THE DRESSING:** Combine the sugar, apricots, pistachios, salt, mustard, vinegar, and ale in a blender and purée. Slowly add the oil with the blender running until the dressing emulsifies. Season with salt and pepper to taste. Store any extra dressing in an airtight container for up to 1 week.

6 **MAKE THE SALAD:** Toss the endive, dandelion greens, and radicchio with the dressing in a large bowl. Season with salt to taste and arrange the greens in the middle of four 10-inch round plates. Top each salad with the Marcona almonds and two slices of the Serrano ham. Place the quartered apricots around the salad, with the rillettes between the apricots. Top the rillettes with dollops of the caramelized Vidalia onions and serve immediately.

Makes 4 servings, with extra dressing and rillettes

Wheat Berry Salad

With a great nutty flavor and chewy texture, wheat berries are a whole-grain alternative to white rice or orzo. This recipe requires some work to cook the wheat berries and prepare the vinaigrette on the front end, but the result is a unique salad with a tangy citrus vinaigrette. The recipe makes plenty of extra vinaigrette; store it in your refrigerator for several days, and use it to dress your favorite green salads. In some cases you might need to soak the wheat berries overnight — consult the packaging before preparing them.

2 cups vegetable broth
2 cups wheat berries

DRESSING
4 garlic cloves
¼ cup orange juice
2 tablespoons lemon juice
2 tablespoons lime juice
½ teaspoon salt
½ teaspoon freshly ground pepper
1 cup vegetable oil

SALAD
3 celery stalks, trimmed and finely diced
1 large carrot, peeled and finely diced
1 Granny Smith apple, peeled, cored, and finely diced
1 small red onion, finely diced (optional)
Fresh arugula

1 Bring the vegetable broth to a boil in a large pot. Add the wheat berries, cover, and cook according to the package instructions until tender but still slightly chewy. Drain any remaining liquid and transfer the wheat berries to a large baking sheet to cool slightly.

2 MAKE THE DRESSING: Combine the garlic, orange juice, lemon juice, lime juice, salt, and pepper in a blender and pulse until the mixture is smooth. With the blender running, whisk in the vegetable oil in a slow stream until the ingredients are combined and the dressing is smooth.

3 MAKE THE SALAD: Combine the wheat berries, celery, carrot, apple, and red onion, if using, in a large bowl and toss with some of the dressing to coat. Place a handful of arugula on each of four salad plates, top with the wheat berry mixture, drizzle with additional dressing as desired, and serve.

Makes 4–6 servings

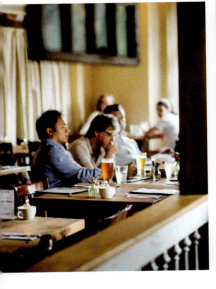
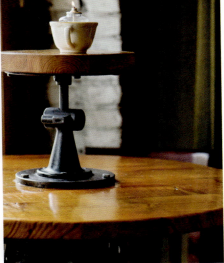

Philadelphia's Earth Bread + Brewery serves perfectly crispy flatbreads and heavenly beers in a casual, artistic atmosphere. Recognizable by its outside full-wall mural of a park scene, the brewery is committed to its neighborhood, carefully sourcing vendors and encouraging customers to bring canned goods with each visit to donate to local food pantries. The space is also a rotating art gallery, with new installations appearing every two months.

Walking the Wissahickon
Designed and Painted by Brian Ames

Durham St
ONE WAY

SUTTER BUTTES BREWING CO.

YUBA CITY, CALIFORNIA

Chopped Reuben Salad with Sweet Sauerkraut Vinaigrette

While a Reuben is one of the world's great sandwiches, this deconstructed recipe adds new dimension to the hearty workhorse. This version replaces Russian (or Thousand Island) dressing with a vinaigrette that adds a sharp kick and nicely blends with the other flavors of the salad; it also lightens things up a bit. This recipe pairs well with golden Belgian ale; the fruity sweet ester is a nice companion to the sour vinegar tang of the salad. A light and refreshing Kölsch would also pair well and provide a perfect summertime finish.

VINAIGRETTE

- ¼ cup packed fresh cilantro leaves
  Juice of ½ orange
- ¼ cup cider vinegar
- ¼ cup red wine vinegar
- 1 tablespoon honey
- 1 tablespoon sugar
- 2 teaspoons German Spice Blend (see box)
- ½ cup extra-virgin olive oil
  Salt and freshly ground black pepper

CROUTONS

- 6 slices rye bread, cut into ½-inch cubes
- 3 tablespoons extra-virgin olive oil
- 1 teaspoon German Spice Blend (see box)

SALAD

- 1 cup chopped romaine lettuce
- ½ cup butter leaf lettuce
- ½ cup chopped red leaf lettuce
- ½ cup grated carrot
- ½ cup shredded Napa cabbage
- ½ cup shredded purple cabbage
- 1½ cups warm shaved pastrami
- ½ cup sauerkraut, seared
- 12 cherry tomatoes, quartered
- 8 slices Swiss cheese, julienned
- ½ bunch cilantro sprigs, for garnish (optional)

Note: Extra dressing may be stored for up to 3 days in an airtight container in the refrigerator.

German Spice Blend

The spice blend is a fragrant and savory enhancement perfect for finishing grilled meats and a variety of salads.

Toast ¼ cup fennel seeds, 2 tablespoons caraway seeds, 2 tablespoons celery seeds, and 2 tablespoons dried onion in a dry skillet over medium heat, stirring occasionally, until golden, about 20 minutes. Allow the spices to cool, and then add 1 tablespoon kosher salt and grind together in a spice grinder or with a mortar and pestle. This seasoning keeps in an airtight container for up to 3 weeks.

1 **MAKE THE VINAIGRETTE:** Blend the cilantro leaves, orange juice, cider vinegar, red wine vinegar, honey, sugar, and spice blend in a blender until combined. With the motor running, slowly add the oil and continue to blend until incorporated. Season with salt and pepper to taste. Set aside.

2 **MAKE THE CROUTONS:** Preheat the oven to 250°F. Toss the bread, olive oil, and spice blend together in a medium bowl. Toast on baking sheets for 10 minutes, toss once, and then bake for 5 minutes longer, or until the bread is nicely browned. Allow to cool.

3 **MAKE THE SALAD:** Combine the romaine lettuce, butter leaf lettuce, red leaf lettuce, carrots, Napa cabbage, and purple cabbage in a large bowl. Divide the greens among four salad plates. Top each plate with equal amounts of the pastrami, sauerkraut, tomatoes, cheese, cilantro sprigs, if using, and 2 tablespoons of the vinaigrette. Top with the croutons and serve immediately.

Makes 4 servings

PROFILE ★ **As one of the only breweries** in its particular region of northern California, **Sutter Buttes Brewing** is all about education. And with its impressive lineup, easy-to-see brewhouse (located just behind the bar), and friendly staff, it's a pretty easy task. Brewery employees are happy to talk with customers about the brewing process, ingredients, and styles. So far, it's paying off with a steady stream of local customers that continues to grow. They also enjoy a great spot downtown that is easily accessible from the highway. Their comfortable dining room gets generous afternoon light from large windows, and the light gleams off the bright tanks holding flavorful ales and lagers (the seasonal stout is a favorite). All this, combined with a solid kitchen and welcoming atmosphere, makes Sutter Buttes the kind of brewpub every city should have.

DRESSING

¾ cup rice wine vinegar
½ cup canola oil
6 tablespoons honey
5 tablespoons ginger purée
5 tablespoons peanut butter
2 tablespoons lemon juice
1 tablespoon finely chopped cilantro leaves
1 tablespoon white pepper
1 teaspoon minced fresh mint
¾ cup extra-virgin olive oil
½ cup sesame oil
Red pepper flakes

SALAD

4–6 ounces fresh, sustainable North Atlantic salmon
3 ounces lo mein noodles
¼ cup shredded carrots
¼ cup shredded red cabbage
¼ cup shredded green cabbage
1 teaspoon black sesame seeds
1 teaspoon white sesame seeds
Wasabi peanuts, scallions, and lemon zest, for garnish (optional)

Note: This recipe makes a lot more dressing than you'll need, but the leftovers can be transferred to an airtight container and stored in the refrigerator for several days.

Asian Grilled Salmon Salad
with Thai Dressing

With its flavors of nuts, spices, citrus, and sweetness, Thai cuisine really stands up to and complements the flavor of fresh salmon. This recipe works well as a starter for two, but it's also great served as the main course for a solo meal. Multiply the ingredients as needed if you plan to serve the recipe as a full meal for more than one person. Pair with a fruity saison, like Fegley's Brew Works Monkey Wrench; the earthiness and spiciness of the beer lifts the oiliness of the salmon.

1 MAKE THE DRESSING: Combine the vinegar, canola oil, honey, ginger, peanut butter, lemon juice, cilantro, white pepper, and mint in a blender and purée until smooth. With the motor running, slowly add the olive oil and then the sesame oil and blend until fully emulsified. Season to taste with pepper flakes.

2 MAKE THE SALAD: Prepare a medium fire in a gas or charcoal grill, and oil the grate. Grill the salmon to desired temperature, flipping once (medium is recommended, and takes 2 to 3 minutes per side). Transfer the salmon to a plate and allow to rest for 5 minutes.

3 Combine the noodles, carrots, red cabbage, green cabbage, black sesame seeds, and white sesame seeds in a bowl and toss with 2 tablespoons of the dressing. Divide the salad between two plates, and top with the salmon, wasabi peanuts, scallions, and a few gratings of lemon zest, if using. Serve immediately, with additional dressing as desired.

*Makes 2 servings
and 2 cups dressing*

PROFILE ★ **When the Fegley family founded their brewery** in the 1990s, they sought to capture the essence of this steel town in eastern Pennsylvania. What customers get today is a respected brewpub with plenty of metal accents that give an industrial feel, while still keeping things comfortable. With expert brewers and accomplished chefs, it's no wonder that *Bethlehem Brew Works* (and its sister location in Allentown) is a local favorite.

Piece Green Salad

All the traditional backyard garden delights are in this salad, but the unexpected sweet crunch from the pecans and the tang of Italian dressing give the ordinary combination a welcome boost.

2 tablespoons sugar
2 tablespoons water
3 tablespoons pecans
5 cups loosely packed mesclun lettuce
5 tablespoons Italian dressing
4 grape tomatoes, sliced in half
1 small cucumber, peeled, seeded, and thinly sliced
¼ cup thinly sliced pear, preferably Anjou
Handful of thinly sliced red onion
1½ ounces Gorgonzola cheese, crumbled

1 Preheat the oven to 450°F. Whisk the sugar and water together in a small bowl until the sugar dissolves. Toss the pecans in the sugar mixture and transfer to a baking sheet. Bake the pecans for 8 to 10 minutes, or until golden brown and toasted. Cool slightly.

2 Meanwhile, combine the lettuce and dressing in a salad bowl and toss until well coated. Top the salad with the tomatoes, cucumbers, pears, onions, Gorgonzola, and pecans. Serve immediately.

Makes 3–4 servings

PROFILE ★ **One of the great culinary combinations** — pizza and beer — has found a perfect home at *Piece Brewery & Pizzeria*. The Chicago brewpub has been serving up award-winning slices and pints since 2001. While the Windy City is known for its deep-dish pizzas, Piece looks to the east and serves up New Haven–style pies with thin, crispy crusts. Popular with residents and tourists alike, Piece has a comfortable trendy atmosphere and a dozen televisions situated throughout, making it a perfect place to watch the local teams in action.

SAINT ARNOLD BREWING COMPANY

HOUSTON, TEXAS

Lady Cream Pea Salad with Gingered Beets

1¼ pounds lady cream peas, shelled
2 quarts water
½ cup chicken demi-glace
1 tablespoon kosher salt
1¼ pounds beets, peeled and diced small
1 (1-inch) piece fresh ginger, peeled
2 tablespoons lemon juice
1½ teaspoons Dijon mustard
Salt and freshly ground black pepper
⅓ cup extra-virgin olive oil
1 bunch scallions, white and light green parts, thinly sliced on the bias

Notes: If you can't find lady cream peas, try this salad with black-eyed peas.

If chicken demi-glace is not available, replace the water and the demi-glace with chicken broth.

When you need a recipe that you can prepare ahead of time for a big party, try this simple pea salad. Lady cream peas are common in Texas but are relatively easy to find even outside the Lone Star State. As their name suggests, the peas are light and sweet in flavor. They balance well with the bold citrus flavors from the vinaigrette. Consider pairing this with a Kölsch, such as Saint Arnold's Fancy Lawnmower. Chef Michael Scott Castell usually serves this recipe in shooter or shot glasses for a new spin on passed hors d'oeuvres. Leftovers make a nice light lunch the following day.

1 Combine the peas, water, demi-glace, and salt in a soup pot and bring to a simmer. Cook until the peas are tender, at least 45 minutes.

2 Drain the peas and then rinse with cold water to cool. Set aside.

3 Put the beets in a saucepan and add water to cover. Bring the water to a simmer and cook until tender, about 15 minutes. Drain the beets, rinse under cold water to cool, and spread on a paper towel to dry.

4 Grate the ginger and measure out 1 tablespoon. Place the remaining ginger on a linen napkin and tightly wring it over a large bowl to capture its juices; discard the grated ginger after juicing. Add the lemon juice, mustard, and salt and pepper to taste. Whisk in the olive oil until the vinaigrette is emulsified.

5 Gently toss the peas in the vinaigrette to coat and add the beets and the reserved tablespoon of ginger. Toss in the scallions, reserving 2 tablespoons for a garnish. Season with salt and pepper to taste and transfer the salad to shot glasses. Garnish with the reserved scallions and serve immediately.

Makes 24–36 shooters or 6 first-course servings

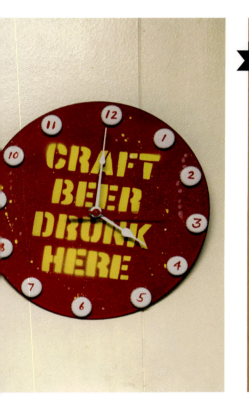

From the outside, Texas's oldest craft brewery doesn't look like much. It's housed in an unassuming red brick building set hard against railroad tracks, and nothing except the name painted along the building's side distinguishes it from anything else in the area. But, as the old saying about a book's cover goes, it is the interior of ***Saint Arnold*** that truly impresses. It's fair to say it has one of the more impressive beer halls to grace the inside of a brewery. The hall is welcoming with rich wood paneling, long Bavarian beer hall–style tables, and a 20-tap-strong bar, complete with views of the brewhouse. It's the type of place that makes visitors envious and locals regulars.

And, as if it couldn't get better, there is the Investors Pub, also inside the same building, a lounge-type space where any gentleman would feel comfortable. That space has high-backed leather chairs, walls painted pool-table green, dart boards, and another bar, of course.

Now, let's talk about the beer. It's good. The brewery has created a lineup of approachable, well-balanced beers that nicely serve the local community and beyond. It has raised the bar and expanded palates in a geographical area where change is hard to come by. Thank the heavens for Saint Arnold.

The Riot Sandwich,
see page 100

Sandwiches and Burgers

Goodness Between Two Slices

½ cup self-rising flour
2 boneless, skinless chicken breasts
  Peanut or canola oil, for frying
2 tablespoons lard
4 tablespoons cayenne pepper
1 tablespoon firmly packed light brown sugar
½ teaspoon garlic powder
½ teaspoon salt
4 slices white bread
  Sliced pickles, for garnish

Nashville Hot Chicken Sandwich

Every city worth its salt has a local delicacy, and Nashville's claim to fame is its hot chicken, put on the culinary map by a local restaurant called Prince's. This is not the restaurant's secret recipe, which is carefully guarded, but it is close. Like the name says, this is a hot, spicy, watery-eyes, reaching-for-a-cool-drink kind of hot. Consider yourself warned. This method of fowl preparation has become so popular that the city now hosts an annual Hot Chicken Festival on the Fourth of July. Local brewery Yazoo is the official beer sponsor, so there is plenty of pale ale available to help soothe the burn.

1 Place the flour in a shallow bowl and dredge the chicken breasts in the flour to coat well. Set aside.

2 Add 4 inches of oil to a deep pot and heat to 375°F. Fry the chicken breasts until golden brown and cooked through, 7 to 10 minutes. Drain on a paper towel–lined plate and keep warm.

3 Microwave the lard in a small bowl for 15 seconds. Mix the cayenne, brown sugar, garlic powder, and salt into the lard until a paste forms.

4 Slather one side of each breast with the paste. Place the sauced side of the chicken breasts on one piece of the bread, and slather the other side of the chicken with the sauce. Top with the pickles and a second slice of bread. Serve immediately.

Makes 2 sandwiches

The people who say that the South can be a tough nut to crack when it comes to craft beer obviously haven't visited Nashville, and they certainly have not tasted anything from *Yazoo Brewing Co.* Founded by Linus Hall, the brewery is often packed with regulars seeking growler refills and visitors lining up for weekend tours.

On several occasions, I've stood shoulder to shoulder with others at the tasting room, where affable bartenders expertly pour pints and answer a lot of questions about the beers. That's a good sign that in the land of Mr. Daniels, people are taking notice and getting interested in craft beer. Yazoo's flagship brew is Dos Perros, a dark brown ale that uses Munich, English pale, and chocolate malts along with Perle and Saaz hops. It gets a refreshing lift from some flaked maize and noble hops added at the end. An endlessly drinkable session beer, it fits in everywhere from a barbecue to the Grand Ole Opry.

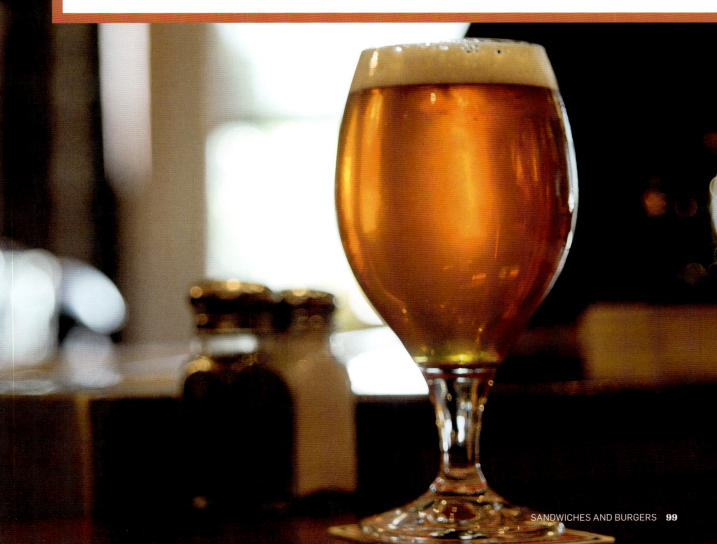

The Riot Sandwich

see photo, page 96

PULLED PORK
- 1 tablespoon firmly packed dark brown sugar
- 1 tablespoon garlic powder
- 1 tablespoon mustard powder
- 1 tablespoon onion powder
- 1 tablespoon paprika
- 1 tablespoon freshly ground black pepper
- 1½ teaspoons kosher salt
- 2½ pounds pork butt
- ½ cup barbecue sauce, plus more for serving

SAUSAGE
- 5 pounds pork butt or shoulder
- ½ pound pork back fat (available from a butcher)
- 5 teaspoons kosher salt
- ¼ cup fennel seeds
- 1 tablespoon minced garlic
- 1 tablespoon brewer's pale malted barley, milled (available from homebrew shops)
- ½ tablespoon brewer's chocolate malted barley, milled (available from homebrew shops)
- ½ tablespoon brewer's dark crystal malted barley, milled (available from homebrew shops)
- ¼ tablespoon cayenne pepper
- 1½ teaspoons freshly ground black pepper
- 3–5 tablespoons extra-virgin olive oil

An indulgence of pork highlighted by complex flavors, this sandwich has many steps — you'll need a smoker and a meat grinder to properly pull it off — but the end result is worth it. The sandwich features a spicy Italian sausage patty, smoked pulled pork, mozzarella, and giardiniera on a brioche bun. This is the perfect alternative to burgers, when you need to feed a lot of people at a big summer gathering. It requires several hours of smoking, so be prepared with enough chips.

A cult classic at the Windy City brewery that created it, this home version has been adapted by brewer Pete Crowley and chef Christopher McCoy. Make it once and your guests will ask for it again and again. Pair with an imperial IPA; Haymarket's Mathias is a perfect choice, giving off hop flavors and aromas of citrus and tropical fruit. The sandwich is messy, spicy, sweet and sour, savory, delicious, and a riot.

1 MAKE THE PULLED PORK: Preheat the smoker to 225°F. Stir the brown sugar, garlic powder, mustard powder, onion powder, paprika, black pepper, and salt together in a small bowl. Rub the mixture all over the pork and place on the smoker. Smoke the pork for 4 to 9 hours, or until the pork reaches an internal temperature of 190°F. Replace the chip plates after 2 hours.

2 MAKE THE SAUSAGE: When the pork is an hour or two from completion in the smoker, mix the pork, back fat, and salt together, and place in the freezer for 30 minutes. (This will help firm up the proteins and keep the fats from breaking down during grinding and mixing.)

3 Remove the pork mixture from the freezer and process it in a meat grinder; the chilled meat should push through easily and pockets of the pork and fat will be visible. Add the fennel seeds, garlic, pale barley, chocolate barley, dark barley, cayenne, and black pepper, and mix in a large bowl until the spices are evenly incorporated into the sausage mixture.

4 Remove the pork from the smoker, set aside, and let cool. Once the pork is cool, shred with two forks to create long strands of meat about ¼ inch thick. Transfer to a large bowl and set aside.

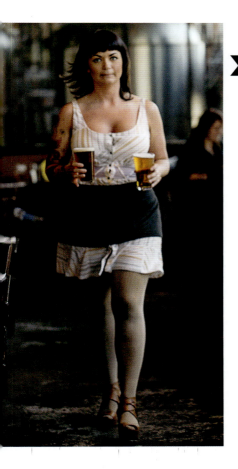

Drinking beer lends itself to writing and quite often writing lends itself to drinking beer. Many great writers have found the muse at the bottom of a glass. For those who put pen to paper, it's nice to know there are places out there that still care about quality pints and treating writers with respect. In Chicago, that place is the ***Haymarket Pub and Brewery***. Those lucky enough to know Pete Crowley, the talented brewer who did his time at other Chicago breweries, say he has been soaring since firing up the kettles in his new place in late 2010. The front bar and dining room is a spacious, light-filled space with warm wood furniture and a dizzying display of televisions broadcasting everything from NASCAR to Cubs' games.

Crowley has a fondness for Belgian beer and has been trying to bring the sensibilities, traditions, and flavors of Belgium into his own recipes. Add in a bit of his creative flair and you will find some fine recipes that everyone should appreciate and enjoy. The back bar is where the writers hang out and has a bookshelf stocked with great works of writing on every subject from Chicago history to, of course, beer.

While it can be easy to get lost in the beers, it's also important to mention the food at Haymarket. Diners rave about the thin-crust pizzas, housemade sausages, and hand-cut fries. In a city that has been blessed with a number of great breweries and beer bars, Haymarket has quickly joined the ranks of a proud tradition.

SANDWICH

- 1 (15-ounce) jar giardiniera
- 15 thin slices mozzarella cheese
- 15 brioche hamburger buns, sliced

Note: Make sure you have plenty of Carolina-style barbecue sauce (spicy, vinegary, and sweet) on hand to top off this sandwich.

5 Form the sausage mixture into 15 3-ounce patties. Heat 2 tablespoons of the olive oil in a skillet over high heat and, working in batches, cook the patties until browned and cooked through; an instant-read thermometer inserted into the center of a patty should reach 150°F. Repeat with the remaining sausage mixture, replacing and reheating the oil in the skillet as needed.

6 ASSEMBLE THE SANDWICHES: Toss the pulled pork with the barbecue sauce. Build each sandwich by placing a layer of the giardiniera, a sausage patty, a slice of mozzarella cheese, and the pulled barbecue pork atop the bottom half of a brioche hamburger bun. Close the sandwich with the bun top and serve immediately with extra barbecue sauce.

Makes 15 sandwiches

BOLERO SNORT BREWERY

RIDGEFIELD PARK, NEW JERSEY

ROASTED CHIPOTLE SALSA

- 7 plum tomatoes, chopped
- 3 dried chipotle chiles, chopped
- ¼ cup minced white onion
- ¼ cup finely chopped fresh cilantro leaves
- 2 garlic cloves, minced
- ½ cup water
- Salt

BURGERS

- 2 pounds lean ground beef
- 1 teaspoon cumin
- 1 teaspoon freshly ground black pepper
- ½ teaspoon garlic powder
- 8 buns
- 8 slices Monterey jack cheese
- 2 ripe avocadoes, pitted and thinly sliced
- Tortilla chips, for serving

A Few Beers to Try with This Recipe

- *Bolero Snort There's No Rye-ing in Basebull*
- *Founders Red's Rye PA*
- *Great Divide Hoss Rye Lager*
- *Sierra Nevada Ruthless Rye*
- *Two Brothers Cane & Ebel*

Roasted Chipotle Salsa Burger

This spicy burger awakens taste buds and adds a kick to any backyard barbecue before calming things down with fresh, ripe avocado. Pair with a rye beer, which enhances some of the spice flavors and quenches a warm-weather thirst.

1 MAKE THE SALSA: Combine the tomatoes, chiles, onion, cilantro, and garlic in a medium saucepan. Cook over medium-high heat, stirring occasionally, until the tomatoes break down and the mixture comes to a simmer.

2 Add the water and bring to a boil. Reduce the heat to low and simmer until the mixture begins to thicken, about 5 minutes.

3 Remove the saucepan from the heat. Mash the ingredients together with a potato masher for a thicker salsa or an immersion blender for a finer salsa, adding salt to taste. Allow the mixture to cool in an airtight container in the refrigerator for at least 1 hour, or for up to 3 days before serving.

4 MAKE THE BURGERS: Mix the beef, cumin, black pepper, and garlic powder together in a large bowl. Form the mixture into eight 4-ounce patties. Transfer the patties to a plate, cover with plastic wrap, and store them in the refrigerator until ready to use, or up to 1 day. (You can also freeze the formed patties, tightly wrapped, for up to 1 month.)

5 Prepare a 450°F fire in a gas or charcoal grill.

6 Transfer the patties to the grill and cook to preferred doneness: for medium burgers cook for 5 minutes, flip once, and cook for 3 to 4 minutes longer. Remove the patties from the grill.

7 Top the bottom half of each bun with a burger patty, slice of cheese, 1 tablespoon of the salsa, and avocado slices. Add the bun tops and serve immediately with tortilla chips and extra salsa on the side.

Makes 8 burgers and 3 cups salsa

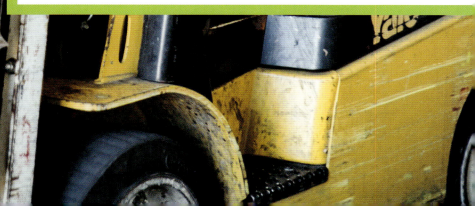

Grilled Lamb Burgers with
Local Chèvre and Mint-Cilantro Aioli

MINT-CILANTRO AIOLI

- 1 cup aioli or mayonnaise
- 1 tablespoon chopped fresh cilantro leaves
- 1 tablespoon chopped fresh mint leaves
- 1½ teaspoons chopped fresh garlic
- Juice of 1 lemon
- ½ teaspoon freshly ground black pepper
- ¼ teaspoon salt

BURGERS

- 3 pounds ground lamb
- 2 eggs
- ¼ cup chopped fresh cilantro leaves
- 1½ teaspoons chopped garlic
- 1½ teaspoons kosher salt
- 1½ teaspoons freshly ground black pepper
- ¼ cup Worcestershire sauce
- 6 ounces fresh chèvre
- 6 brioche or burger buns
- 1 head green or red leaf lettuce
- 2 ripe tomatoes, sliced
- 1 red onion, sliced

Using ground lamb rather than the more traditional beef in a burger adds a juicier flavor, especially if you're using naturally raised young spring lamb. Many farms offer lamb of this quality, and butcher shops will probably offer a better selection than the meat aisle of your local grocery store. Eggs help the burger mixture bind together and cook more evenly. The addition of cilantro to the burger mixture and cilantro and mint to the aioli gives the dish a pop of vibrant flavor. Pair with a fortifying amber ale that allows malts and hops to mingle harmoniously.

1 **MAKE THE AIOLI:** Whisk the aioli, cilantro, mint, garlic, lemon juice, black pepper, and salt together in a small bowl to fully incorporate the ingredients. Cover and refrigerate until ready to serve.

2 **MAKE THE BURGERS:** Mix the lamb, eggs, cilantro, garlic, salt, pepper, and Worcestershire in a large bowl until combined. Form the burger mixture into six 7-ounce patties, transfer to a plate, cover with plastic wrap, and store them in the refrigerator until ready to use, or up to 1 day.

3 Prepare a medium-high fire in a gas or charcoal grill.

4 Transfer the patties to the grill and cook until medium-well, 5 to 6 minutes per side. Remove the patties from the grill. Top the burgers with the chèvre, dividing the cheese equally. Let the patties rest for 1 minute.

5 Spread the aioli on the bottom halves of the buns, and then top with the lettuce, tomato, and onion. Add the burger patties and top halves and serve immediately.

Makes 6 burgers

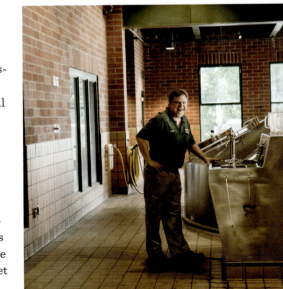

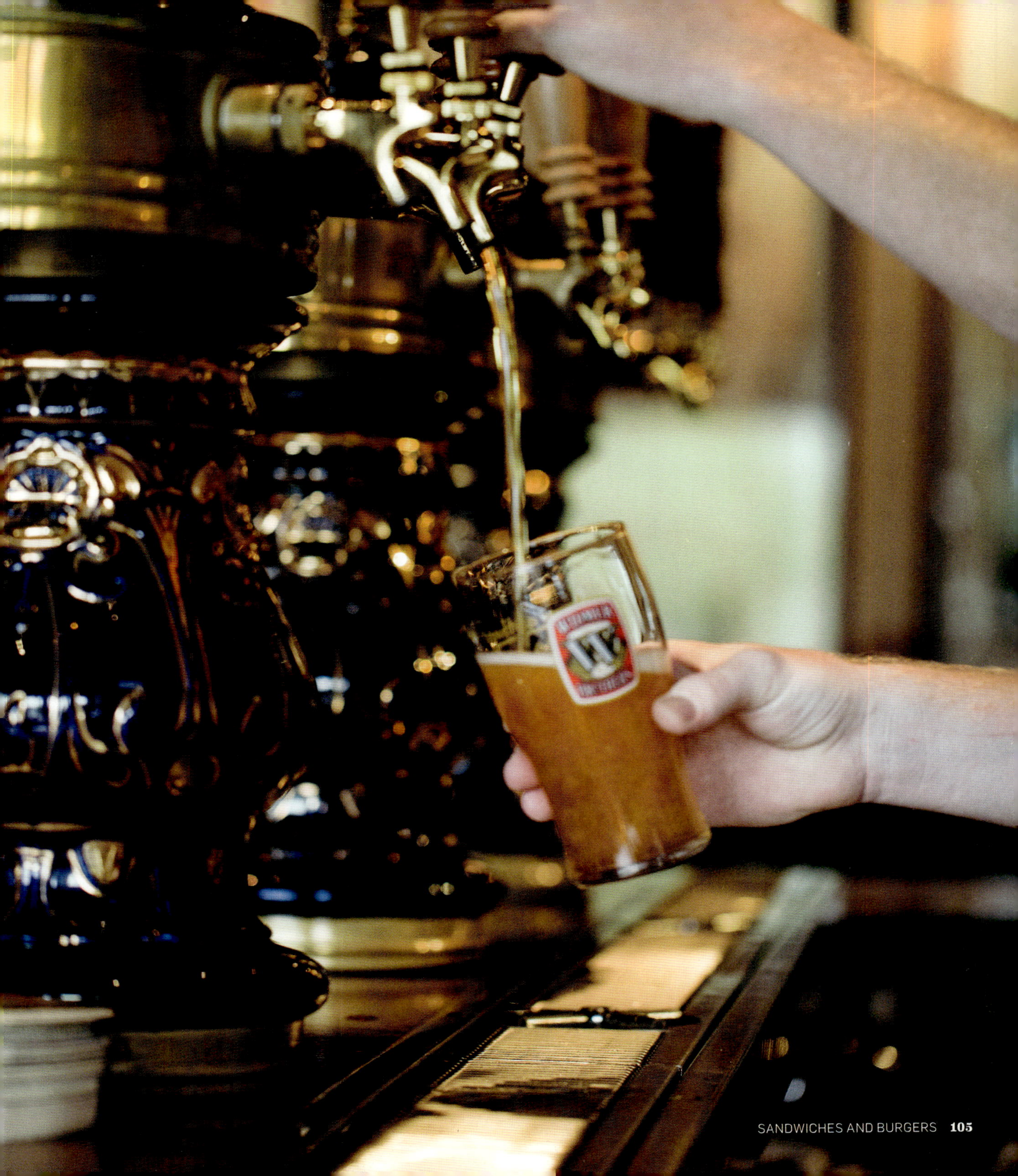

It seemed like a simple enough idea at the time. The affable Kurt and Rob Widmer were homebrewers who went pro in the early pioneer days of the Oregon beer scene. At first they offered two beers on tap — an alt-bier and a weizenbier — but when one of their favorite accounts asked for a third offering, the brothers faced a problem. They only had two fermenters, which limited the quantities of beer they could produce. To remedy the situation, they decided to let the weizenbier sit in the fermenter a little longer and then serve it unfiltered. The golden hazy concoction is credited with being the first "American hefeweizen" and it helped put the brothers and the brewery on the craft beer map.

Today, *Widmer* produces a stunning array of widely available beers that are deeply flavorful and strong on creativity. The hefeweizen remains the most popular in the lineup; served with a lemon, or not, it's an American classic that inspired future brewers to join the trade.

Hot Tea Sandwich

Jimmy Carbone is one of New York City's great men of beer, serving customers an ever-changing selection of draft and bottled beers, many of them local, at his restaurant, Jimmy's No. 43. He has created an environment where simple yet flavorful dishes and craft brews are eaten and appreciated together. This comfort-food sandwich, according to Jimmy, is an homage to Elvis. The banana esters that emerge from the yeast strain used in hefeweizen make the beer an ideal match for this sandwich. And while it might seem strange, do not skip the sea salt, as it adds great flavor. Jimmy urges chefs to cook with local ingredients and free-trade bananas when possible to make this relatively simple dish. Multiply the ingredients to make additional sandwiches if cooking for a crowd.

2 tablespoons almond butter
  Brioche or thin white sandwich bread, such as Pepperidge Farm
1 banana
2 teaspoons honey
  Smoked sea salt
1 tablespoon unsalted butter

1 Spread the almond butter on the inside of one slice of the bread, thoroughly coating.

2 Mash the banana with a fork and spread it on the second slice of bread. Drizzle the honey over the almond butter and banana. Sprinkle the sandwich filling with the smoked sea salt. Combine the two slices into a sandwich.

3 Heat a cast iron (or similar) skillet over medium heat and then melt the butter. Grill the sandwich in the skillet until one side is golden, about 2 minutes. Flip the sandwich and cook until the second side turns golden brown, about 2 minutes longer. Remove the sandwich from the skillet, cut into triangles, and serve immediately.

Makes 1 sandwich

PROFILE ★ **Follow the steep staircase** down to the entrance of this basement bar in Manhattan's East Village and open the wooden door. There you find a cozy spot filled with the aromas of a slow-food-minded kitchen, the sounds of excited but relaxed conversation, and the general warmth that comes from a quality bar. Jimmy Carbone, the generous and gregarious owner of *Jimmy's No. 43*, keeps a good variety flowing through his taps, and his staff is knowledgeable, helping new customers and established patrons alike find the perfect pint.

Pork Tenderloin Sandwich

- 4 (8-ounce) boneless pork top loin chops
- 1 cup all-purpose flour
- ½ cup buttermilk
- 2 cups panko breadcrumbs
  Salt and freshly ground black pepper
  Garlic powder
- 2 tablespoons canola oil
- 4 white sandwich buns

In certain parts of the country a pork tenderloin sandwich is a source of pride that can spark a fierce debate among aficionados. Making this sandwich at home can jolt you out of a burger rut. Pounding out the meat not only speeds up cooking time, it also adds to the overall presentation, with the meat stretching well beyond the borders of its bun. Garnish with lettuce, tomato, onion, pickles, and a spicy mustard (try Bell's Spicy Two Hearted Mustard on page 71), and enjoy with an American wheat or pale ale.

1 Place the pork chops on a cutting board and cover each chop with a piece of plastic wrap. Evenly pound each chop with a kitchen mallet until it is 8 to 10 inches in diameter.

2 Put the flour in a shallow bowl. Pour the buttermilk into another shallow bowl, and put the breadcrumbs, seasoned with salt, pepper, and garlic powder to taste, in a third shallow bowl.

3 Dredge each chop first in the flour, then in the buttermilk, and finally in the breadcrumb mixture.

4 Heat the oil in a deep skillet. Add the pork chops, one at a time, to the skillet and fry for 3 to 5 minutes, or until cooked through. Remove and drain on a paper towel–lined plate. Garnish with condiments of choice and serve on sandwich buns.

Makes 4 sandwiches

PROFILE ★ **On the outskirts of Omaha,** big things are happening in a small brewery. Kim and Paul Kavulak have created a beer destination that's celebrated countrywide by those in the know. This is thanks in part to their welcoming and enthusiastic attitude toward the industry and their customers, and also because of their special beer releases, such as Mélange A Trois, a barrel-aged strong Belgian-style blonde ale; HopGod, an IPA sometimes aged in French oak chardonnay barrels; and Black Betty, a Russian imperial stout. While their beer is available in select cities and markets outside their native plains, their **Nebraska Brewing Co.** is great to visit in person thanks to a restaurant menu that satisfies hearty appetites and curious thirsts with brews only available on site.

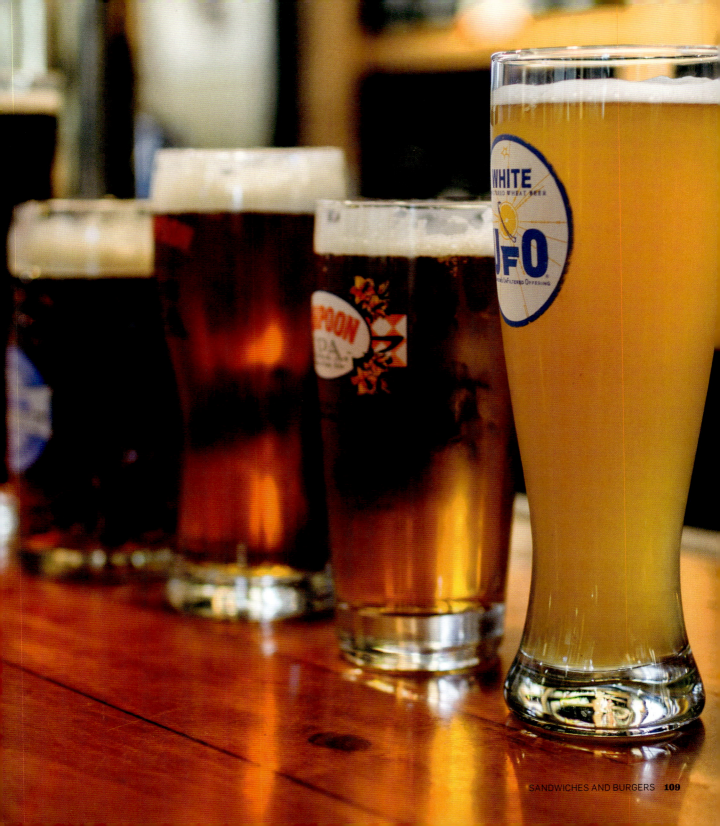

Barley-Crusted Tuna Sandwich with Remoulade

BARLEY CRUST

- 1⅓ cups pale malted barley
- ⅔ cup light brown sugar
- 1 tablespoon ground coriander
- 1½ teaspoons kosher salt
- 1 teaspoon freshly ground black pepper

REMOULADE

- 2 anchovy fillets, minced
- ¼ cup mayonnaise
- ¼ cup sweet relish
- 1 tablespoon lemon juice
- 1 tablespoon Worcestershire sauce
- 1 tablespoon finely chopped scallions
- 1½ teaspoons Dijon mustard
- 1½ teaspoons extra-virgin olive oil
- 1 teaspoon finely chopped fresh Italian parsley leaves
- ½ teaspoon garlic powder Freshly ground black pepper

SANDWICH

- 1 pound albacore tuna loins
- ¼ cup extra-virgin olive oil
- 4 hamburger buns
- 4 green leaf lettuce leaves
- 4 slices fresh tomato
- 4 thin slices red onion
- 4 lemon wedges

Even if you're not a brewer, you can easily obtain malted barley at homebrew supply shops and online. (Do **not** substitute malted barley flour; it will not give you the texture you want for the crust.) The barley crust on the tuna gives a satisfying crunch to this meaty sandwich, and the tangy, salty remoulade brings an additional layer of flavor; the sauce is also great as a dip for a side of French fries. With the crispy, malty crust, you'll want to drink a malty beer. Rogue suggests its single-malt ale, made with malts grown micro floor-malted and kilned at its own facility. Other brewers are experimenting, with single-malt beers, so consult your local brewpub or bottle shop for additional suggestions.

1 MAKE THE BARLEY CRUST: Pulse the malted barley in the bowl of a food processor until it reaches a medium-fine coarseness. Add the brown sugar, coriander, salt, and pepper, and mix until well combined. Spread the mixture onto a large plate and set aside.

2 MAKE THE REMOULADE: Combine the anchovies, mayonnaise, relish, lemon juice, Worcestershire, scallions, mustard, olive oil, parsley, garlic powder, and black pepper in a medium bowl and mix until fully incorporated. Set aside.

3 MAKE THE SANDWICHES: Coat the tuna with 2 tablespoons of the olive oil and press each piece into the crust mixture, turning to thoroughly coat all sides. Set the coated tuna on a plate.

4 Warm the remaining 2 tablespoons olive oil in a skillet over medium heat. Add the tuna to the hot oil and cook until the barley browns, about 2 minutes per side. (The tuna should remain pink on the inside.)

5 Spread the remoulade on the bottom halves of the buns, reserving any extra remoulade for another use. Layer the lettuce, tomato, onion, and tuna on top of the bun. Add the top halves and serve immediately, garnished with the lemon wedges.

Makes 4 sandwiches

½ cup raw unsalted
   pistachios, finely chopped
¼ cup panko breadcrumbs
4 (6-ounce) fresh salmon
   fillets
½ cup (1 stick) unsalted butter
¼ cup hefeweizen
½ Meyer lemon, zested, then
   peeled and segmented
   Salt and white pepper
2 tablespoons canola or other
   light salad oil
4 soft sandwich rolls
4 butter lettuce leaves

A Few Beers to Try with This Recipe

- *Flying Dog In-Heat Wheat*
- *Saint Arnold Weedwacker*
- *Shiner Hefeweizen*
- *Sierra Nevada Kellerweis Hefeweizen*
- *Yazoo Hefeweizen*

Pistachio-Crusted Salmon Sandwich with Meyer Lemon Butter

The satisfying, nutty crunch from the salmon's crust yields to the sweet, soft, and flaky fish, and the whole thing gets a zing of flavor from the tart lemon butter. A hefeweizen or summer beer is the perfect accompaniment.

1 Combine the pistachios and bread-crumbs in a shallow baking dish. Press each salmon fillet into the crust mixture, turning once to coat both sides. Put the coated salmon on a plate, cover with plastic wrap, and set aside in the refrigerator for 1 hour.

2 Whip the butter with a whisk in a small bowl until smooth. Add the beer, lemon zest, and lemon segments, and mash together to fully combine. Season with salt and pepper to taste.

3 Warm the oil in a large non-stick skillet over medium heat. Working in batches, sauté the salmon on one side for 2 to 3 minutes. Turn and cook until the salmon is cooked through, about 10 minutes total per inch of thickness of the fillet.

4 Spread the rolls with the Meyer lemon butter. Top each roll with a fillet and butter lettuce and serve.

Makes 4 sandwiches

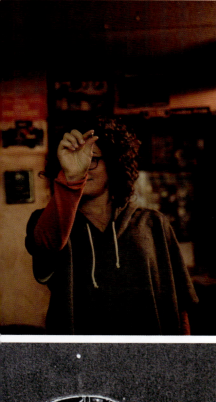

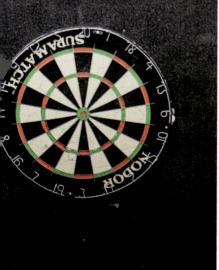

Ken Grossman was operating a homebrew shop in Chico in the late 1970s when he caught wind of a small brewery that had opened in Sonoma. He took a drive, checked it out, and realized that what that brewer — Jack McAuliffe — had created was a new brewery with a mix of repurposed equipment. Grossman, who had always been handy and had a keen engineering mind, realized he could do the same thing. So he did, and the *Sierra Nevada Brewing Company* was born. Today it's one of the largest craft breweries in the country and its flagship Pale Ale, with its distinctive green label, is one of the most recognized craft beers.

The once small brewery has grown into a sprawling campus where some of the best beer in the country is produced around the clock and shipped around the world. Tourists line up to get a firsthand look at the immaculately clean brewery and its facilities, including one of the most impressive waste management systems anywhere. Most visitors stop at the great restaurant for their fill of any number of hearty and innovative dishes (look around and try to find the hidden Bigfoot likenesses while you dine) before heading to the gift shop for those much-needed logo items.

Sierra Nevada is heading into its second generation of family ownership, and all of its employees are vested in the company and understand that the company's success is good for everyone. To that end, it's rare to meet an employee who is not smiling and happy to be a part of the brewery. Of course, when you work around beer of Sierra Nevada's quality, inventiveness, and taste, it's hard not to be pleased.

Business has been so strong and demand so great that Sierra Nevada recently announced that it would build a second brewery on the East Coast. The 184-acre site is 12 miles south of Asheville, North Carolina, in the Henderson County town of Mills River along the French Broad River. Similar to its northern California counterpart, the new facility will be a full-production brewery with plans for an on-premises restaurant and gift shop. The initial design calls for a capacity of up to 300,000 barrels, with room for expansion. The added barrelage will accommodate wider production of seasonal beers and bottled specialties when it opens to the public in 2014.

Black Bean Sliders

4 cups cooked black beans, drained
6 medium white mushrooms, chopped
1 medium carrot, peeled and chopped
½ medium white onion, diced
2 teaspoons chili powder
2 teaspoons kosher salt
1 garlic clove, crushed
1 jalapeño pepper
1 egg
¼ cup heavy cream
4 cups panko breadcrumbs
1 cup all-purpose flour
   Canola oil, for frying
   Miniature kaiser rolls, lightly toasted
   Cheese of your choice for serving (optional)
   Pico de gallo, for serving
   Guacamole, for serving

This is not your average veggie burger. Packed with flavor, easy to make, and satisfying for even the heartiest of carnivores, this is one of the most popular items at Elysian. One bite and you'll see why. The spice level is up to you — for milder patties remove the seeds from the jalapeño. Top with your choice of cheese, pico de gallo, and guacamole, and then pair with a flavorful lager.

1 Purée the beans, mushrooms, carrot, onion, chili powder, salt, garlic, jalapeño, egg, and cream in the bowl of a food processor until smooth.

2 Transfer the mixture to a large bowl and mix in the breadcrumbs. Let the mixture sit at room temperature for 10 minutes.

3 Place the flour in a small bowl and heat about ⅛ inch of oil in a large skillet. Portion the bean mixture into ten 3- to 4-ounce balls, flatten into puck-shaped disks, and dip in the flour to coat all sides. Knock off any excess flour, and pan-fry the patties until browned, about 2 minutes per side.

4 Place a patty on each roll and garnish with cheese, pico de gallo, and guacamole before serving.

Makes 10 sliders

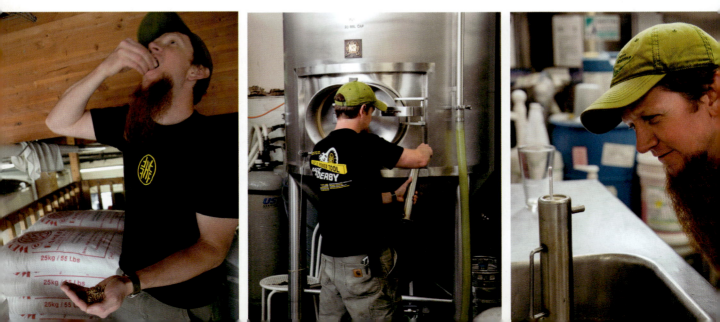

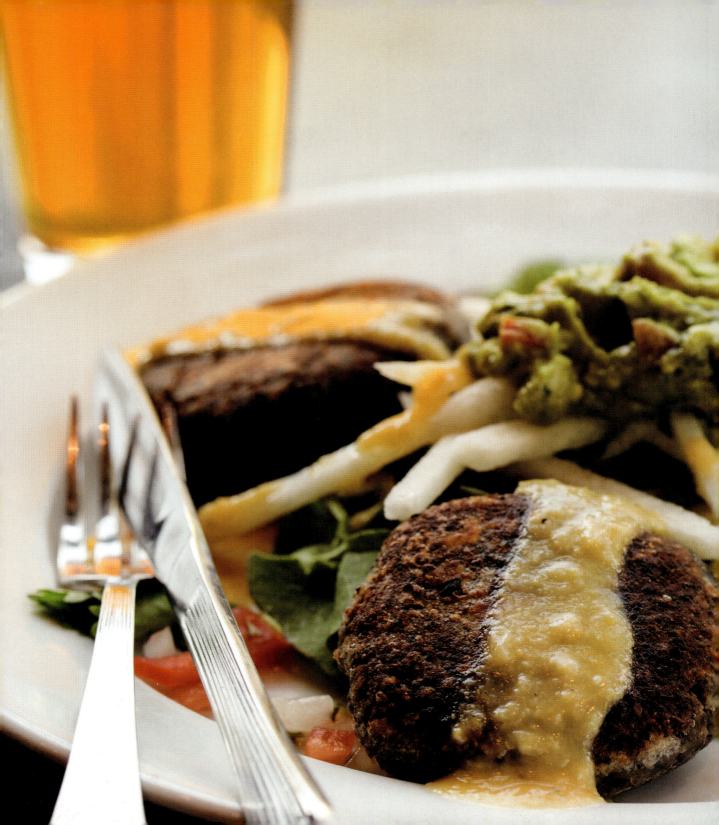

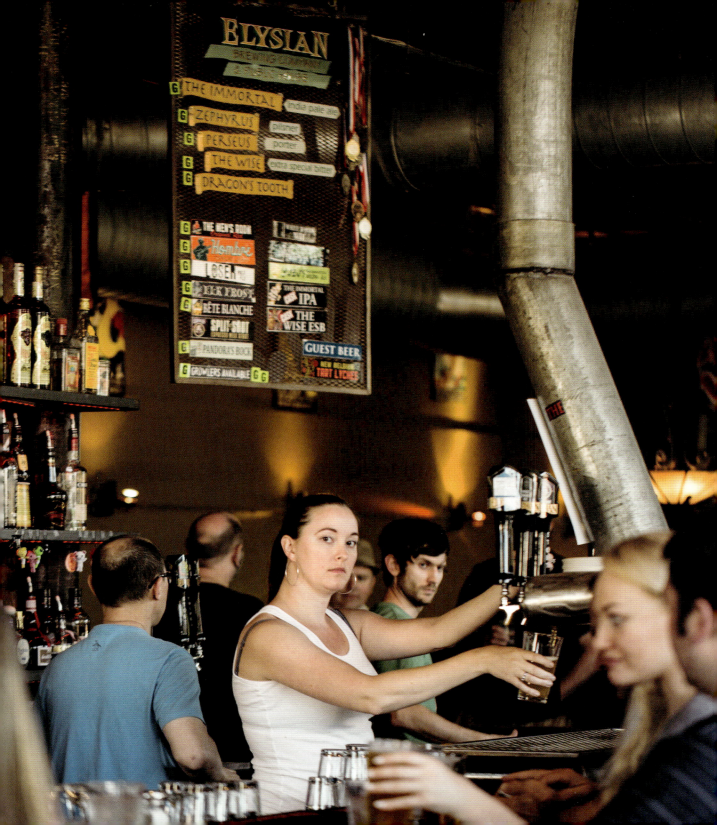

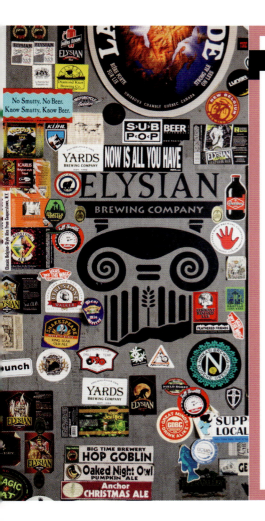

Elysian is many good things, but it is certainly a prince of the pumpkins. As beers using the gourd became more popular, the Seattle-based brewery separated itself from the pack.

Dark O' the Moon is one of three Elysian beers that are bottled and distributed, and each year the brewery makes at least two more on draft. Dick Cantwell, an owner and the head brewer at Elysian, said the company has probably made 20 different pumpkin beers over the years. Elysian's love of the round orange squash is so great that each October the brewery hosts a two-day event called the Great Pumpkin Beer Festival. It features more than 30 pumpkin beers, food fit for cooler weather, pumpkin carvings, and the release of Elysian's Great Pumpkin Ale, at 8.1 percent ABV. The brewery describes the beer as "deep copper with a ghostly white head. Intense pumpkin, sugar, and spice on the nose with a nice bready and malty backdrop to tame all those autumn spices into a remarkably smooth, balanced, and delectable fall treat."

The festival is the brewery's biggest day of the year, and Elysian always finds new ways to cram in even more pumpkin flavor, including filling a huge pumpkin full of pumpkin-conditioned beer (secondary fermentation takes place in the pumpkin).

Elysian was founded in 1995 by principals Dick Cantwell, Joe Bisacca, and David Buhler, and their first location — ambitious for a start-up — was a 220-seat beer hall in Seattle's Capitol Hill neighborhood. It's since grown to several more locations, including a large production facility. Elysian routinely releases unique brews that earn the respect and notice of peers and customers.

Grilled Italian Sando

Combining many flavors commonly found in rustic Italian cooking yields this light and flavorful sandwich. Thick focaccia makes all the difference in this handheld beauty; its texture allows the bread to absorb the oil, balsamic vinegar, and natural juices from the veggies. Enjoy with a side salad or French fries and a lighter beer, such as a pale ale.

8 thin slices eggplant

8 thin slices yellow squash

　Olive oil, to coat vegtables

　Salt and freshly ground
　　black pepper

1¼ cups balsamic vinegar

1 loaf focaccia bread, about
　　10 × 15 inches

　Garlic oil

4 ounce garlic cream cheese

6 ounces roasted red pepper

8 slices fresh tomato

4 slices raw red onion

1　Prepare a medium fire in a gas or charcoal grill. Brush the eggplant and squash with olive oil and season with salt and pepper to taste. Grill, turning once, until the slices are soft and show a little char from the grill, 5 to 7 minutes.

2　Put the balsamic vinegar in a small saucepan and bring to a boil over medium-high heat. When the vinegar begins to boil, reduce it to a simmer, and cook until the liquid is reduced by half, 4 to 6 minutes.

3　Cut the focaccia in half lengthwise and drizzle the inside with garlic oil. Grill the halves, cut side down, until lightly browned. Cut each half into quarters.

4　Spread one-quarter of the cream cheese on one of the bottom-half quarters of focaccia. Top with 2 slices of squash, a few pieces of red pepper, 2 slices of eggplant, 2 slices of tomato, a slice of onion, and a drizzle of the balsamic reduction. Top the fillings with the second slice of bread. Repeat to make three more sandwiches and serve.

Makes 4 sandwiches

PROFILE ★　**A leader in the hop-forward thinking** that has made California breweries famous, ***Bear Republic*** does not disappoint when it comes to lupulin. Beers such as Racer 5 IPA, Hop Rod Rye, XP Pale Ale, Black Racer, and Racer X all showcase the hop bite one would want and expect from a California craft brewer. Bear Republic's other offerings, from brown ales to stouts, also pack a considerable hop kick.

While its beers are great for home consumption, check out Bear Republic's brewpub for the full experience. The pub, which features a full menu and friendly atmosphere, is a family affair owned by Richard R. Norgrove (behind the bar) and his wife, Sandy (greeting you at the door), and Richard G. Norgrove (son and brewmaster) and his wife, Tami (handling the books). Factor in the other employees who are like family and you have a great place to enjoy a fun night out.

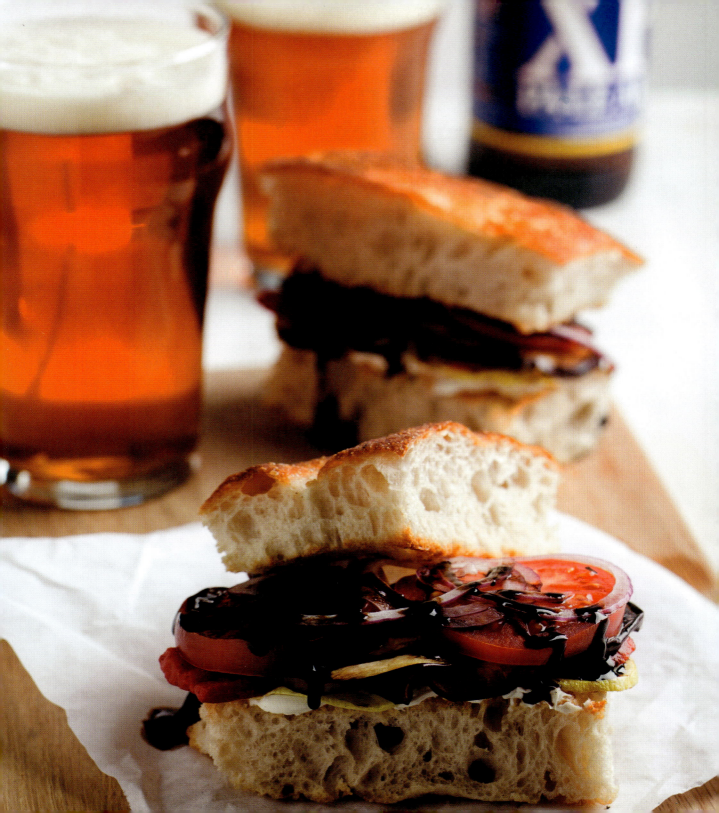

Potato Chip Chicken Sandwich

1 cup mayonnaise
1 bunch scallions, roughly chopped
2 teaspoons freshly ground black pepper
1 teaspoon salt
2 teaspoons fresh lemon juice
1 (14.5-ounce) bag potato chips
1 teaspoon ground coriander
1 teaspoon paprika
4 eggs
1 tablespoon water
1 cup all-purpose flour
4 boneless, skinless chicken breasts
  Vegetable oil, for cooking
4 sandwich rolls

This is a pairing that allows many flavors and textures to play in harmony. The sandwich harkens back to school days, when placing chips on a sandwich felt like culinary innovation. But serving pale ale on the side is decidedly adult. The pale ale is still light enough to allow the mayonnaise and fried chicken their palate dominance, but a hop varietal — like Zythos — with citrus and pine notes stands up to the grassy sharpness of the scallions. Serve the sandwich on a hearty roll and garnish with a cheese of your choice and other sandwich fixings.

1 Pulse the mayonnaise, the scallions, 1 teaspoon of the black pepper, the salt, and the lemon juice in the bowl of a food processor until the scallions are finely ground, 1 to 2 minutes. Cover and refrigerate until ready to use.

2 Make a small opening in the bag of chips to let the air out, and then crush the potato chips inside the bag. Pour the crumbs into a shallow baking dish and add the remaining 1 teaspoon black pepper, the coriander, and the paprika, and set aside. Whisk the eggs and water together in a separate shallow bowl and set aside. Pour the flour into a third shallow bowl and set aside.

3 Pound the chicken breasts to a thickness of about 1/2 inch. Dredge the chicken breasts in the flour, shake off the excess, and then dip them into the egg. Finally, dip the breasts into the potato chip mixture, pressing firmly and turning to thoroughly coat the chicken with the chips.

4 Heat 1/2 inch of oil in a large skillet over medium-high heat. Pan-fry the chicken breasts in batches until golden brown, 5 to 7 minutes per side. Remove, and drain any excess oil on a paper towel–lined plate.

5 Spread the scallion mayonnaise on the top half of the inside of the rolls. Add a chicken breast to each roll, top with desired accoutrements, and serve.

Makes 4 sandwiches

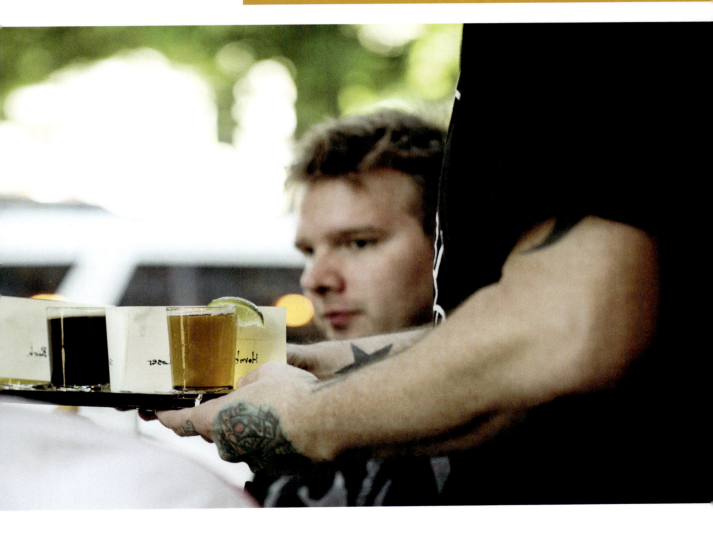

FOUNDERS BREWING COMPANY

GRAND RAPIDS, MICHIGAN

Devil Dancer Chicken Sandwich

Chipotle mayonnaise, purchased or homemade (see box)
1 French roll, halved and toasted
½ chipotle pepper in adobo, thinly sliced
½ jalapeño pepper, thinly sliced
½ banana pepper, thinly sliced
2 slices Muenster cheese
¼ pound leftover roast chicken
2 thin slices red onion
2 slices pepper jack cheese

This spicy-hot sandwich is perfect for those afternoons when the leftovers from last night's roast chicken are calling your name. This sandwich pairs very well with an aggressively hopped IPA. You should look for a beer with big aromatics to complement the spicy notes of the peppers. So, do you dare to dance with the devil? If it's a sandwich this good, yes. Multiply ingredients as needed to make additional sandwiches.

Spread the mayonnaise on each side of the roll to taste. Layer the peppers, Muenster, chicken, onion, and pepper jack on the bottom half of the roll. Close the sandwich and serve.

Makes 1 sandwich

Chipotle Mayonnaise

Put 1 cup mayonnaise and 2 chipotle peppers in adobo sauce in the bowl of a food processor, and blend until combined.

PROFILE ★ **Founders Brewing Company** has a beer-brewing philosophy that is displayed at its brewery: "We don't brew beer for the masses. Instead, our beers are crafted for a chosen few, a small cadre of renegades and rebels who enjoy a beer that pushes the limits of what is commonly accepted as taste. In short, we make beer for people like us."

So, who are they? Mike Stevens and Dave Engbers were guys with steady jobs who wanted to chase their dreams. They found their fulfillment the day they opened their brewery. They started with safe, true-to-style beers but quickly reconsidered their direction and began brewing complex, in-your-face ales with huge aromatics, bigger body, and tons of flavor. That was the ticket!

Now rated among the best breweries in the world, Founders has a solid lineup of respected, sought-after big beers — perhaps none more than its Kentucky Breakfast Stout, an imperial stout that is cave aged in oak bourbon barrels for 1 year. It makes an appearance just once a year in March and quickly sells out. In fact, its release each year brings fans from around the country to the brewery to line up early for that first sip.

Portabella Sub

A little work goes a long way with this sandwich. Marinating the mushrooms before cooking and then finishing the sandwich with a drizzle of beer glaze brings a flavorful boost to the humble fungi. Pair this warm sandwich with a crisp pale ale, and you'll have a combo to remember.

LONG TRAIL BREWING COMPANY

BRIDGEWATER CORNERS, VERMONT

2 cups balsamic vinegar
1 (12-ounce) bottle Long Trail Ale, or similar altbier
1 tablespoon light brown sugar
8 whole portabella mushrooms, cleaned and sliced into ½-inch slices
4 garlic cloves, minced
½ cup extra-virgin olive oil
1 teaspoon salt
1 teaspoon freshly ground black pepper
1 cup roasted red peppers, slivered
6 French sandwich rolls, sliced in half lengthwise and toasted
12 slices cheddar cheese

1 Bring the vinegar, beer, and brown sugar to a boil in a saucepan over medium heat and boil, stirring occasionally, until reduced by half, about 30 minutes.

2 Toss the mushrooms, garlic, olive oil, salt, and black pepper together in a medium mixing bowl.

3 Preheat the oven to broil.

4 Sauté the mushrooms and red peppers in a large skillet over medium-high heat until softened, 5 to 7 minutes. Fill each roll with the mushroom-pepper mixture, drizzle with the glaze (about ¼ cup per sandwich), and top with the cheese.

5 Transfer the sandwiches to a baking sheet and broil until the cheese melts. Cut in half and serve immediately.

Makes 6 sandwiches

PROFILE ★ **Long Trail has been encouraging customers** to "Take A Hike" since its founding. Its logo depicts a trekker, stick in hand, taking to the trails, and it's the brewery's commitment to and fondness for nature that has brought many fans to this flavorful brand. Long Trail's visitor center is modeled after the famed Hofbrauhaus in Munich, and the large yet cozy space — with a restaurant that specializes in and celebrates local food — makes it hard to leave and get back on the trail.

Marie's Turkey Sandwich

Mayonnaise
2 slices fresh sourdough
   bread
4 slices all-natural oven-
   roasted turkey
2 red leaf lettuce leaves
2 slices fresh tomato
2 slices thick-cut bacon,
   cooked until crispy
2 slices smoked cheddar
   cheese

The simple pleasure of a great sandwich is made possible by quality ingredients and proper construction. This sandwich combines familiar flavors in a working collaboration that never goes out of style. Serve with a pale wheat ale or a summer brew, any lighter beer with a zest of flavor. It is easy to double the ingredients if making more than one sandwich at a time.

Spread the mayonnaise on the inside of each slice of bread to taste. Layer the turkey, lettuce, tomato, bacon, and cheese on the bottom slice. Top with the second slice of bread and serve.

Makes 1 sandwich

A Few Beers to Try with This Recipe

- *Big Sky Montana Trout Slayer Wheat Ale*
- *Jackie O's Orange Oak*
- *Lagunitas Little Sumpin' Sumpin' Ale*
- *Southern Tier Hop Sun*
- *Stevens Point Nude Beach Summer Wheat*
- *Three Floyds Gumballhead*
- *Wolaver's Wildflower Wheat*

PROFILE ★ **In 1997, Wolaver's became the first** organic brewer certified by the United States Department of Agriculture. The brewery model perfectly fit the organic lifestyle many Vermonters love, and it quickly gained a following. Wolaver's later merged with Otter Creek, and the two used organic barley and worked with farmers in the area to create an "organic beer market." Since Wolaver's, a number of other breweries around the country have followed suit by producing their own organic beers.

Pickled Jalapeño Turkey Sandwich

The earthiness of sprouts blends well with the tang from the cream cheese and cheddar in this sandwich. With a little heat from the hot sauce (a vinegar-based blend is best for this recipe) and the coolness of the turkey and cucumber, this sandwich uses simple ingredients to pack a lot of flavor. Try pairing it with a Vienna lager. Multiply ingredients as needed to make additional sandwiches.

1 kaiser roll, split open
2 tablespoons cream cheese
Hot sauce
2 ounces alfalfa sprouts
4 slices roasted turkey breast
2 slices sharp cheddar cheese
4 slices cucumber
3–5 thin slices pickled jalapeños

1 Spread the bottom half of the roll with the cream cheese and drizzle the hot sauce over the top to taste.

2 Layer the sprouts, turkey, cheese, cucumber, and jalapeños on the bottom half of the roll. Top with the other half of the roll, slice in half, and serve.

Makes 1 sandwich

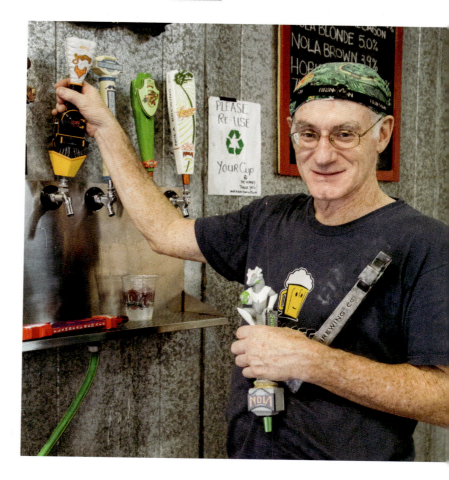

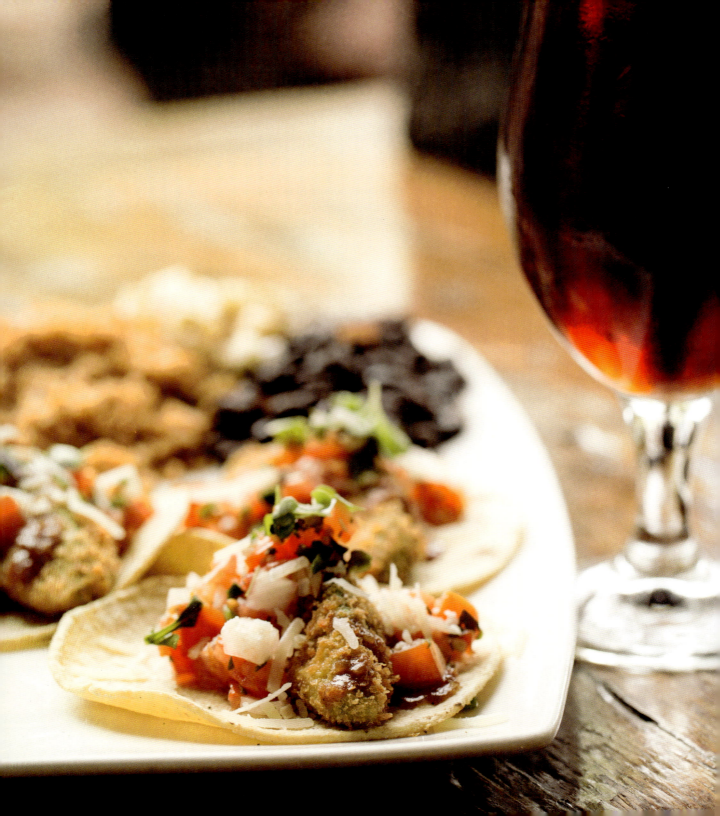

Arrogant Bastard Ale Avocado Tacos

STONE BREWING CO.
ESCONDIDO, CALIFORNIA

The Stone Brewing Co. is very vegetarian friendly, and this recipe from the Southern California brewery offers strong proof. Nor does the brewery do anything half-assed, and again this recipe is proof. What follows is the how-to for preparing and assembling Stone's avocado tacos, including the batter and salsa fresca recipes. Stone recommends using its barbecue sauce (available on its website), or you may substitute another natural sauce. Vegetarian tacos are a great alternative to meat-laden variations, and all the fresh ingredients in this recipe really bring a pop of flavor. If frying is not your thing, the avocados can be served fresh. Accompany the tacos with black beans, Spanish-style rice, and an American strong ale like Arrogant Bastard Ale, which has a smack of hop bitterness.

SALSA FRESCA

- 1½ cups seeded and diced plum tomatoes
- ¼ cup diced yellow onion
- ¼ cup seeded and finely diced jalapeño peppers
- ¼ cup lime juice
- 2 tablespoons finely chopped fresh cilantro leaves
- Salt and freshly ground black pepper

ARROGANT BASTARD ALE BATTERED AVOCADOS

- 2 cups Stone Arrogant Bastard Ale, chilled
- ¾ teaspoon Cajun spice blend
- ½ teaspoon ground dried chipotle chiles
- ½ teaspoon granulated garlic
- ½ teaspoon kosher salt
- ½ teaspoon smoked paprika
- 1 cup all-purpose flour
- 1 teaspoon baking powder
- 4½ ripe avocados, peeled, pitted, and quartered
- 2 cups panko breadcrumbs
- Salt

TACOS

- 1 cup Stone Levitation Ale BBQ Sauce, or similar barbecue sauce
- 18 small corn tortillas
- 1 cup grated Asiago cheese
- Microgreens or chopped fresh parsley, for garnish

1 MAKE THE SALSA FRESCA: Combine the tomatoes, onion, jalapeños, lime juice, and cilantro in a bowl and stir to combine. Season with salt and pepper to taste. Cover the bowl with plastic wrap and refrigerate for at least 30 minutes or up to 3 days to allow the flavors to mingle.

2 MAKE THE BATTER: Pour the ale into a narrow high-sided container. Stir in the Cajun spice blend, chiles, garlic, salt, and paprika.

3 Sift the flour and baking powder together in a small bowl, then add them to the beer mixture slowly, whisking well until the ingredients are thoroughly incorporated. Add more flour if necessary to create a tempura-style batter for coating the avocados. Set the batter aside.

4 Preheat the oven to 200°F. Prepare a deep fryer or pour 2 to 3 inches of oil into a deep cast iron or heavy pot that is at least 4 inches deep. Heat the oil to 360°F. Pour the breadcrumbs into a shallow dish.

recipe continues on next page

5 Use tongs to grab the avocado quarters and dunk them in the prepared batter. Shake off any excess and roll the avocados in the breadcrumbs to coat all sides. Fry the avocados in batches until golden brown, 1 to 2½ minutes each. (Do not overcrowd the pot, as this will lower the temperature of the oil significantly.)

6 Transfer the cooked avocados to a parchment paper–lined baking sheet. Season with a sprinkling of salt and keep them in the oven until the entire batch is ready.

7 **ASSEMBLE THE TACOS:** Heat the barbecue sauce in a medium saucepan over medium-low heat, stirring occasionally, until heated through. Warm the tortillas on a griddle or in the oven, if desired.

8 Place one avocado quarter on each of the tortillas. Top each avocado with the warm barbecue sauce, salsa, cheese, and microgreens. Serve immediately.

Makes 6–8 servings

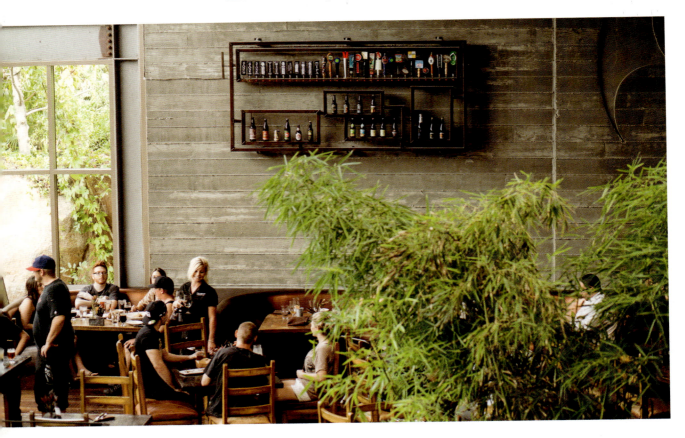

PROFILE ★ **Stone Brewing Co.** is home to some of the most assertive, cocksure, unapologetic, and respected beers in the country. From its perch in Southern California, Stone has slowly been taking over the country with the goal of replacing fizzy yellow beer with concoctions of substance. A forward-thinking brewery, Stone uses as many locally sourced ingredients as possible for its Stone Brewing World Bistro and Gardens restaurant. The company is also known for its philanthropy and being a leader in collaboration brews. It's staffed with cunning linguists, so be sure to carefully read their labels, and try to keep up.

Croque Monsieur with Blackberry Onions

1 teaspoon extra-virgin olive oil

½ yellow onion, thinly sliced

4 blackberries or 2 tablespoons blackberry jam

2 slices hearty sourdough bread

4 slices Serrano ham, Iberico ham, or prosciutto

1 slice Gruyère cheese Mayonnaise or Dijon mustard (optional)

A hot topping on a common sandwich adds a certain fanciness without much work. In this case, sautéed onions and blackberries mirror the saltiness of the ham and the nuttiness of the cheese; the tang of the sourdough bread brings it all together. Pair with a bière de garde that has a slightly sour taste with some sweet undertones, such as Domaine DuPage from Two Brothers.

1 Heat the oil in a large skillet over medium heat until shimmering. Add the onions and cook, stirring occasionally, until they begin to soften, about 5 minutes. Add the blackberries, reduce the heat to medium-low, stir well, and cook until the berries break down and the mixture is the consistency of jam, 5 to 10 minutes longer.

2 Preheat the oven to 250°F. Top one slice of the sourdough with the ham, then the cheese, and then the blackberry onions. Spread the mayonnaise or mustard, if using, over the inside of the second slice of the bread, close the sandwich, place on a baking sheet, and bake for 3 to 5 minutes, flipping once. Remove from the oven, slice, and serve.

Makes 1 sandwich

There is no sibling rivalry at *Two Brothers Brewing Company*, as brothers Jim and Jason Ebel have brought individual strengths and passions to the brewery they cofounded in 1995. Both brothers had spent time in Europe, where they learned about beer styles and culture while expanding their own tastes. After returning home, Jim took up homebrewing and soon brought Jason into his hobby. Before long, beer and brewing were all they could talk about, and it became a foregone career choice.

Together they opened a homebrew (and wine) shop called the Brewer's Coop in 1993. Jason eventually moved to Colorado to begin work as a brewer, and Jim enrolled in law school and kept the shop going (with the help of his wife and mother). But as the interest in homebrewing grew, so did business, and soon Jason moved back to help out with the shop and work as a brewer at a local pub.

Soon the idea began to ferment that the brothers should open their own place, and one night their mother had the final say. "You guys either need to open a brewery or shut up about it 'cause you're driving me crazy," the brothers recall her saying. Thus, Two Brothers was born, and it has grown tremendously since then as customers have embraced its ales of all styles. Several expansions later, the brewery is still 100 percent family owned and now includes a brewpub, a separate restaurant, and a large brewery.

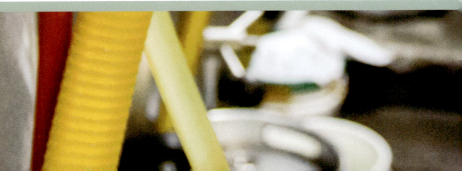

Vegetarian Green
Chili, see page 134

Soup, Stew, and Chili

Everything You Need and Want in One Bowl

Vegetarian Green Chili

see photo, page 132

1 cup canola oil
2 medium yellow onions, diced
6 garlic cloves, minced
1½ cups all-purpose flour
1 pound green Anaheim chiles, diced
1 pound plum tomatoes, diced
½ bunch fresh cilantro, finely chopped, plus more for serving
1 jalapeño pepper, diced
1 tablespoon dark chili powder
1 tablespoon ground cumin
1½ teaspoons cayenne pepper
9 cups vegetable broth
  Kosher salt
  Tortilla chips and sour cream, for serving

Colorado seems to be the epicenter of green chili. The dish draws the name from the color of peppers used. This vegetarian option has a nice kick and is great on its own; you can also serve it with pinto beans, tortillas, cheddar cheese, and scallions or use it as a topping for sandwiches and burgers.

1 Heat the oil in a soup pot over medium heat until shimmering. Add the onions and garlic and cook, stirring frequently, until translucent, about 4 minutes. Add the flour and cook, stirring constantly, until the mixture is golden brown.

2 Add the chiles, tomatoes, cilantro, jalapeño, chili powder, cumin, cayenne, and broth to the pot. Season with salt to taste. Cook the chili over low heat, stirring occasionally, until the tomatoes begin to break down, about 1½ hours.

3 Taste and adjust seasonings again.

4 Serve in a bowl topped with tortilla chips, sour cream, and fresh cilantro, if desired. The chili is also great with eggs or as a burger topping.

Makes 8–10 servings

PROFILE ★ **Denver is a beer lover's paradise,** and **Wynkoop**, the oldest brewpub in the city, is on everyone's must-visit list. Founded in the late 1980s by a group of young urban industry pioneers, the brewery has consistently served well-crafted pints and superb food that hits all the right notes. Its welcoming bar area and tables on the first floor are great places to gather with friends for conversation or to soak up the local scene. Upstairs is a billiards hall where friendly competition offers stress relief.

Wynkoop is also home to great events each year — like the Pints for Prostates fund-raiser, held when the Great American Beer Festival rolls into town. And while many will caution against mixing beer and politics, it's worked out quite nicely for one of the founders, John Hickenlooper, who was a successful mayor of Denver before ascending to the statehouse.

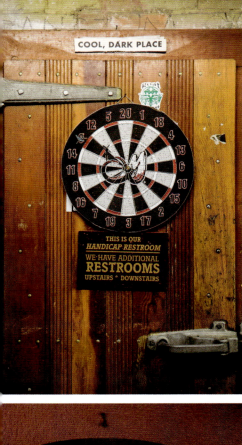

COOL, DARK PLACE

THIS IS OUR
HANDICAP RESTROOM
WE HAVE ADDITIONAL
RESTROOMS
UPSTAIRS • DOWNSTAIRS

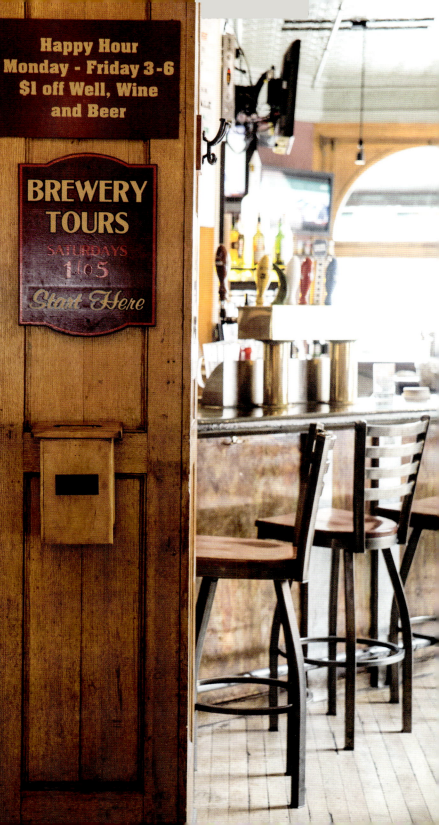

Happy Hour
Monday - Friday 3-6
$1 off Well, Wine
and Beer

BREWERY
TOURS
SATURDAYS
1:05
Start Here

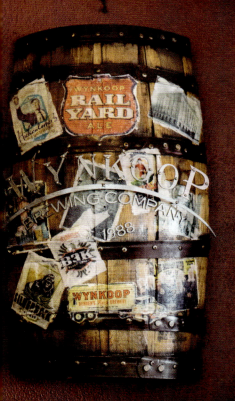

EPIC BREWING COMPANY

SALT LAKE CITY, UTAH

Curried Pumpkin Chicken Soup

- 2 boneless, skinless chicken breasts
- 2 teaspoons Madras green curry powder
- 1 teaspoon ancho chile powder
  Salt
- ¼ pound pork chorizo, ground
- ½ medium red onion, chopped
- 1 small tomato, chopped
- ¼ orange or yellow bell pepper, cored, seeded, and finely chopped
- 2 Gala apples
- 2 pounds unseasoned pumpkin purée
- 6 cups chicken broth
- 1 cup soy milk

A Few Beers to Try with This Recipe

- *Cape Ann Fisherman's Pumpkin Stout*
- *Elysian Dark o' the Moon*
- *Epic Fermentation without Representation Porter*
- *Saint Arnold Pumpkinator Imperial Pumpkin Stout*

This unique soup blends two great autumn bounties: apples and pumpkins. Curry powder and other spices give the vibrancy of the apples and the rich flavor of the pumpkin a subtle kick. A pumpkin stout or porter, with its malt roastiness and notes of cinnamon and allspice, rounds out the pumpkin experience.

1 Prepare a hot fire in a gas or charcoal grill. Season the chicken breasts with 1 teaspoon of the curry powder, the ancho chile powder, and salt to taste. Grill the chicken breasts until cooked through, 8 to 10 minutes per side. Transfer the chicken breasts to a cutting board to rest for 4 minutes, then dice the chicken into small pieces and set aside.

2 Brown the chorizo in a large soup pot over high heat. Add the red onion and sauté, stirring occasionally, until the chorizo is browned and the onions are well cooked, 5 to 6 minutes. Reduce the heat to medium-low.

3 Add the grilled chicken, the remaining 1 teaspoon green curry powder, the tomato, and the bell pepper to the pot. Cook, stirring frequently, until the tomato juice is cooked off, 10 to 15 minutes.

4 Remove the pot from the heat. Core and finely chop one of the apples. Add the chopped apple, pumpkin purée, chicken broth, and soy milk to the pot, set it back over high heat, and bring to a low boil. Cook, stirring often, until the soup has a nice, semi-thick consistency, just short of the consistency of applesauce, about 20 minutes.

5 Core and thinly slice the remaining apple. Ladle the soup into eight bowls, and garnish with the apple slices. Serve immediately. Store any leftovers in an airtight container in the refrigerator for up to 3 days or for up to 1 month in the freezer.

Makes 8 servings

WIENER MALZ

MÜNCHNER MALZ

ENBRAUMALZ HELL

NBRAUMALZ DUNKEL

ROGGENMALZ

CARAPILS ®

CARAHELL ®

ARAMÜNCH ®

ENCARAMELMALZ

CARAFA ®

AFA ® SPEZIAL

ENRÖSTMALZ

After Utah relaxed some of its strict alcohol rules in 2008, a few entrepreneurs — namely David Cole and Peter Erickson — saw an opportunity to open the kind of brewery they had long dreamed of running. ***Epic Brewing*** burst onto the scene with a bevy of ales and lagers that started in the 5 percent ABV range and rose from there. Offerings include pale ales, porters, and a particularly delightful sour-apple saison. They are gaining traction across the country, meaning you don't have to go to Utah to get Epic, but the brewery is certainly worth an in-person visit to see brewing passion at work.

Black Bean Soup

Hearty and delicious, this soup is a meal in itself and is even better a day or two after being made, when the flavors have had a chance to mingle. A hoppy amber or red ale is the perfect accompaniment, adding some heft, spice, and sweetness to the smoky rich soup.

2 tablespoons corn oil
1 yellow onion, diced
4 celery stalks, diced
1 carrot, peeled and cut into small coins
2 garlic cloves, minced
2¼ teaspoons ground cumin
1½ teaspoons garlic salt
1 teaspoon minced fresh oregano
1 teaspoon red pepper flakes
4 (15-ounce) cans black beans, with their liquid
1 (14.5-ounce) can fire-roasted tomatoes
1½ cups chicken broth
1½ cups water

1 Heat the oil in a large soup pot over medium heat. Add the onion, celery, and carrot, and sauté, stirring occasionally, until soft, 5 to 7 minutes.

2 Add the garlic to the pot and sauté, stirring occasionally, for 2 to 3 minutes longer. Stir in the cumin, garlic salt, oregano, and pepper flakes, and sauté for 1 minute longer.

3 Add the beans, tomatoes, chicken broth, and water, and bring to a simmer over medium heat. Reduce the heat and simmer the soup, stirring frequently, for 40 minutes over low heat so the beans do not stick. Serve hot.

Makes 8–10 servings

A Few Beers to Try with This Recipe

- *Hoppy Stony Face Red Ale*
- *Ithaca Cascazilla*
- *Karl Strauss Off the Rails*
- *Moab Derailleur Ale*
- *Oskar Blues G'Knight Imperial Red Ale*
- *Peak Organic King Crimson*
- *Terrapin Big Hoppy Monster*

PROFILE ★ **Moab Brewery calls itself** an "oasis in the desert," and for those traversing the dusty (but beautiful) landscape of eastern Utah, it certainly is. The brewery serves flavorful food and pints in a roadhouse-style setting just south of Arches National Park. It is a delightful spot to unwind after a day of outdoor activities.

Pork Green Chili

The addition of pork to this pepper-heavy chili creates a hearty texture and even adds a slight bit of sweetness. Roasting the whole pot in the oven draws out extra flavor and adds an earthy depth that you can't quite achieve on the stovetop. Serve with a light lager that can stand up to the heat and quench your thirst at the same time.

BLUE STAR BREWING COMPANY

SAN ANTONIO, TEXAS

2½ pounds pork, cut into 1-inch cubes (choose Boston butt, picnic shoulder, or boneless country-style spareribs, or pre-cut stew meat)
Salt and freshly ground black pepper
1 teaspoon granulated garlic
1 cup diced onion
½ cup all-purpose flour
1½ cups canned diced mild green chiles
1 large tomato, diced
¼ cup chicken bouillon base dissolved in 3 cups water
1–2 tablespoons diced pickled jalapeño peppers
Tortilla chips or corn bread, for serving

1 Preheat the oven to 350°F.

2 Combine the pork, salt and pepper to taste, and garlic in a Dutch oven or similar pot. Bake, stirring once, for 20 minutes.

3 Add the onions to the pot, stir, and bake for 20 minutes longer.

4 Stir in the flour. Add the chiles, tomato, and chicken bouillon base in water, and mix thoroughly. (The chicken bouillon base and flour should make a mixture with the consistency of a gravy.) Bake, stirring every 10 minutes, for 30 minutes.

5 Add the jalapeños and bake for 5 minutes longer. Remove from the oven and serve with tortilla chips or corn bread.

Makes 8 servings

PROFILE ★   **Blue Star is a comfortable neighborhood** bar that frequently sees foot traffic from out-of-town visitors and the arts crowd. Owned and operated by Joey and Maggie Villarreal, the brewpub has been around since 1996, making it an established brewery in the River Walk City. Located inside the Blue Star Arts Complex — a home for contemporary art — the brewery is reliving history in a sense: its building was once a beer storage warehouse.

BOULDER BEER COMPANY

BOULDER, COLORADO

Planet Porter Bison Stew

Bison is a lean and flavorful red meat, and in this hearty dish it stands out while absorbing and working with the vegetables in the pot. Brown porter adds roasty flavors and even some grain or bread notes that present an earthy aroma and depth to the finished stew. Other red meats such as beefsteak will work in this recipe if bison is not available in your area. This stew is great fresh but even better a day later, after the flavors have really had some time to marry.

5 tablespoons vegetable oil

1 large red onion, finely chopped

8 garlic cloves, minced

½ tablespoon finely chopped fresh rosemary leaves

½ tablespoon salt, plus more for seasoning

½ tablespoon coarsely ground black pepper, plus more for seasoning

1 pound bison steak, cut into 1-inch cubes

4 cups (1 quart) Boulder Planet Porter, or similar porter

4 cups beef broth

4 carrots, peeled and sliced ¼ inch thick

4 celery stalks, trimmed and chopped

2 russet potatoes, peeled and diced into ½-inch cubes

2 bay leaves

3 tablespoons white roux (see box)

A Few Beers to Try with This Recipe

- *Anchor Porter*
- *Boulder Planet Porter*
- *Deschutes Black Butte Porter*
- *Great Lakes Edmund Fitzgerald Porter*
- *Sierra Nevada Porter*
- *Upland's Bad Elmer's Porter*
- *Wasatch Polygamy Porter*

1 Heat 3 tablespoons of the vegetable oil in a large cast iron skillet over medium-high heat. Add the onion, and sweat, stirring occasionally, until translucent, about 5 minutes. Add the garlic, rosemary, salt, and pepper, and cook, stirring often so the garlic doesn't burn, for 5 minutes longer. Transfer the onion mixture to a 5-quart soup pot and set aside.

2 Toss the bison with the remaining 2 tablespoons vegetable oil in a medium bowl and season with salt and pepper to taste.

3 Reheat the skillet over medium-high heat. When the skillet is hot, add the bison, working in batches if necessary to prevent overcrowding. Cook the bison, stirring occasionally, until browned on all sides. (Allow the fond to build up on the bottom of the skillet. The more you can brown the meat, the richer the flavor of your stew.) Transfer the bison to the pot with the onions.

4 Deglaze the skillet with ³/₄ cup of the Planet Porter, scraping the fond into the liquid. Transfer the beer and fond mixture to the pot and add the remaining 3¼ cups porter.

5 Bring the stew to a simmer over medium-high and cook for 15 minutes. Add the beef broth, carrots, celery, potatoes, and bay leaves, and return the stew to a boil over medium-high heat. Reduce the heat and simmer until the vegetables are soft, about 30 minutes.

6 Stir the white roux into the pot and simmer for 30 minutes longer to thicken the stew. Remove the bay leaves and serve hot.

Makes 4–6 servings

White Roux

Combine 2 tablespoons softened unsalted butter, 1 tablespoon corn flour, and 1 teaspoon all-purpose flour in a small bowl. Mash with a fork to create a fine paste; use this mixture to thicken stews and sauces.

Leading the charge in what has become one of the great brewing regions, ***Boulder Beer*** was the first microbrewery to open in Colorado way back in 1979. The brainchild of two University of Colorado professors, it was originally housed on a small goat farm on the outskirts of town. It would later move to a larger space and expand several times, from a one-barrel system to one that can turn out more than 43,000 barrels per year. A true American original, Boulder Beer releases a variety of well-respected brews, and its restaurant and taproom serve up tasty meals that complement every flavor.

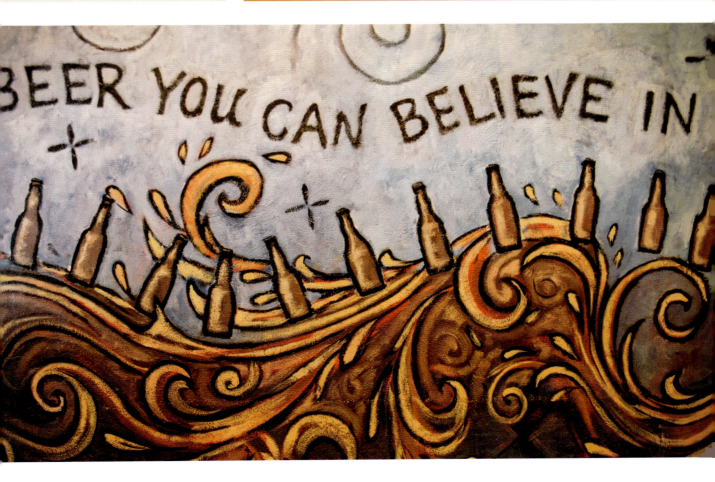

Chicken and Sausage Jambalaya

- 1¾ cups chicken broth
- 5 tablespoons unsalted butter
- 1 bay leaf
- ½ teaspoon salt
- 1 cup uncooked medium-grain or long-grain rice
- 1 medium onion, chopped
- ½ bell pepper, cored, seeded, and chopped
- 1 celery stalk, chopped
- 1 tablespoon minced garlic
- ½ pound smoked sausage, sliced into ¼-inch rounds
- ⅛ teaspoon freshly ground black pepper
- 1 (14.5-ounce) can stewed tomatoes
- ½ teaspoon Tabasco sauce
- ½ pound cooked chicken, roughly chopped or shredded
- 1 cup sliced scallions, white and light green parts only
- Finely chopped fresh parsley, for garnish

Jambalaya is an economical, one-pot Creole meal and in southern Louisiana, it's served at everything from black-tie political fund-raisers to afternoons when you need to feed a group of friends. Traditionally it's made with rice, tomatoes, and whatever leftover meat or seafood is on hand — shrimp, ham, chicken, crawfish, shredded pork, sausage, oysters, or pretty much anything else available. It can be especially wonderful with smoked duck. This recipe from Bayou Teche Brewing pairs well with a pale ale and very well with the brewery's LA-31 Bière Pâle, a take on a Belgian-style pale ale. *Ça c'est bon!*

1 Combine the chicken broth, 1 tablespoon of the butter, the bay leaf, and the salt in a medium saucepan and bring to a boil. Add the rice, reduce the heat to low, and when the rice is at a very gentle simmer, cover and cook until the rice is cooked and the broth is absorbed, about 20 minutes. Remove the saucepan from the heat and set aside.

2 Melt the remaining 4 tablespoons butter in a Dutch oven over medium heat. Add the onion, bell pepper, and celery, and sauté, stirring occasionally, until soft, about 10 minutes. Add the garlic and sauté for 1 minute longer.

3 Stir in the sausage, black pepper, stewed tomatoes and their juices, and Tabasco, reduce the heat to low, and simmer, uncovered, until the soup thickens, about 20 minutes.

4 Add the chicken and scallions, and cook for 5 minutes longer. Mix the cooked rice into the tomato mixture until combined.

5 Divide the jambalaya among bowls, garnish with the parsley, if desired, and serve.

Makes 8–10 servings

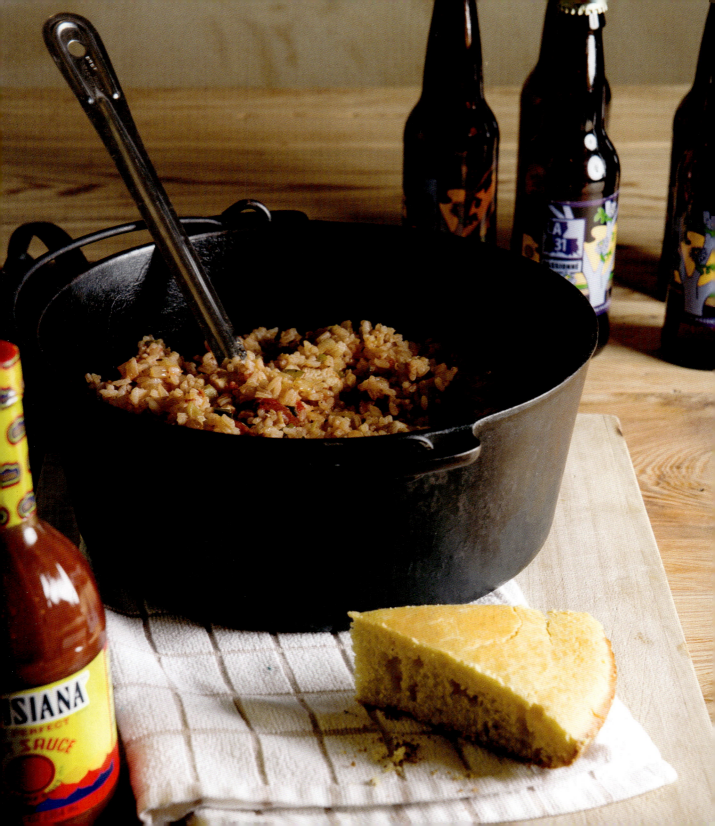

Bayou Teche's brewer, Karlos Knott, began his love affair with beer while serving overseas in the Army. After returning stateside, he was stationed in the Pacific Northwest — the fertile crescent of microbreweries — where his education continued. When he returned to his ancestral homeland of southern Lousiana (his family arrived there in the 1700s and put down serious roots), Karlos joined forces with his brothers, Byron and Dorsey, and launched a brewery inside an abandoned rail car. The car has been remodeled and now resembles a traditional Acadian-style home, complete with a tasting porch. This brewery embodies the spirit of southern Louisiana, and it's just what the craft beer world needs.

Cheddar Ale Soup

A version of this soup is a staple at many brewpubs across the country. The combination of sharp cheese, sweet malt, and smoky notes is a winner. On a cold day, this soup will stick to your ribs and bring a smile to your face. While there is porter in the soup, I suggest drinking a cream ale or golden ale with it, something with a refreshing taste that will let the cheddar reveal its flavor without too much hop smack getting in the way. Consider adding smoked sausage or sliced scallions as a garnish.

2 tablespoons unsalted butter
⅓ cup all-purpose flour
2 cups whole milk
2 cups chicken broth
1¼ pounds sharp cheddar, shredded (5 cups)
3 garlic cloves, minced
1 cup smoked porter

1 Melt the butter in large soup pot and add the flour as the butter begins to bubble. Cook over medium heat, whisking constantly to prevent burning, until browned, about 5 minutes.

2 Whisk in the milk about ½ cup at a time, adding more milk when it becomes absorbed into the roux. When the roux reaches a thick sauce-like consistency, start adding the chicken broth ½ cup at a time, whisking frequently.

3 Add the cheese to the soup one handful at a time. Stir until the cheese is combined and fully melted before adding more cheese. Reduce the heat to low, add the garlic and beer, and simmer for 15 minutes, stirring frequently.

4 Divide the soup among bowls and serve immediately.

Makes 6-8 servings

A Few Beers to Try with This Recipe

- *Anderson Valley Summer Solstice Cerveza Crema*
- *Laughing Dog Cream Ale*
- *New Glarus Spotted Cow*
- *O'Fallon Gold*
- *Sixpoint Sweet Action*
- *Terrapin Golden Ale*

PROFILE ★ **With a commitment to local ingredients** and flavorful beers, **O'Fallon** has gained a reputation among beer drinkers as a solid yet inventive brewery that never disappoints. With its brews available in a growing number of states, the brewery, helmed by Brian Owens, has won numerous awards and delights fans each year with seasonal releases like O'Fallon Cherry Chocolate, O'Fallon Black Hemp, and O'Fallon Pumpkin Beer.

Festbier Cheddar Bisque

Although this soup calls for Victory's Oktoberfest offering, the chef who designed the recipe, Eric MacPherson, describes the bisque as "an easy and hearty soup for all seasons." Victory's Festbier lager uses whole German hops and generous amounts of German pilsner, Munich, and Vienna malts; that beer adds a richer flavor to the bisque.

2 cups (4 sticks) salted butter

2 cups all-purpose flour

1 tablespoon canola oil

1 tablespoon extra-virgin olive oil

1 medium yellow or white onion, minced

3 large celery stalks, minced

8 strips bacon, cooked and diced

1 garlic clove, minced

2 cups Victory Festbier, or similar German lager

2 cups heavy cream

8 ounces cheddar cheese, shredded (2 cups)

Salt and freshly ground black pepper

Tabasco sauce, or similar hot sauce

Finely chopped chives, for garnish

1 Melt the butter in a large skillet over medium-high heat, and then whisk in the flour. Toss the roux mixture in the skillet so it folds over itself. Continue to fold until the starch cooks out of the flour and the roux smells like toasted almonds, about 3 minutes. Spread the roux on a baking sheet to cool.

2 Warm the canola oil and olive oil in a soup pot over medium-high heat. Add the onions and celery, and sauté, stirring occasionally, until the vegetables are translucent, 4 to 6 minutes. Add the bacon and garlic to the pot and sauté, stirring occasionally, until the mixture is aromatic, about 2 minutes.

3 Deglaze the pan with the beer, stirring the brown bits up from the bottom of the pot. Stir in the cream. Add the reserved roux to the pot, and stir constantly until the soup is thick enough to coat the back of a spoon, about 3 minutes.

4 Stir the cheese into the pot, one handful at a time, to incorporate. Bring the soup to a simmer over medium-high heat.

5 Season with salt, pepper, and Tabasco to taste. Garnish with the chives and serve hot.

Makes 8–10 small servings

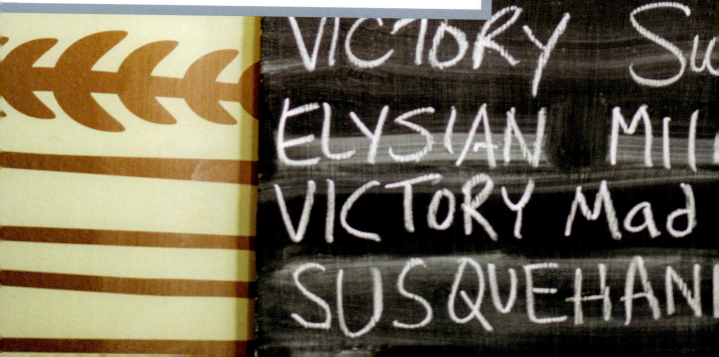

Bill Covaleski and Ron Barchet met as elementary school students in the early 1970s and became fast friends. As they grew older, Covaleski's father introduced him to homebrewing and he later brought Barchet into the fold. From there, it's a story heard all over the country, but one that never gets old. As the men started careers in the "working world" they grew disillusioned with the rat race and began to talk of becoming brewers. Barchet went first, winding up at a Baltimore brewery and moving on to brewing school in Germany. When Barchet went overseas, Covaleski took his place in Baltimore. Fast-forward a few years of education, recipe tweaking, and learning from mistakes, and the lifelong friends were ready to hang their own shingle.

They opened the doors of **Victory Brewing Company** in early 1996 in what used to be a Pepperidge Farm factory. With an attached restaurant that has since grown so much in size that a second full-prodcution brewery is being constructed, with an opening planned for 2014, Victory has become a destination for those who have come to know and enjoy the fruits of the friends' labor.

3 tablespoons extra-virgin olive oil

3 pounds beef stew meat, cut into ½-inch cubes

3 yellow onions, chopped

3 cups Cigar City Big Sound Scotch Ale, or similar Scotch ale

3 cubes chicken or beef bouillon, preferably Maggi brand

2 bay leaves

1 teaspoon fresh thyme leaves

Freshly ground black pepper

4–5 baguette slices

Dijon mustard

2 tablespoons sugar

Minced fresh parsley leaves, for garnish

A Few Beers to Try with This Recipe

- *Captain Lawrence Rosso E Marrone*
- *Deschutes The Dissident*
- *Jackie O's Chunga's Old Bruin*

Carbonnade à la Big Sound Scotch Ale

A carbonnade is a traditional beef and onion stew with roots in Belgium. Adding a full-bodied and boozy Scotch ale gives this recipe lots of deep flavor. Simple boiled potatoes and a green salad make fine accompaniments to this rich dish. As delicious as it is immediately after cooking, save some for leftovers and appreciate how the flavors mingle after a day or two, creating a whole new taste profile.

While the recipe calls for Cigar City's Scotch ale (a spring seasonal release) as an ingredient, I suggest drinking a Flanders brown ale/oud bruin, a Belgian style that has received some solid American treatment in recent years. With its strong malt backbone and notes of fruit, chocolate, and even a little sherry, this ale gives the comforting stew some welcome company.

1 Heat the oil in a large soup pot. Add the beef, and cook, working in batches if necessary, until brown on all sides, about 5 to 8 minutes total. Drain any excess liquid out of the pot, transfer the beef to a medium bowl, and set it aside.

2 Add the onions to the pot and cook, stirring occasionally, until browned, 7 to 10 minutes. Return the beef to the pot and add the beer, bouillon cubes, bay leaves, thyme, and black pepper.

3 Coat the baguette slices with a generous slather of mustard and stir the whole slices into the pot. Add the sugar and bring the stew to a boil. Reduce the heat to medium-low and simmer the stew, uncovered, stirring every 30 minutes, until the beef is fork-tender, 2 to 3 hours.

4 Divide the stew among six bowls. Garnish with the parsley and serve immediately.

Makes 6 servings

In a state known for theme parks, *Cigar City Brewing* has become a major attraction for those who appreciate and seek out excellent beer. It opened with a flourish and spread its reach quickly, appealing to both hardened beer geeks and brew novices with eyebrow-raising flavors and commitment to quality. Capitalizing on the Latin culture and tobacco-manufacturing history of Tampa Bay, Cigar City highlights those strengths on its labels and in its beer names and recipes. Many of the beers it produces — Jai Alai IPA, Improv Oatmeal Rye India-Style Brown Ale, Cubano-Style Espresso Brown Ale — reflect the sensibilities and ingredients of Florida. Dedicated fans flock to the ever-expanding brewery each March for the one-day release of Hunahpu's Imperial Stout. The 11 percent ale is aged on cacao nibs, Madagascar vanilla beans, ancho chiles, pasilla chiles, and cinnamon. Line up early to get a bottle; it's the best attraction in all of Florida.

Khmer Wild Boar Curry

2 pounds wild boar
  Kosher salt or 2 tablespoons soy sauce
2–3 tablespoons extra-virgin olive oil or sunflower oil
4 garlic cloves, thinly sliced
½ pound eggplant, cubed into bite-size pieces
3 large carrots, peeled and sliced
2 medium potatoes, cubed into bite-size pieces
1 (4-inch) piece fresh ginger, peeled and thinly sliced
¼ cup yellow curry paste
1 cup coconut milk
¼ cup grated coconut
1 tablespoon palm sugar
2 ounces tamarind paste
1 teaspoon fish sauce
1 teaspoon freshly ground black pepper
¼ teaspoon ground cloves
  Thai or hot red chile peppers
10–12 large fresh Thai basil leaves, chopped

Don't be daunted by the long list of ingredients. This is a relatively simple recipe that, once prepped, takes care of itself in a smoker and then a soup pot. It is a wonderful combination of game-hunting flavors from the western United States and Southeast Asian ingredients; it is also pretty versatile. You can substitute pork for the boar, chile sauce for the fresh hot peppers, and Italian basil for the Thai basil (just add a few extra leaves to boost the flavor). Pair this lipsmacking dish with an American pale ale that not only quenches but adds some additional hop bite.

1 Rub the boar all over with salt, cover, and refrigerate for 1 hour. Alternatively, rub the boar with the soy sauce, cover, and refrigerate for 4 hours.

2 Prepare your smoker to between 120 and 140°F. Place the boar on the smoker and smoke for 2 to 3 hours. Remove from the smoker and cut the boar into 1/4-inch cubes.

3 Heat the olive oil in a large skillet or wok over high heat. Add the boar, and cook, stirring occasionally, until brown, 12 to 15 minutes. Add the garlic to the skillet halfway through.

4 Transfer the boar to a large pot and add the eggplant, carrots, potatoes, ginger, curry paste, coconut milk, grated coconut, sugar, tamarind paste, fish sauce, black pepper, cloves, and chile peppers to taste. Bring the curry to a boil over high heat. Reduce the heat to low and simmer until the boar is very tender, 2 to 4 hours.

5 Garnish with the basil and serve hot.

Makes 8–10 servings

The Anderson Valley Brewing Company has come a long way since it was founded in 1987. After outgrowing its original 10-barrel brewhouse, it expanded to a 30-barrel system and then to one with 100-barrel and 85-barrel brew kettles. With an impressive lineup of beer, AVBC turns out a staggering number of ales and supplies much of the country with flavorful recipes. Brewery founder Ken Allen turned the business over to Trey White, who brought back Fal Allen (no relation to Ken) to serve as brewmaster. The resulting beer has been a welcome sight on shelves, and the brewery shows no signs of slowing down.

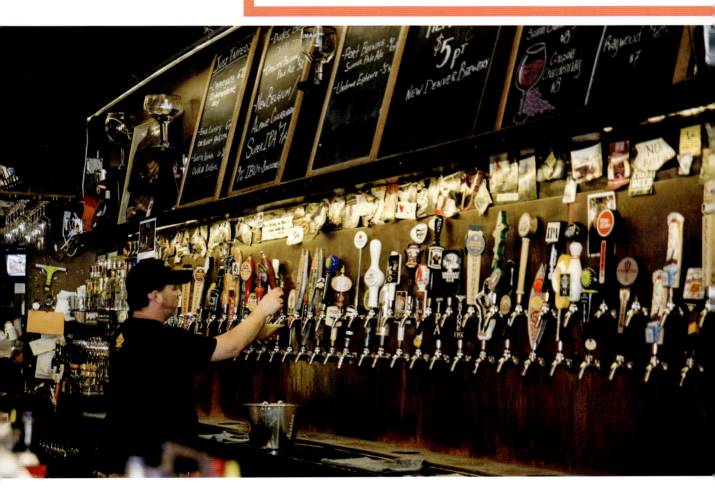

Brew Free! Chili

For many, making chili is a sacred art. A prized recipe might be tweaked to perfection over many years, with tiny changes involving mere pinches and dashes. For those who consider chili a religion (and many do) the precise ingredients in these batches are meticulously chosen and guarded. For the rest of us, there is this recipe from 21ST Amendment. Its beauty is its simplicity — classic meat chili ingredients and clearly defined measurements. Use this recipe over and over again with confidence, or begin to add your own ingredients — a pinch of this or that as you get more comfortable. It's great for weekends and tailgating. When choosing a beer, follow your heart. Chili is a versatile dish. It goes well with pale ales, IPAs, stouts, porters, and lighter beers. Experiment and find one that fits your palate.

- 3 tablespoons extra-virgin olive oil
- 1½ pounds ground beef
- 2 large yellow onions, diced
- 3 large carrots, peeled and diced
- 4 celery stalks, diced
- 4 garlic cloves, chopped
- 2 tablespoons tomato paste
- 2 (12-ounce) cans 21ST Amendment Brew Free or Die IPA, or similar American IPA
- ⅓ cup chili powder
- 2 bay leaves
- 1 tablespoon finely chopped fresh thyme leaves
- 1 tablespoon Tabasco sauce
- 1 tablespoon Worcestershire sauce
- 1 (15-ounce) can red beans, drained and rinsed
- Salt and freshly ground black pepper

Makes 8–10 servings

1 Heat the olive oil in a soup pot over medium heat; add the beef, and cook, stirring to break up the meat, until browned, 7 to 10 minutes. Add the onions, carrots, celery, and garlic, and cook, stirring often, for about 5 minutes longer.

2 Add the tomato paste, and stir to incorporate. Pour in the beer, and add enough water to cover the beef mixture. Add the chili powder, bay leaves, thyme, Tabasco, and Worcestershire, and bring to a boil. Reduce the heat to low and simmer the chili, stirring occasionally, for 1 hour.

3 Add the beans to the pot and simmer for 15 minutes longer. Season with salt and pepper to taste and adjust any other seasonings as desired before serving.

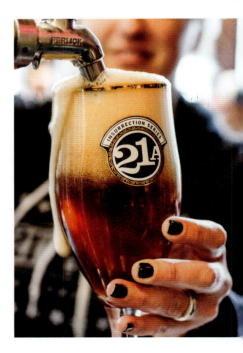

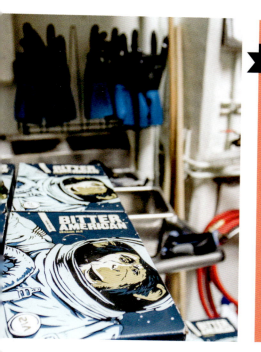

PROFILE ★ **For beer drinkers,** the Twenty-First Amendment remains one of the most important and favorite of the Constitutional amendments. It was ratified on December 5, 1933 by President Franklin D. Roosevelt, repealing the Eighteenth Amendment and ending Prohibition. It was a day to celebrate the return of legal alcohol, but Prohibition had done and would long continue to do damage to the country's breweries. This was true in San Francisco, where the brewing scene was nearly decimated, but it came back strong with the craft renaissance five decades later.

When Shaun O'Sullivan and Nicco Freccia opened their *21ST Amendment Brewery* brewpub in what's now the city center, they reached back and named their venture after that important piece of legislation. Their stylish two-level pub is a great spot to gather, drink, and discuss events of the day and life in general. Their beers are also canned and available throughout the country. With offerings like Hell or High Watermelon, Fireside Chat, and Back in Black, we should all be grateful that the noble social experiment came to an end.

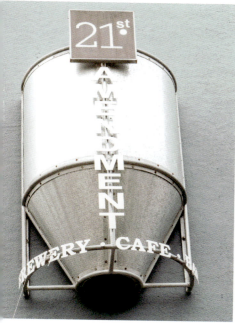

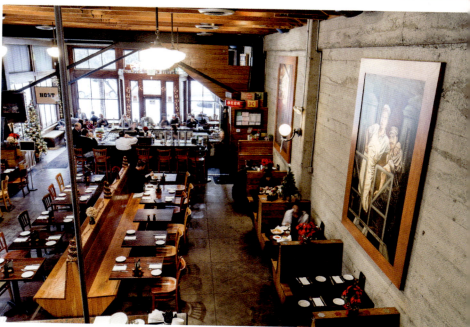

Rhode Island Clam Chowder

1 pound shucked clams
2½ cups chicken broth
2½ cups clam juice
1 cup Narragansett Lager Beer, or similar lager
¼ cup unsalted butter
2 medium white onions, diced
2 large celery stalks, chopped
1 pound fingerling potatoes, quartered
3 tablespoons dried dill weed
2 tablespoons freshly ground black pepper
1 teaspoon salt
Pinch of cayenne pepper
2 drops hot pepper sauce (optional)
¼ cup chopped fresh parsley

A Few Beers to Try with This Recipe

- *Big Sky Summer Honey Ale*
- *Gray's Honey Ale*
- *Narragansett Light*
- *Rapscallion Honey*

Some might argue that this dish perfectly represents the Ocean State — salty, hearty, reliable, and a little fiery. This broth-based chowder occupies the middle ground between New England (cream-based) and Manhattan (tomato-based) chowder varieties and is sometimes known as clear. Enjoy this chowder and its Atlantic flavors anywhere with an ale brewed with honey to balance some of the saltiness and accentuate the sweetness of the clams.

1 Bring the shucked clams, chicken broth, clam juice, and beer to a simmer in a large pot over medium-high heat. Reduce the heat to medium-low and simmer for 15 minutes.

2 Meanwhile, melt the butter in a large skillet over medium heat. Stir in the onions and celery, and cook, stirring occasionally, until the vegetables are tender, 5 to 7 minutes. Stir the vegetable mixture into the clam mixture and add the potatoes.

3 Add the dill weed, black pepper, salt, cayenne, and hot pepper sauce, if using, to the pot. Simmer for 15 minutes longer. Divide the chowder among bowls and sprinkle with the parsley before serving.

Makes 8–10 servings

PROFILE ★ **In certain parts of the East, Narragansett** was the traditional local brew, one of those heritage brands that was such a part of family life and gatherings that locals often spot it when looking through grandparents' photo albums. But, like so many before it, the brewery fell on hard times and was forced to close for a while. In the late 2000s it reopened with new owners who don't just rely on the name to sell "nostalgia beer." The flavorful lager produced by Gansett is refreshing on a hot day (or any day), and the brewery has been releasing a number of seasonal offerings, giving today's generation additional choices.

Venison Stew

DESCHUTES BREWERY AND PUBLIC HOUSE

BEND, OREGON

Generally, deer-hunting season begins as the temperatures dip in fall and winter and delivers plenty of venison to use in cold-weather recipes like this. The venison in this recipe is balanced by fresh herbs that bring a rich, floral aroma sure to permeate your house with earthy warmth. Pair with a winter warmer beer, one with a high alcohol content, strong malt backbone, and even a touch of sweetness.

4 tablespoons salted butter
2 pounds venison stew meat
¼ cup all-purpose flour
2 garlic cloves, chopped
2 tablespoons dried thyme
  Needles from 1 rosemary
    sprig, finely chopped
½ cup dry red wine
1 large yellow onion, diced
4 large carrots, peeled and
    sliced into 1-inch rounds
3 celery stalks, thinly sliced
1 pound fingerling potatoes,
    sliced into 1-inch rounds
6 cups beef broth
½ cup Deschutes Obsidian
    Stout, or similar stout
  Sea salt and freshly ground
    tellicherry pepper

1 Melt the butter in a soup pot over medium-high heat. Add the venison and sauté, turning once, until the meat has browned slightly, about 5 minutes. Add the flour and stir to incorporate thoroughly.

2 Add the garlic, thyme, rosemary, and wine, and cook for 30 seconds, stirring constantly. Add the onion, carrots, celery, potatoes, and broth to the pot and bring to a boil over high heat.

3 Reduce the heat to low and simmer the stew, stirring every 15 minutes, until the venison is fork-tender, about 2 hours.

4 Add the beer to the stew and salt and pepper to taste. Serve hot.

Makes 8–10 servings

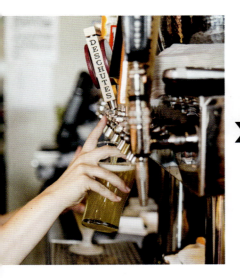

PROFILE ★ **Deschutes Brewery exists** to "profitably deliver the finest beers in the world and cultivate extraordinary experiences." No small task, but it's one Deschutes has successfully lived up to since the business was founded in 1988. The visually stunning brewery overlooks the Deschutes River and can be both a raucous and tranquil place to enjoy an expertly made beer. An Oregon institution, Deschutes has a number of locations, such as the always-packed Portland brew-pub. It's a great and popular place for people who can't make it to Bend.

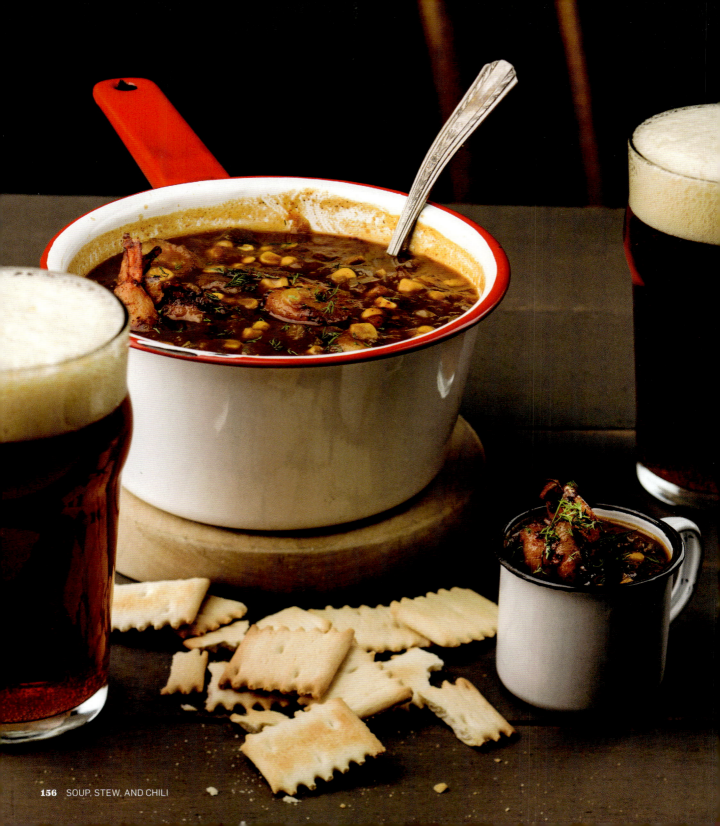

Blackened Shrimp and Corn Chowder

This satisfying chowder can restore even the most waterlogged sailor. Fresh-from-the-sea shrimp adds a salty kick. Pair with an amber ale, like Gritty's Red Claws Ale, to fortify yourself against the elements and whatever's coming next. Serve with oyster crackers, tortilla chips, corn bread, or another bread of your choice.

- 2 tablespoons extra-virgin olive oil
- 1 medium Spanish onion, finely chopped
- 2 celery stalks, finely chopped
- 2 medium banana peppers, finely chopped
- ½ cup red or amber ale
  Salt and freshly ground black pepper
- 1 pound fresh shrimp, peeled and deveined, preferably Maine-harvested
- 2 teaspoons chili powder
- 2 teaspoons smoked paprika
- 1½ cups fresh or frozen corn
- 4 cups fish broth
- 1 large sweet potato, baked and mashed
  Fresh dill, finely chopped

1 Heat 1 tablespoon of the olive oil in a soup pot over medium heat. Add the onion, celery, and banana peppers, and cook, stirring occasionally, until the onions are translucent, 5 to 7 minutes. Add the ale and salt and pepper to taste. Reduce the heat to medium-low and continue cooking and stirring until the beer's foam subsides and the liquid reduces by half, about 5 minutes.

2 Rinse the shrimp under cold water and pat dry with a paper towel. Toss the shrimp, chili powder, and paprika together in a bowl, coating thoroughly. Heat the remaining 1 tablespoon olive oil in a cast iron skillet. Add the shrimp and cook, stirring once, until nicely seared, about 2 minutes.

3 Immediately transfer the shrimp to the soup pot, and then stir in the corn and broth. Bring the mixture to a light boil over medium-high heat and add the mashed sweet potato. Reduce the heat to low, and cook, stirring occasionally, for 20 minutes longer.

4 Divide the soup among bowls and top with the fresh dill before serving.

Makes 8–10 servings

PROFILE ★ **Founded in 1988, Gritty McDuff's Portland** location was the first brewpub to open in Maine since Prohibition. The comfortable spot in the historic Old Port district hosts a mix of locals and visitors coming together over good beer and food. Gritty's operates two other locations: one in Freeport, a town famous for its factory outlet stores, where tired shoppers come to rest their weary feet, and the other on the banks of the Androscoggin River in Auburn, offering great views and the same quality food and beer that has regularly won the brewery awards in both state and national competitions.

New Mexican Posole

This classic stew relies on hominy, or posole (pronounced poh-SOH-leh), and is popular in New Mexico, where it is traditionally served on Christmas Eve to celebrate life's blessings. But it is great for any time of year and pairs well with an IPA that can stand up to the heat from the chiles. New Mexico Chimayo chiles work well in this recipe, but you can choose a variety that fits your tolerance level. Serve with sour cream, queso, and fresh tortillas.

1 pound dried blue corn posole (hominy)
2 quarts vegetable broth
2 quarts water
2 pigs' feet
½ cup New Mexican roasted red chili powder
2 pounds boneless pork butt, diced into bite-size pieces
1 large yellow onion, chopped
6 garlic cloves, minced
Salt and freshly ground black pepper
Sour cream, queso asadero, and flour tortillas, for serving

Note: This recipe requires overnight preparation.

A Few Beers to Try with This Recipe

- Bell's Two Hearted Ale
- Cigar City Jai Alai IPA
- Coast HopArt IPA
- La Cumbre Elevated IPA
- Odell IPA
- Russian River IPA or Blind Pig IPA
- Sierra Nevada Torpedo
- Smuttynose Finest Kind IPA
- Surly Furious

1 Place the posole in a soup pot and cover with room-temperature water the night before preparing the dish. Cover the pot and refrigerate overnight.

2 Strain the posole, thoroughly rinse, and set aside.

3 Combine the broth and water in a soup pot and bring to a boil over high heat. Reduce the heat to medium and add the reserved posole, pigs' feet, and 4 tablespoons of the chili powder; bring to a slow boil. Reduce the heat to low, cover the pot, and simmer for 3 hours.

4 Add the pork butt and onion to the pot and simmer over low heat for 1 hour longer.

5 Add the garlic, the remaining 4 tablespoons chili powder, and salt and pepper to taste. Simmer for 30 minutes.

6 Serve in soup terrines with sour cream, queso asadero, and fresh tortillas, if desired.

Makes 10 servings

PROFILE ★ **Jeff Erway was a music teacher** who hadn't given any thought to brewing before a vacation brought him to Arizona back in 2002, and he found himself in a homebrew shop. There, he bought one of the most famous how-to tomes on the subject: John Palmer's *How to Brew*. From there, Erway was off like a shot. After a few years brewing for family and friends, he went pro, wound up at New Mexico's busiest brewpub, won several awards, and finally felt comfortable starting his own brewery. *La Cumbre Brewing Co.* is a celebration of all things New Mexico, and Erway has continued his medal-winning streak, recently earning gold at the Great American Beer Festival for his Elevated IPA.

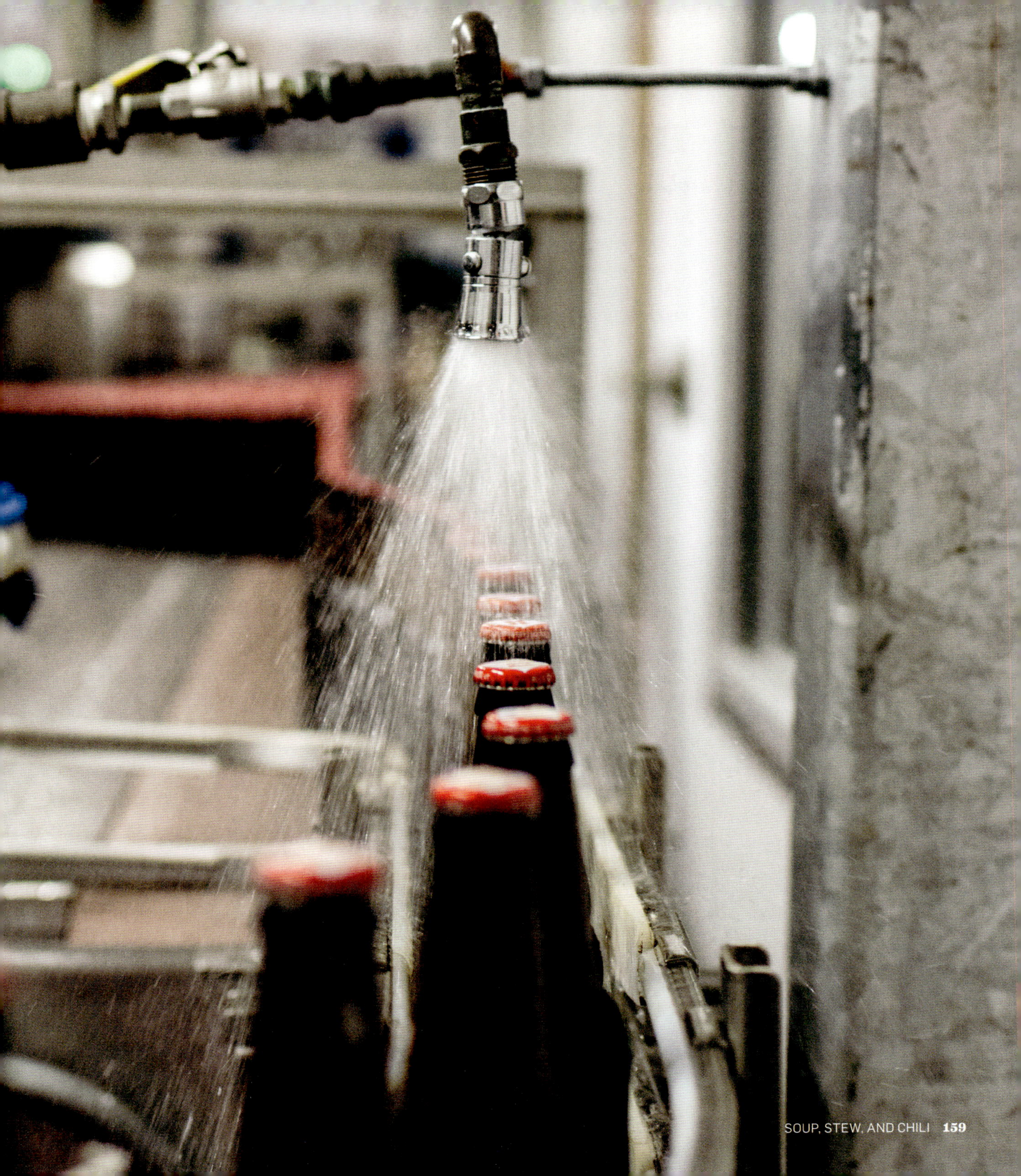

FISH STOCK

- 3 tablespoons olive oil
- 1 pound fish bones (available at most fish markets and some supermarkets)
- 1 medium onion, chopped
- 1 carrot, peeled and chopped
- 3 stalks celery, chopped
- 2 bay leaves
- 1 bunch fresh thyme
- ½ gallon water

BROTH

- 3 tablespoons butter
- 1 medium onion, thinly sliced
- 1 fennel bulb, cored and thinly sliced
- 1 leek, washed well and thinly sliced, white and pale green part only
- 3 garlic cloves, minced
  Salt and freshly ground black pepper
- ½ cup tomato paste
- 2 tablespoons chopped fresh thyme
- ½ gallon fish stock (see above)
- ½ gallon water
- 3 medium russet potatoes, peeled and diced into 1-inch cubes
- 1 cup heavy cream

Bouillabaisse

Making your own bouillabaisse is a rewarding culinary experience, and the homemade base adds a true taste of home to this stew. Taking care not to overcook the ingredients is the name of this game — when making the stew, watch the shellfish carefully and follow the timing in the recipe. The result is a delicate and flavorful bowl of soup featuring seafood cooked the way it should be. On the side, enjoy a French baguette, lightly grilled with a brushing of olive oil. To make this a truly traditional dish, you can spread the bread with a simple aioli of red peppers and mayonnaise known as "rouille." A tripel pairs well with this dish; it complements the roasted flavors the shrimp and cod acquire under the broiler.

1 **MAKE THE FISH STOCK:** Heat the olive oil in a soup pot over medium-high heat. Add the fish bones and cook, stirring constantly with a wooden spoon, just until the bones turn white, 2 to 3 minutes. Add the onion, carrot, celery, bay leaves, and thyme, sauté for 2 minutes, and then add the water all at once. Bring the mixture to a boil, reduce the heat to low, and simmer for 30 minutes. Strain through a fine-mesh sieve or a kitchen towel and discard the solids.

2 **MAKE THE BROTH:** Melt the butter in another large pot over medium heat until it foams. Add the onion, fennel, leek, and garlic, season lightly with salt and pepper, and sweat until the vegetables are tender, about 5 minutes.

3 Stir in the tomato paste and thyme and stir vigorously for a minute or two to cook the paste and remove some of the sharp, acid taste. Add the fish stock, the water, and the potatoes, bring to a boil, reduce the heat to low, and simmer until the potatoes are cooked through, about 30 minutes.

4 At this point, you can purée the broth if you like, but it is equally good left chunky. If you do decide to purée it, work in batches in a blender and add a little of the cream to each blenderful. If you leave the broth chunky, add the cream all at once. Then adjust the seasoning, and store the broth, covered, in the refrigerator until you're ready to assemble the stew. (It will develop a more complex flavor if you make it ahead and leave it to sit for a day in the refrigerator.)

STEW

- 12 large shrimp, peeled and deveined
- 1 pound whitefish (cod works very well)
- 2 tablespoons olive oil
  Salt and freshly ground black pepper
- 1 pound mussels, cleaned and debearded
- 1 pound Manila clams
- 1 fennel bulb, cored and thinly sliced
- 1 leek, washed well and thinly sliced, white and pale green part only
  Seafood broth (see above)
- 1 baguette, sliced and grilled or toasted with olive oil (optional)

5 **MAKE THE STEW:** Preheat the broiler to high.

6 Lightly brush the shrimp and fish with 1 tablespoon of the olive oil, season with salt and pepper, and spread in a single layer on a roasting pan or baking sheet. Broil for about 2 minutes, flip the shrimp and fish, and broil for about 2 minutes more.

7 Heat a large skillet over medium-high heat, add the remaining 1 tablespoon olive oil, and sauté the mussels and clams for a minute or so to start them cooking. Add the fennel and leek, and sauté until the vegetables begin to soften, about 2 minutes. Add enough broth to the pan to cover the shellfish, reduce the heat to low, and cook the shellfish in the broth just until they open. If you continue to cook your shellfish after they have opened your mussels and clams will be tough and dry.

8 To assemble the stew, divide the shrimp and fish equally among six shallow soup bowls, ladle broth and shellfish over the top. Serve with a piece of grilled baguette, if desired.

Makes 6 servings and 2½ quarts broth

BLACK SWAN BREWPUB

PLAINFIELD, INDIANA

Butternut Squash Soup

1 (2- to 3-pound) butternut squash, halved and seeded
1 teaspoon ground cumin
¼ teaspoon freshly ground nutmeg
Salt and freshly ground black pepper
1 medium onion, peeled and halved
2 medium carrots, scrubbed
2 tablespoons unsalted butter
6 cups chicken or vegetable broth
½ cup heavy cream
1 teaspoon fresh thyme leaves
1–2 teaspoons good-quality aged sherry vinegar

There is a misconception that great soup can be made by simply throwing ingredients into a pot and letting them simmer. In this recipe, roasting the vegetables before adding them to the soup pot results in a deeper and more rounded flavor in the bowl. An optional garnish such as fresh thyme leaves, fried sage leaves, or a cranberry compote enhances not only the presentation but the autumnal flavor. A malty brown ale adds additional heft to the taste experience.

1 Preheat the oven to 400°F. Place the squash cut side up on a baking sheet. Sprinkle with the cumin, nutmeg, and salt and pepper to taste. Add the onion and carrots to the baking sheet and roast until the vegetables are tender and starting to caramelize on the outside, 20 to 30 minutes.

2 Allow the vegetables to cool slightly, and then finely chop them. (You may remove any peel from the squash that comes off easily, but it isn't necessary to get it all.)

3 Transfer the vegetables to a soup pot over medium-low heat. Add the butter and cook, stirring, until the vegetables have softened,

3 to 5 minutes. Add the broth, bring to a simmer, and cook for 20 minutes longer.

4 Add the cream and thyme to the pot and simmer for 30 minutes longer. Cool slightly, and then purée the soup in a blender until smooth. Adjust the consistency of the soup with additional broth, if needed, and then add the sherry vinegar and additional cumin, if needed, to taste. Season with salt and pepper to taste.

5 Divide the soup among warm bowls and serve immediately with desired garnishes.

Makes 6–8 servings

Before he opened his own brewpub, D.J. McCallister came up through the brewing ranks from the very bottom. His first brewing job was washing kegs. From there he graduated to emptying the mash tun and "general sanitation," as he calls it. Soon enough, however, he was brewing. He cut his teeth at breweries around Indiana, and when it came time to open *Black Swan* he promised a "no-holds-barred" approach. He takes the title of craftsman seriously, and both his beers and the food from his kitchen prove that. With innovative food and drink recipes, Black Swan has a dedicated following that grows with each new visitor.

Cauliflower Lavender Soup

Too often lavender is relegated to perfumes and soaps and doesn't find its way into the kitchen. Here it adds a subtle fragrance to an otherwise earthy and savory soup. This soup pairs well with a saison or a Belgian wit, a brew with depth and a floral character.

2 tablespoons unsalted butter or duck fat
½ cup chopped shallots
3 garlic cloves, minced
½ cup dry vermouth
1 small head cauliflower, chopped
1 cup chopped celeriac
1 cup peeled and roughly chopped potatoes
1 bay leaf
4 cups chicken broth
1 tablespoon dried lavender
½ cup heavy cream
Freshly ground nutmeg
Salt and freshly ground white pepper
Juice from ½ lemon (optional)
Fresh herbs, for serving

1 Melt the butter in a soup pot; add the shallots and garlic and sauté for 1 minute before adding the vermouth. Bring the vermouth to a boil and add the cauliflower, celeriac, potatoes, bay leaf, and chicken broth. (Add more broth to completely submerge the vegetables if needed.) Reduce the heat to a simmer and cook until the vegetables are tender, about 15 minutes.

2 Add the lavender to the pot, and then remove from the heat. Let cool slightly and purée in a traditional blender or with a handheld immersion blender.

3 Pass the soup through a coarse strainer back into the pot. Press the soup through the strainer with a flat wooden spatula or similar utensil. Discard the fibrous pulp left in the strainer.

4 Place the pot back on the stove and bring the soup to a simmer over low heat. Stir in the cream, and then season with nutmeg, salt, and white pepper to taste; stir to incorporate. Stir in the lemon juice, if using, and additional lavender, if desired.

5 Serve the soup in preheated bowls and garnish with a pinch of your favorite chopped fresh herbs, such as parsley, tarragon, thyme, or chives.

Makes 8–10 servings

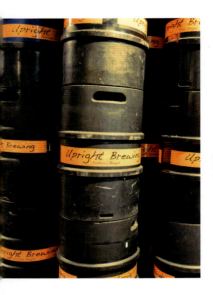

PROFILE ★ **Upright is one of those inventive breweries** that takes the tradition of an established beer country (Belgium) and infuses those tried-and-true beer recipes with a healthy dose of good old-fashioned American ingenuity. Upright's hybrid styles are a marriage of tradition and whimsy. In case you were wondering, the brewery takes its name from the upright bass, played by Charles Mingus, a musician who also fused styles to create unique artistic offerings.

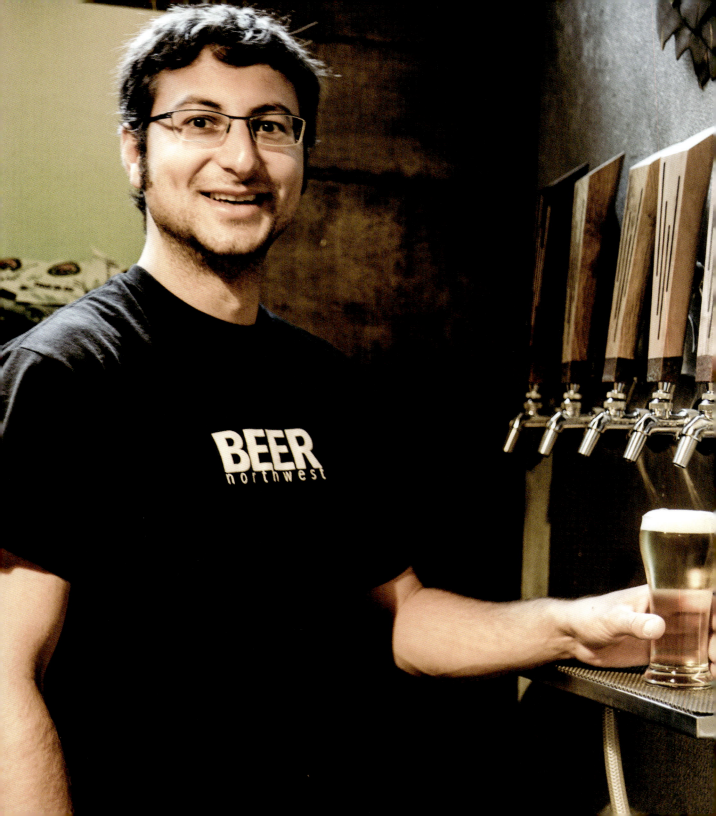

Irish Lamb Stew

2 tablespoons beef base
10 cups water
2 cups peeled and diced russet potatoes
2 cups diced yellow onions
2 cups peeled and diced carrots
3 celery stalks, trimmed and diced
½ pound turnip, peeled and diced
3 pounds lamb meat, diced into ½-inch pieces
¼ cup pearled barley
1 tablespoon finely chopped fresh rosemary leaves
1 teaspoon dried basil
1 teaspoon dried thyme
   Salt and freshly ground black pepper

Savory, hearty, and satisfying, this classic stew will fill the house with herbal and meaty aromas long before it's ready to serve. Take that time to set the table and enjoy the company of family, all while building up an appetite for a warm, comforting meal. This stew — a meal in one bowl — encourages long conversations and drinking a pint with good friends and family. A heads-up: Chances are folks will be craving another bowl while the last drop still lingers on the tongue! The intricate flavors come to life when paired with an Irish red ale or a Scotch ale.

1 Preheat the oven to 450°F. Combine the beef base and water in a large bowl and set aside to dissolve.

2 Combine half of the potatoes, onions, carrots, celery, and turnips in a Dutch oven or similar pot. Layer the lamb on top of the vegetables, and then top with the remaining mixed vegetables. Add the barley, rosemary, basil, thyme, and salt and pepper to taste, and then add enough of the beef-based water to just cover all the ingredients.

3 Cover the pot with aluminum foil and the lid. Cook in the oven for 3 hours, or until the lamb and vegetables are fork-tender. Remove the stew from the oven and serve immediately.

Makes 6–8 servings

A Few Beers to Try with This Recipe

- *Blacktooth Bomber Mountain Amber*
- *Boulevard Irish Ale*
- *Harpoon Celtic Ale*
- *Hook and Ladder Pipe and Drum Irish Ale*
- *Karl Strauss Red Trolley Ale*
- *Moylan's Danny's Irish Style Red Ale*
- *Short's the Magician*
- *Wachusett Quinn's Amber Ale*

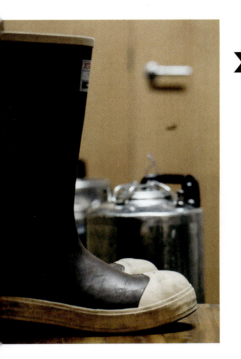

PROFILE ★
One of the Golden State's great breweries was inspired by an early pioneer. Brendan Moylan had been a homebrewer when he visited the venerable Buffalo Bill's Brewing and realized that he wanted to be a part of a larger brewery. So, he became a founding partner in the Marin Brewing Company in 1989, took additional brewing classes, and immersed himself in the waters of beer. Soon he was ready to have a place of his own, and in 1995 he opened *Moylan's*, a beer drinker's haven. It is a comfortable spot where families gather and friends catch up, and, like its Irish pub ancestors, it is a hub for community conversation. There is much to like about the well-appointed, well-decorated brewpub, but its reading room is particularly special. Filled with beer books and periodicals, the room is a wonderful place to enjoy a pint, sit by the fireplace, or throw a game of darts. Weather permitting, move the party outside to the cozy garden patio, or just hang out at the nearly 60-foot bar. There is something for everyone — and that includes beer. Under the direction of brewmaster Denise Jones, Moylan's has released a number of traditional award-winning ales available at the pub and in 22-ounce bottles around the country.

Moroccan-Cured Duck Breasts, see page 192

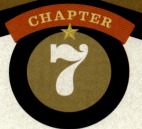

Entrées

The Main Event from Steak and Poultry to Pizza and Tacos

Rolling Chicken with Beurre Blanc

Making a beurre blanc for the first time (or even the second or third time) can be a daunting task. One key to getting this creamy delicate sauce just right is to make sure that the butter is cold when you add it to the sauce, and then whisk constantly until it is fully incorporated. This dish pairs well with a dortmunder gold lager or a hefeweizen; both have hearty flavors that can stand up to the goat cheese in the chicken.

SAUCE

- 1 cup dry white wine
- ½ cup white wine vinegar
- 1 tablespoon finely chopped shallots
- ½ cup heavy cream
- 2 cups (4 sticks) cold unsalted butter, cold, cut into ½-inch pieces
- Kosher salt

CHICKEN

- ⅔ cup sundried tomatoes
- ⅔ cup fresh goat cheese
- 2 tablespoons dried thyme
- 2 tablespoons dried basil
- 2 tablespoons dried oregano
- ⅔ cup pilsner
- 1 pound boneless skinless chicken breasts, pounded flat
- Salt and freshly ground black pepper
- Chopped fresh parsley, for garnish

1 MAKE THE SAUCE: Combine the wine, vinegar, and shallots in a saucepan. Bring to a boil, and then lower the heat and simmer, stirring occasionally, until the liquid has reduced to 2 tablespoons, about 10 minutes. Strain the sauce and discard the shallots. Return the pan to high heat, add the cream, and bring to a boil.

2 Lower the heat to a light simmer and begin adding the butter cubes one at a time, whisking rapidly with a wire whisk. As the butter melts and incorporates, add more butter and continue whisking. When only 2 to 3 butter cubes remain, remove the sauce from the heat, and then whisk in the last few cubes. Continue to whisk 1 to 2 minutes longer, until the sauce is thick and smooth. Season to taste with kosher salt and transfer to a thermos until ready to serve.

3 Preheat oven to 350°F degrees. Lightly grease a baking sheet.

4 MAKE THE CHICKEN: Place the tomatoes in a blender and process into small pieces. Add the goat cheese, thyme, basil, and oregano, and blend together. Slowly add the beer and continue to blend into a spreadable filling for the chicken.

5 Cut the chicken into four pieces and season with salt and pepper to taste. Spread one-quarter of the cheese mixture on each piece of chicken and roll the meat into a tube (with filling on the inside); secure in place with a toothpick.

6 Place the chicken rolls on the prepared baking sheet and bake for 8 to 10 minutes, or until cooked through. Remove the toothpicks, plate, and cover the stuffed chicken with beurre blanc. Sprinkle with parsley and serve hot.

Makes 4 servings

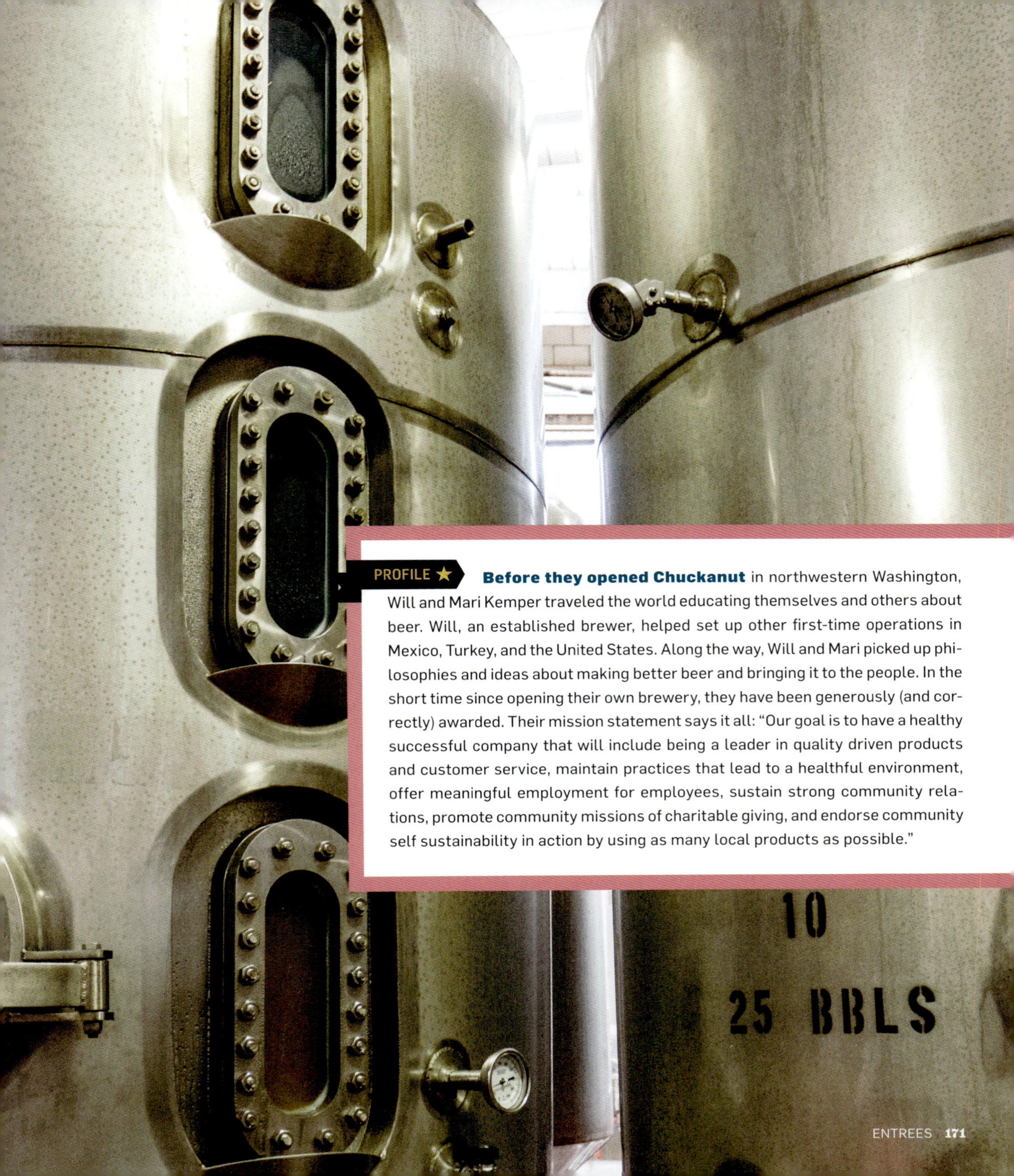

Before they opened Chuckanut in northwestern Washington, Will and Mari Kemper traveled the world educating themselves and others about beer. Will, an established brewer, helped set up other first-time operations in Mexico, Turkey, and the United States. Along the way, Will and Mari picked up philosophies and ideas about making better beer and bringing it to the people. In the short time since opening their own brewery, they have been generously (and correctly) awarded. Their mission statement says it all: "Our goal is to have a healthy successful company that will include being a leader in quality driven products and customer service, maintain practices that lead to a healthful environment, offer meaningful employment for employees, sustain strong community relations, promote community missions of charitable giving, and endorse community self sustainability in action by using as many local products as possible."

10

25 BBLS

½ teaspoon fennel seed
½ teaspoon coarse salt
2 teaspoons unsweetened
    cocoa powder
1 teaspoon hot paprika
1 (1½-pound) pork tenderloin
¼ cup extra-virgin olive oil
2 sweet potatoes, peeled and
    thinly sliced
2 tablespoons minced fresh
    rosemary leaves
  Salt
½ cup Bavarian black lager
1 tablespoon brown sugar
¾ cup light cream

A Few Beers to Try with This Recipe

- *Full Sail Session Black Lager*
- *Gordon Biersch Schwarzbier*
- *Samuel Adams Black Lager*
- *Sprecher Black Bavarian*

Cocoa-Crusted Pork Tenderloin

This hearty and savory recipe combines many strong flavors that compete for the attention of your taste buds. The unsweetened cocoa powder is an unexpected but delicious addition, and the fennel adds a slight bite to the pork loin. Pair the pork with a Bavarian Schwarzbier or black lager in which the malts have a slight chocolate taste that brings out interesting flavors with each bite and sip. Though the brewery is now closed and the beer gone, this recipe remains.

1 Preheat the oven to 350°F.

2 Grind the fennel seed and coarse salt together in a mortar and pestle until finely ground. Mix in the cocoa powder and paprika. Pat the pork dry with a paper towel, and coat well on all sides with the cocoa mixture.

3 Heat 2 tablespoons of the olive oil in a large skillet, and sear the pork until browned on all sides, about 5 minutes per side. Place the pork in a baking dish and transfer to the oven to cook for 25 to 30 minutes, or until the pork forms a dark crust and reaches an internal temperature of 165°F.

4 Toss the sweet potatoes with the remaining 2 tablespoons olive oil and the rosemary in a medium bowl. Spread them out on a baking sheet, sprinkle with salt to taste, and bake for 30 minutes, turning once after 15 minutes, until lightly browned and slightly crispy.

5 Deglaze the skillet with the black lager, stirring up the browned bits in the pan. Add the brown sugar and simmer until the liquid gets thick and sticky, about 20 minutes. Reduce the heat to low and add the cream slowly while briskly stirring to avoid curdling. Continue to cook and stir until the sauce is smooth, brown, and slightly thick, about 5 minutes. Remove from the heat and cover to keep warm.

6 Allow the pork loin to rest for 5 minutes after removing it from the oven. Spoon the sauce onto a serving platter and arrange pork slices and sweet potatoes on top. Serve with extra sauce as desired.

Makes 4–6 servings

Imu Pork

Lest you think it is a specific breed, *imu* is actually the name for the pit oven used in Hawaii to steam whole pigs. This traditional recipe has been adapted for a standard oven, set at a very high temperature, to re-create the authentic island flavor. Pork is versatile and can be paired with any number of beers, including porters, pale ales, red ales, and lagers. If you cannot locate ti leaves (check your local florist), banana leaves are an acceptable substitute. This recipe yields a large amount of pork — perfect for your at-home luau or any large gathering.

KONA BREWING COMPANY

KAILUA KONA, HAWAII

1 (8- to 10-pound) pork butt
2 tablespoons kosher salt
2 tablespoons taco seasoning
¼ cup Kona Castaway IPA
  or Fire Rock Pale Ale, or
  similar pale ale
3 tablespoons liquid smoke
1 cup water, plus more as
  needed
  Ti leaves, as needed
½ cup chopped cabbage
12–15 kaiser rolls
  Barbecue sauce
  Shredded cheddar cheese
  (optional)

1 Preheat the oven to 500°F. Pat the pork butt dry with paper towels. Cut several long shallow cuts into the pork to let the spices and liquids penetrate the flesh, and then cut the pork in half.

2 Place the pork in two separate baking dishes, fat side up. Rub the pork with the salt and taco seasoning.

3 Combine the beer and liquid smoke in a measuring cup, and then divide the liquid equally between the two baking dishes. Add just enough water to each pan to come halfway up the pork butt. Layer the ti leaves over the pork butt and then cover the pans tightly with foil.

4 Bake for 45 minutes, and then reduce the heat to 350°F and cook for 3 hours longer or until fork-tender.

5 Remove the pork from the oven and shred it using two forks. Drain off any excess liquid and mix all the pork with the cabbage in a large bowl. Serve with rolls and bowls of barbecue sauce and shredded cheese.

Makes 12–15 servings

PROFILE ★   **Aloha. Since 1994, Kona Brewing Company** has been bringing a taste of the fiftieth state to the rest of the country, using local lore, imagery, and even local ingredients in its beers. Some of its beer is made at partner breweries on both coasts; brewing technology allows the mainland breweries to match the mineral content of Hawaii's water. Committed to environmental causes that work to keep the islands pristine, Kona showcases those initiatives along with its beers during the tour at its Big Island home.

Roasted Venison Saddle with Samuel Adams Chocolate Bock Mole

- 1 (12-ounce) bottle Samuel Adams Chocolate Bock, or similar chocolate bock
- ¾ cup chicken broth
- ½ tart apple, peeled, cored, and chopped
- ¼ cup raisins
- 3 pitted prunes
- 1 tablespoon raw pumpkin seeds
- 1 tablespoon raw slivered almonds
- 1 tablespoon honey
- 1 dried ancho chile, lightly toasted
- 1 dried pasilla chile, lightly toasted
- 1 cinnamon stick
- 1 clove
  Kosher salt and freshly ground black pepper
- 2 tablespoons canola oil
- 4 (6-ounce) venison steaks
- 1 tablespoon unsalted butter
- 1 teaspoon dried thyme

Many people think venison tastes gamey, but if it is handled properly and cooked correctly this lean meat can take on a velvety texture and mild flavor. Many venison recipes rely on long simmering times or braising to coax the meat toward tenderness and allow seasonings to be absorbed. This recipe highlights the true taste of the meat, complemented by an original take on mole, a traditional Mexican sauce. Serve with a chocolate bock, where cocoa and malt live in harmony and lift this dish to new heights.

1 Combine the bock, broth, apple, raisins, prunes, pumpkin seeds, almonds, honey, ancho chile, pasilla chile, cinnamon stick, and clove in a large saucepan. Bring the mixture to a boil over medium-high heat, and then immediately reduce the heat to medium. Cook at a gentle simmer, uncovered, for about 1 hour to give the flavors time to blend. Do not let the liquid boil after the first time.

2 Remove and discard the cinnamon stick and clove from the mole sauce using a slotted spoon. Transfer the mole to a blender or the bowl of a food processor and blend until smooth. Season with salt and pepper to taste and set aside.

3 Heat a large skillet and, when very hot, add the canola oil. Sear the venison steaks in the hot oil until medium-rare, about 5 minutes on the first side and 6 minutes on the second side. Add the butter and thyme to the skillet during the last minute of cooking and baste the steaks with the pan juices. Remove the steaks from the skillet and set aside on a plate.

4 Reheat the mole sauce on the stovetop, if needed. Spoon about ¼ to ½ cup of mole sauce on each of four dinner plates and set a venison steak atop each puddle of mole. Serve immediately. You might have a little extra mole left over; if you're thinking about tomorrow's dinner it goes great with grilled chicken or burgers.

Makes 4 servings

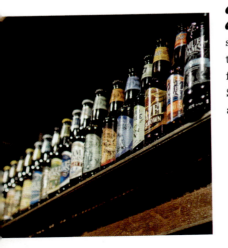

As the largest craft brewery in the country, *Samuel Adams* has been instrumental in reinvigorating the industry. Led by its flagship Boston Lager, the brewery is continually creating and releasing beers that cover every conceivable beer category and has even created a few styles of its own. Founded in 1984 by fifth-generation brewer Jim Koch, the brewery swiftly rose to the top. When he first started the company, Koch peddled homebrewed batches to bars throughout Boston. As interest grew, the brewery began contracting through a larger facility and was able to quickly gain ground in the marketplace.

Today, Samuel Adams has a small pilot brewery in Boston where its brewers create many new recipes and barrel-aged brews. Breweries in Pennsylvania and Ohio produce the bulk of its more than two million barrels of beer. With its television commercials and other advertising, Samuel Adams has helped stem the flow of larger breweries and guided craft beer to a stronger foothold in the market. Thanks to its flavorful beers using premium ingredients, Samuel Adams has welcomed scores of new beer drinkers who have eschewed pale watery lagers in favor of beers with more taste.

Braised Beef Short Ribs

The Belgian dark strong ale in this recipe gives the beef and vegetables a rich sweetness and fruity undertones of cherry and fig. Serve the ribs over polenta or potatoes with a vegetable side of your choice and a glass of the ale to drink.

2 tablespoons black peppercorns

2 tablespoons yellow mustard seeds

2 teaspoons salt

½ teaspoon cayenne pepper

5 pounds beef short ribs

3 tablespoons extra-virgin olive oil

2 large onions, chopped

2 carrots, peeled and diced

2 celery stalks, diced

1 head garlic

2 cups beef broth

1 cup North Coast Brother Thelonious ale, or similar strong ale

1 (6-ounce) can tomato paste

¼ cup red wine vinegar

3 tablespoons honey

2 tablespoons beef base
Fresh thyme sprigs, for garnish

1 Crush the peppercorns and mustard seeds together using a mortar and pestle. Blend in the salt and cayenne.

2 Preheat the oven to 350°F. Pat the short ribs dry with paper towels and rub all over with the spice mixture.

3 Warm the olive oil in a large skillet over high heat. When the oil begins to smoke, place the beef short ribs in the skillet and cook until brown on all sides, about 3 minutes per side. Transfer the ribs to a large Dutch oven.

4 Add the onions, carrots, and celery to the skillet and stir. Separate and peel the garlic cloves. Cut each clove in half and add all the garlic to the skillet. Cook, stirring frequently, until the vegetables are golden brown, 5 to 7 minutes. Transfer the mixture to the Dutch oven.

5 Deglaze the skillet with the beef broth, beer, tomato paste, red wine vinegar, honey, and beef base, and bring to a simmer over medium heat. Add the beer mixture to the Dutch oven, cover, and bake for 2½ hours, or until the beef is tender.

6 Remove the meat from the Dutch oven and keep warm. Heat the sauce in the pan to a boil over medium-high heat and reduce to the desired thickness. Nestle the ribs in creamy polenta or serve alongside boiled potatoes, and dress everything with the sauce. Garnish with fresh thyme and serve immediately.

Makes 6–8 servings

A Few Beers to Try with This Recipe

- *Allagash Black*
- *Dogfish Head Raison D'etre*
- *Lost Abbey Judgment Day*
- *North Coast Brother Thelonious*
- *Russian River Salvation*
- *Tröegs Mad Elf*

North Coast Brewing Company is a California brewery that walks the walk, talks the talk, and produces strong and flavorful beers worthy of your time and glass. Take for example the Brother Thelonious used in the short ribs recipe. Not only is the 9 percent dark strong ale everything one would want from the style, it is named after the late jazz master, Thelonious Monk, and a portion of the sales goes to benefit a charity in his name. The affable and knowledgeable Mark Ruedrich heads the brewery and has been an advocate for bringing new beers to market while honoring the past of craft brewing. For example, North Coast has resurrected the Acme Beer name — a California brewing staple dating back to the 1800s. Visit the brewery and attached taproom and restaurant for a true taste of California with some genuine brewer hospitality.

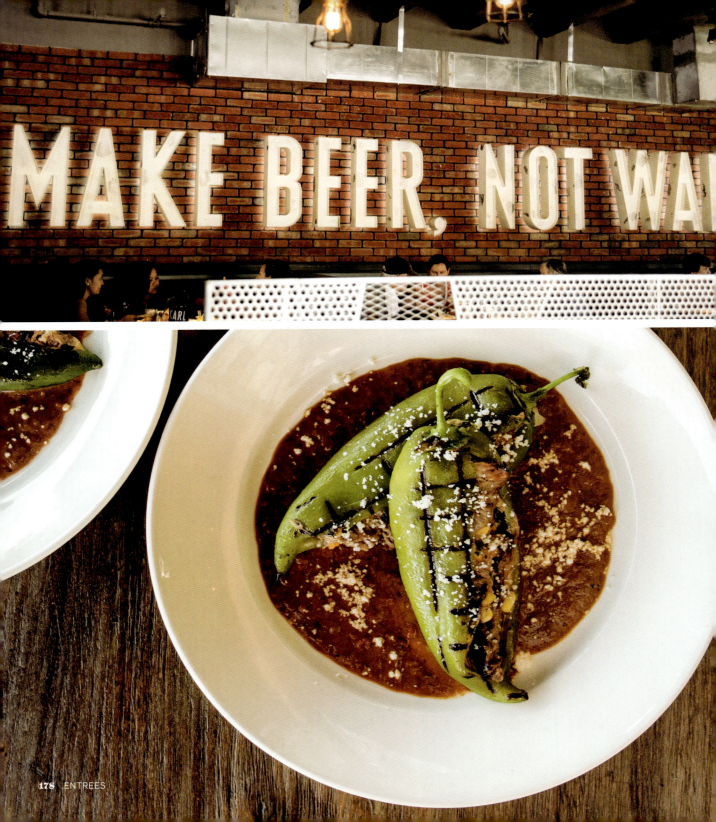

Duck Chiles Rellenos

KARL STRAUSS BREWING COMPANY

SAN DIEGO, CALIFORNIA

Rellenos are stuffed peppers, and this recipe combines a multitude of flavors for those who enjoy spicy heat. Anaheim chiles are sometimes called California or Magdalena chiles and rank among the lowest on the heat scale. Chicken may be substituted for duck, but this dish gets a lot of additional flavor from the waterfowl. Use a bold red ale heavy on the caramel malts (like the Karl Strauss Red Trolly Ale) for the cooking and pair the end result with a hoppy red ale.

1 **MAKE THE SAUCE:** Heat the olive oil in a large saucepan. Add the onions and garlic and cook until translucent, about 5 minutes. Add the chiles, sugar, cinnamon, salt, black pepper, chicken broth, beer, and vinegar to the saucepan. Bring to a simmer and cook until the chiles are soft, about 30 minutes.

2 Add the pineapple and banana and cook the sauce for 10 minutes

longer. Remove the sauce from the heat and let cool slightly. Transfer the sauce to a blender and purée until smooth. Strain the sauce through a medium-fine strainer, pushing the solids against the sides of the strainer until dry; discard the dry solids. Adjust the thickness of the sauce to that of thick cream with water if needed. Cover and set aside.

recipe continues on next page

ANCHO CHILE SAUCE
- 1 tablespoon extra-virgin olive oil
- 1 medium yellow onion, diced
- 2 garlic cloves, minced
- 4 dried ancho chiles
- 1 tablespoon sugar
- ½ teaspoon cinnamon
- ½ teaspoon salt
  Freshly ground black pepper
- 1 cup chicken broth
- 1 cup Karl Strauss Red Trolley Ale, or similar ale
- 1 tablespoon cider vinegar
- 1 cup crushed pineapple
- 1 banana, peeled and thinly sliced
  Water, if needed

SHREDDED DUCK MEAT FILLING
- 2 duck legs
- ½ cup Karl Strauss Red Trolley Ale, or similar ale
- 2 tablespoons unsalted butter
- ¼ cup canola oil
- 1 teaspoon salt
- ¼ teaspoon freshly ground black pepper
- 2 ounces pepper jack cheese, shredded (½ cup)
- ¼ cup sweet corn kernels, fresh or frozen and defrosted
- 1 tablespoon chopped cilantro leaves

- 2 Anaheim chiles
  Cotija cheese, for serving

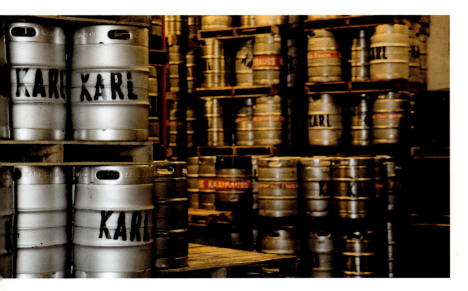

3 **MAKE THE FILLING:** Preheat the oven to 300°F. Place the duck legs in a single layer in a baking dish. Add the beer, butter, oil, salt, and black pepper, cover with aluminum foil, and bake until the duck is tender and easily pulls away from the bone, about 90 minutes.

4 Remove the dish from the oven and remove the duck legs from the baking dish to cool. (Discard any fat in the baking dish.) Once cool, remove and discard the skin and bones and shred the duck meat. Place the shredded duck meat in a medium bowl and gently mix in the cheese, corn, cilantro, and 1/2 cup of the ancho chile sauce.

5 **ASSEMBLE THE CHILES RELLENOS:** Prepare a hot fire in a gas or charcoal grill or preheat the oven to broil. Roast the Anaheim chiles, turning occasionally, until the skins start to blister and char. Remove the chiles from the heat and let cool to room temperature. Peel the skin from the cooled chiles and rinse under cold water.

6 The chiles will be fragile at this point, so carefully cut a slit into one side of each chile and, if desired, gently remove its seeds with a spoon. Stuff the chiles with the shredded duck meat mixture, dividing it equally between the two chiles.

7 Place the stuffed chiles on a medium-hot oiled grill and cook

for 1 minute. Once grill marks appear, turn the chiles over and cook on the other side until hot, about 2 minutes longer.

8 Rewarm the remaining ancho chile sauce on the stovetop or in a microwave. Place 1/2 cup of the sauce in the center of a serving plate. Place the rellenos atop the sauce, sprinkle with the cotija cheese, and serve immediately.

Makes 2 servings and 1¼ cups sauce

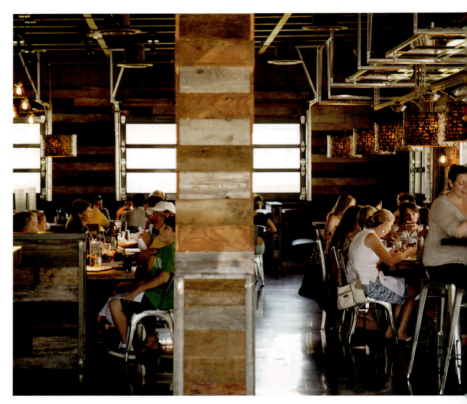

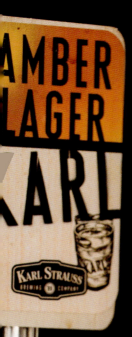
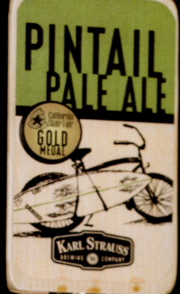

AMBER
LAGER
KARL

PINTAIL
PALE ALE

GOLD
MEDAL

KARL STRAUSS
BREWING COMPANY

WINDANSEA
WHEAT

KARL STRAUSS
BREWING COMPANY

WOODI
GOL

KARL STRAUSS
BREWING COMPANY

PROFILE ★ **Chris Cramer and Matt Rattner were pioneers** in what is now a celebrated beer destination. Opening the first microbrewery in San Diego since Prohibition, the duo successfully navigated outdated laws and red tape to bring locals *Karl Strauss Brewing Company*. Chris's cousin Karl M. Strauss, a successful and celebrated brewmaster who trained at Weihenstephan and had a career at Pabst, lent his name and expertise to the new venture. The response was immediate and strong, and the brewery grew. In addition to their large production brewery, the two friends own eight brewery restaurants and boast an impressive lineup of annual beers, special releases, and fun events.

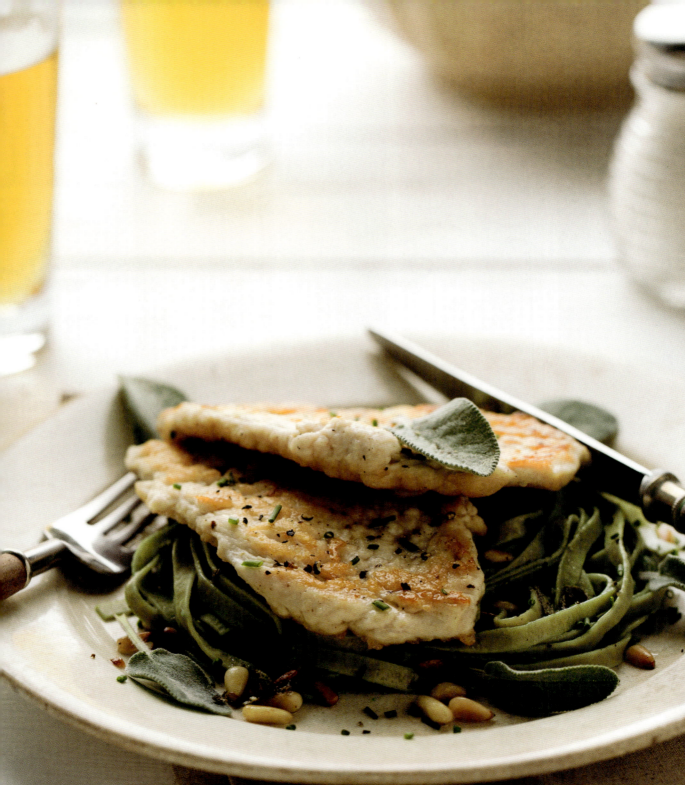

Sage Veal Medallions

This tasty recipe, which owes much of its flavor to pine nuts and fresh herbs, is as great for weeknight dinners as it is for fancier weekend meals. For the wary: Many butchers now sell humanely raised veal. Consult the package label or talk to your butcher before purchasing the veal. Pair this dish with a saison, such as Willimantic's Flowers Infusion, which has many botanical notes that draw out the flavors of the dish.

WILLIMANTIC BREWING COMPANY

WILLIMANTIC, CONNECTICUT

3 tablespoons all-purpose flour
Salt and freshly ground black pepper
2½ pounds veal medallions, pounded thin
3 tablespoons extra-virgin olive oil
½ cup fresh lemon juice
4 tablespoons unsalted butter
½ cup pine nuts, toasted
6 whole sage leaves plus 1 tablespoon thinly sliced fresh sage leaves
3 garlic cloves, minced
1½ pounds dried spinach fettuccine
12 fresh chives, thinly sliced

1 Combine the flour with salt and pepper to taste in a medium bowl. Dredge the veal in the seasoned flour, shaking off any excess, and set aside.

2 Warm the olive oil in a large skillet. Add the veal and pan-sear for 1½ minutes; flip and cook for 1 minute longer. Transfer the veal to a plate to rest.

3 Return the skillet to the heat, add the lemon juice, and cook, stirring up the browned bits in the pan. Add the butter and stir into the lemon juice; allow to melt and thicken slightly. Add the pine nuts, the tablespoon of sliced sage, the garlic, and salt and pepper to taste.

4 Meanwhile, bring a large pot of salted water to a boil. Cook the fettuccine to desired doneness according to the package instructions. Drain the pasta, and then spin the fettuccine into the sauce with tongs.

5 Transfer the pasta to a large round plate and top with the veal medallions. Garnish with the whole sage leaves and chives and serve immediately.

Makes 6 servings

PROFILE ★ **Housed inside a decommissioned post office** in central Connecticut, *Willimantic Brewing Company* is a perennial award winner that draws both locals and those from the nearby University of Connecticut. While some renovations have been made to the 1909 building, to the delight of philatelists it retains much of its postal heritage. The menu features some unexpected surprises, and the staff is as welcoming to visitors as to regulars. Thanks to the bevy of beers made on premises, the locals have plenty of reasons to make the brewery a regular stop.

Imperial Meat Pie

There are everyday ho-hum meat pie or shepherd pie recipes. Then there is this impressive version from Schlafly that uses a generous pour of the brewery's Imperial Stout to bring some bite and sweetness to the filling. Stouts and porters pair well with this dish, but consider a malty doppelbock as an accompaniment to the rich toasty flavors as well.

2 tablespoons vegetable oil
2½ pounds beef stew meat, cubed
1 teaspoon dried thyme
Salt and freshly ground black pepper
1½ pounds baby red potatoes, quartered
2 medium carrots, peeled and diced
2 medium yellow onions, diced
½ pound cremini mushrooms, quartered
1 tablespoon chopped garlic
1 cup Schlafly Imperial Stout, or similar stout
¼ cup red wine vinegar
1 tablespoon Dijon mustard
2 tablespoons dark brown sugar
⅓ cup brown roux (see box)
4 cups beef broth
1 pound prepared biscuit dough

Brown Roux

Melt 4 tablespoons of unsalted butter in a small skillet over medium heat. Whisk in 2 tablespoons of flour, reduce the heat to low, and cook, stirring often, until the color is similar to that of milk chocolate, about 45 minutes.

1 Heat the oil in a large Dutch oven over medium-high heat. Season the beef with the thyme, salt, and pepper and sear it in the skillet until brown on all sides, about 2 minutes per side. Transfer the beef to a plate or bowl and set aside.

2 Put the potatoes in a large saucepan and cover with water. Bring to a boil and cook until tender, about 7 minutes. Drain and set aside.

3 Add the carrots, onions, mushrooms, and garlic to the pan in which you browned the beef. Sauté over medium heat until tender, 5 to 7 minutes. Deglaze the pan with the stout and cook, stirring up the browned bits, until half of the liquid has evaporated. Add the vinegar, mustard, and brown sugar and simmer, uncovered, for 15 minutes.

4 Whisk in the roux until combined. Slowly whisk in the broth and continue to simmer, stirring occasionally, until you have a rich stew, about 30 minutes.

5 Preheat the oven to 375°F.

6 Season the broth mixture to taste with salt and pepper and add the beef and potatoes to the pan. Stir gently to combine, and then transfer the beef mixture to a 9- by 13-inch casserole dish. Top the casserole with the biscuit dough, poking holes in the top with a fork for ventilation. Bake for 15 to 20 minutes, until the crust is golden brown and the filling is bubbling. Serve hot with a crisp green salad.

Makes 6–8 servings

Two decades ago, when the founders of *Schlafly* opened their business in Saint Louis, there were locals who questioned why a small upstart would try to challenge the king. The city was, of course, synonymous with Budweiser. But the founders were determined to bring flavorful beer to the lager-choked market, and after a long uphill climb, they have established themselves as a solid brewery known for flavorful brews that have converted even the most stubborn of company men. Schlafly's must-visit taproom is a charming location housed inside a building that's on the National Register of Historic Places; it boasts a sure-fire kitchen staff that expertly highlights the joys of beer and food pairing.

Kilt Lifter Mac & Cheese

The childhood staple has grown up. Thanks to a generous upgrade of flavors (including a dash of Scotch ale) this gooey and creamy delight explodes with flavor and will fill you up right. A dish this good is worth a little extra preparation effort and will make you rethink reaching for that packaged product in the future. While this recipe suggests serving the mac and cheese in individual ramekins, it can also be baked in a large baking dish for a more homestyle presentation. Try pairing with a cream ale, which complements the cheddar and does not overpower the other flavors.

- 4 tablespoons butter
- ¼ cup flour
- ½ cup vegetable or chicken broth
- 1 cup whole milk
- ¼ cup Scotch ale
- 2 garlic cloves, minced
- 1 teaspoon dry mustard
- ⅛ teaspoon cayenne pepper
- 1 teaspoon salt
- 8 ounces sharp cheddar cheese, grated (2 cups)
- 1½ pounds elbow macaroni, or other small-shape pasta of your choice

1 Preheat the oven to 375°F and begin heating a large pot of salted water to a boil for the pasta.

2 Melt the butter in a saucepan over medium heat. Add the flour, stir to combine, and cook for about 2 minutes, taking care not to brown the flour. Add the broth and bring to a simmer, stirring to prevent lumps. Reduce the heat to medium-low, add the milk and ale, and bring the mixture back to a simmer, stirring frequently. Add the garlic, mustard, cayenne, and salt, stirring to incorporate.

3 Add 1½ cups of the cheese, a handful at a time, stirring to make sure the cheese melts evenly and is fully incorporated before adding the next handful. Remove the pan from the heat and set aside, covered.

4 Cook the pasta in the boiling water according to the directions on the package, or until al dente. Drain well and combine with the slightly cooled sauce.

5 Divide the macaroni and cheese mixture into individual ramekins, divide the remaining ½ cup cheese over the tops of the casseroles, and bake for 10 minutes, until the sauce is bubbly and the top is browned. Serve hot.

Makes 6–8 servings

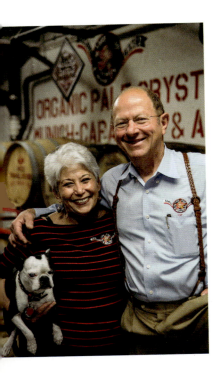

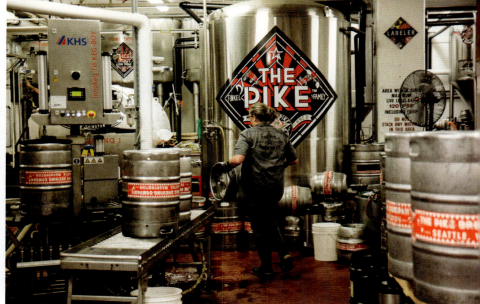

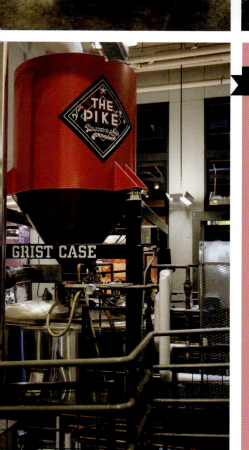

PROFILE ★ **The importance of Charles and Rose Ann Finkel** on America's contemporary beer scene cannot be overstated. In the 1970s, they were already firmly ensconced in the wine industry but had a fondness for beer and wanted to bring many of the world's great beers to American shores, where the majority of drinkers had been deprived of real flavors. Together they founded Merchant du Vin, an importing company that featured — and still does — some of the more established and respected brands from overseas. Settling in Seattle, the couple purchased a homebrew supply store at Pike Place Market in 1989 and quickly installed a small brewing system on the premises, from which they turned out flavorful brews to an appreciative local clientele. The endeavor was, obviously, called *Pike Place Brewery*. The Finkels also cultivated a lot of brewing talent: quite a few of the country's leading brewers got their start at Pike. The business grew, and a larger setup was installed and a restaurant added when they moved to a bigger location. In the late 1990s they were offered a chance to sell their businesses, and they took the opportunity. Less than a decade later, however, they found themselves missing the brewpub and repurchased the Pike, coming back to the business with all cylinders firing. There is no mistaking their influence on today's beer scene, as referenced by the countless awards and recognitions, the revered tones in which they are mentioned by those in the industry, and the regular customers who came to know good beer at the Pike. Many of those customers continue to call the brewpub their home away from home.

DOUGH

- ½ teaspoon active dry yeast
- ¼ cup warm water (100–110°F), plus additional tablespoons as needed
- 4½ cups all-purpose flour
- ½ teaspoon salt
  Nonstick cooking spray
  Cornmeal

SAUCE

- 1 (15-ounce) can tomato sauce
- 1 (6-ounce) can tomato paste
- 2 teaspoons dried basil
- 2 teaspoons dried oregano
- 2 teaspoons freshly ground black pepper
- 1 teaspoon salt
- 1 teaspoon granulated garlic
- ½ teaspoon granulated onion
- 1 tablespoon extra-virgin olive oil

PIZZA

- 2 ounces whole-milk mozzarella cheese, shredded (½ cup)
- 1 ounce provolone cheese, shredded (¼ cup)
- 1 ounce white cheddar cheese, shredded (¼ cup)

Cheese Pizza

There is no need for delivery when you have a recipe like this to make at home. A fresh-from-the-oven classic cheese pizza (add toppings of your choice) requires a little more work than dialing a phone number, but it's worth the extra effort. With each saucy and cheese-filled bite comes a feeling of satisfaction and the desire for another slice. Pair with any number of beers, but pale ales, traditional lagers, and even hoppy red ales work quite well. It is okay to substitute a premade crust, but if you do make the dough, use a pizza stone and make sure that it's fully heated before baking the pizza. An inverted baking sheet can also work in a pinch. This recipe makes more sauce than you will need, but it freezes well and can be used in other dishes such as pasta.

1 **MAKE THE DOUGH:** Dissolve the yeast in the warm water in a small bowl. Let sit for 5 minutes.

2 Combine the flour and salt in the bowl of a food processor. Pulse two times. With the processor running, add the yeast mixture. Add additional water with the motor running, 1 tablespoon at a time, as needed until the dough forms a ball. Process for 30 seconds.

3 Turn the dough onto a lightly floured surface and knead four or five times. Place the dough in a bowl coated with nonstick cooking spray and cover with a damp towel. Let the dough rise until doubled in size, about 1 hour. Punch the dough down, cover, and let rest for 5 minutes.

4 **MAKE THE SAUCE:** Combine the tomato sauce, tomato paste, basil, oregano, black pepper, salt, garlic, onion, and olive oil in a medium bowl and stir until the ingredients are incorporated.

5 **MAKE THE PIZZA:** Place a pizza stone on the lowest rack of the oven and preheat the oven to 500°F.

6 Dust a pizza peel with cornmeal. Roll the dough into a 10-inch circle on a lightly floured surface and then transfer the dough to the prepared peel. Spread ¼ cup of the pizza sauce over the dough. (Refrigerate any remaining pizza sauce for another use; it will keep for up to 1 week.) Top the pizza with the mozzarella, provolone, and cheddar.

7 Transfer the pizza to the pizza stone and bake for 8 minutes, or until the cheese is melted and the crust turns golden brown around the edges. Remove the pizza from the oven and let stand 1 minute before slicing and serving.

Makes 1 (10-inch) pizza

PROFILE ★ **Pizza and beer are a classic combination**, and in San Antonio, the two have come together in spectacular fashion. Founder Scott Metzger had the idea to open a place of his own while sitting at another brewpub, enjoying a beer. He thought, why not bring good beer to south-central Texas and add some quality pizza along with it? Three years later *Freetail* (which is named after the state's official flying mammal, the Mexican free-tailed bat) opened, and it has been serving pies and pints to an eager crowd ever since.

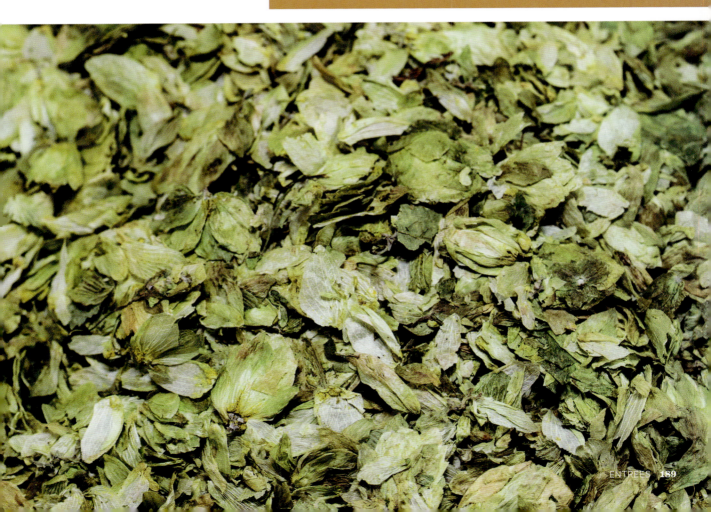

Hanger Steak
with Gorgonzola Sauce

With just a modest amount of prep work, this recipe delivers a flavorful, powerful dish. Using Old Brown Dog or a similar brown ale to marinate the meat gives it a hearty flavor and breaks down some muscle tissue, resulting in a more tender texture. Gorgonzola, part of the blue cheese family, is a dominating flavor, so pairing this dish with an assertively hoppy India pale ale is a smart bet.

HANGER STEAKS

- 2 tablespoons light brown sugar
- 1 shallot, minced
- 2 fresh thyme sprigs, leaves removed and minced
- 2 fresh rosemary sprigs, leaves removed and minced
- 1 garlic clove, minced
- 1 teaspoon freshly ground black pepper
- Red pepper flakes
- 1 cup Smuttynose Old Brown Dog, or similar brown ale
- ¼ cup extra-virgin olive oil
- 2 tablespoons tamari
- 2 tablespoons Worcestershire sauce
- 1 tablespoon Dijon mustard
- 4 (10-ounce) hanger steaks, or beef tips

GORGONZOLA SAUCE

- 2 cups heavy cream
- 3 ounces Gorgonzola cheese, crumbled
- 1 teaspoon fresh lemon juice
- 1 dash Worcestershire sauce
- 1 dash Tabasco sauce
- Freshly ground black pepper

1 MARINATE THE STEAKS: Combine the brown sugar, shallot, thyme, rosemary, garlic, black pepper, a pinch of pepper flakes, beer, olive oil, tamari, Worcestershire, and mustard in a large bowl, and mix well. Put the steaks in an airtight container and pour the marinade on top. Cover and refrigerate for at least 8 hours or up to 2 days, turning the steaks occasionally.

2 MAKE THE GORGONZOLA SAUCE: Reduce the heavy cream by half over medium-high heat in a small saucepan, about 10 minutes. Whisk in the cheese, and then remove the saucepan from the heat just as it has melted. Whisk in the lemon juice, Worcestershire, Tabasco, and black pepper to taste.

3 GRILL THE STEAKS: Prepare a hot fire in a gas or charcoal grill. Remove the steaks from the marinade and pat dry with paper towels; discard the marinade. Place the steaks at least an inch apart on the grill and cook on one side until a dark crust forms on the underside, 3 to 5 minutes. Turn them over and grill 3 to 5 minutes longer for medium-rare. The steaks will have shrunk a bit and they will feel slightly firm to the touch.

4 Transfer the steaks to a cutting board to rest for several minutes before slicing and serving with warm Gorgonzola sauce.

Makes 4 servings

Immediately recognizable by its logo featuring a common harbor seal, the *Smuttynose Brewing Co.* is named after the third largest island of the archipelago that lies off the coast of New Hampshire and Maine. Aside from its world-class beer, another thing that sets this established New England brewery apart is the use of photos, not illustrations, on its beer bottles. Old Brown Dog features a photo of the now-departed Olive, who was, in fact, a brown Brittany Spaniel and Weimaraner mix, and the brewery's IPA shows two older New England gentlemen, Cy and Paul, sitting on lawn chairs with a garden gnome lurking in the background. The photos are fun and kitschy and often evoke a smile.

Founded by Peter Egelston, his sister (who also owns the wonderful Northampton Brewery in western Massachusetts), and a few others, the brewery today has a dedicated staff who would love to show you around should the spirit move you to visit their Granite State brewery.

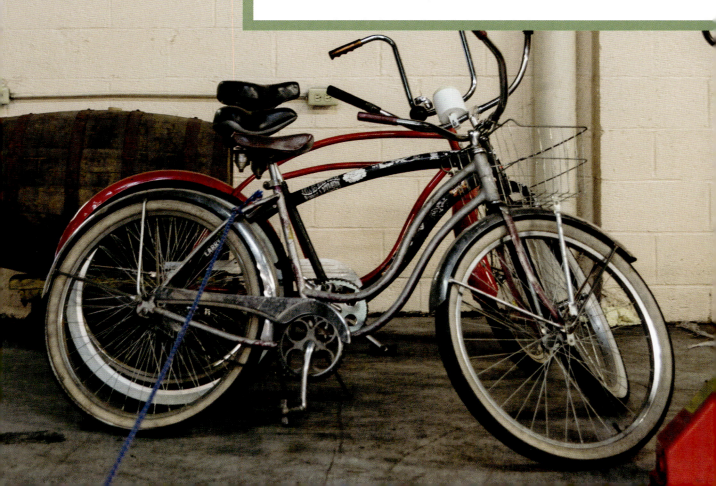

Moroccan-Cured Duck Breasts with Pomegranate, Prune, and §ucaba Sauce and Black Beluga Lentils

Moroccan flavors highlight the dark chocolate, vanilla-bourbon, and slight cherry notes of the §ucaba (Firestone Walker's English barley wine) used in the sauce for this dish. The flavors in this dish unfold slowly with each bite: the rich, meaty duck breasts followed by the sweet and savory spices. What better to stand up to the meat than the earthy lentils and the tart/sweet barley wine sauce? Courtesy of Sean Z. Paxton, a culinary and beer wizard (and friend of the brewery) who is known and celebrated for his stunning presentation and blending of flavors, this recipe is ambitious but worth the time.

DUCK BREASTS

- 2 teaspoons kosher salt
- 2 tablespoons soft candi sugar, such as Brun Foncé Dark, or brown sugar
- 1 teaspoon ground Ceylon cinnamon
- 1 teaspoon ground coriander
- 1 teaspoon ground ginger
- 1 teaspoon dried orange peel
- 4 boneless skin-on duck breasts

SAUCE

- 2¾ cups Firestone Walker §ucaba, or a similar English barley wine
- ½ cup pitted and finely chopped prunes
- 4 Medjool dates, pitted and finely chopped
- 3 tablespoons unsalted butter
- 3 shallots, minced
- ½ cup chicken or vegetable broth
- 3–4 tablespoons pomegranate molasses, plus more as needed

LENTILS

- 2 tablespoons unsalted butter
- 2 shallots, minced
- 2 garlic cloves, minced
- 1 cup black beluga lentils
- 1½ cups fresh carrot juice
- 1 (12-ounce) bottle IPA
  Salt and freshly ground black pepper

Note: Pomegranate molasses can usually be found in the specialty aisle of a grocery store or at a Mediterranean market.

1 SEASON THE DUCK BREASTS: Whisk the salt, soft candi sugar, cinnamon, coriander, ginger, and orange peel together in a medium bowl until combined. Reserve 2 teaspoons of the spice blend for the sauce.

2 Pat the duck breasts dry with paper towels. Score the skin in a square or diamond pattern, being careful not to cut all the way through the skin. (This step will help render the fat from the duck and create a pattern on the breast for presentation.)

3 Divide the spice mix into four equal portions, and evenly sprinkle a portion on both sides of each duck breast; rub the spice mix into the skin and meat. Place the duck breasts in an airtight container and refrigerate for at least 4 hours or up to overnight to lightly cure.

4 MAKE THE SAUCE: Pour the barley wine down the inside of a lidded quart-size jar, limiting the foamy head. Add the prunes and dates, seal, and refrigerate for at least 4 hours or up to overnight to rehydrate and soften the fruit.

5 When you are ready to prepare dinner, melt the butter in a medium saucepan over medium heat; let it begin to foam and turn a light brown color to create a brown butter. Add the shallots and sauté until they just start to caramelize, 5 to 6 minutes. Add the reserved 2 teaspoons of the Moroccan spice blend and cook for 1 minute longer to toast the spices.

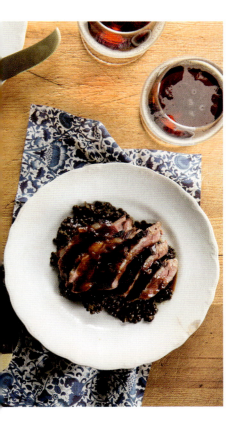

6 Add the marinated fruit mixture, broth, and pomegranate molasses to the saucepan. Bring the mixture to a boil and simmer, uncovered, until the sauce has thickened and reduced by half and the fruit is falling apart, 25 to 30 minutes. (If the fruit remains intact, purée one-third of the sauce in a blender and add it back to the saucepan.) Season with additional pomegranate molasses to taste and keep warm until ready to serve. (This sauce can be made in advance and rewarmed if needed.)

7 **MAKE THE LENTILS:** Melt the butter in a medium pot over medium heat. Add the shallots and cook, stirring occasionally, until caramelized, 6 to 7 minutes. Add the garlic and cook for 1 minute longer.

8 Add the lentils to the saucepan, stirring to evenly coat in the butter-shallot mixture, and lightly toast for 2 to 3 minutes. Add the carrot juice and IPA, and bring to a boil. Reduce the heat to low, cover with a lid, and simmer. Cook the lentils until they are tender but not falling apart and most of the liquid is absorbed, 30 to 40 minutes. Add a little water if needed to finish cooking. Season with salt and pepper to taste.

9 **PREPARE THE DUCK BREASTS:** Remove the duck breasts from the refrigerator and pour off any juice that might have collected. Place the duck breasts, skin side down, in a cold skillet. Turn the heat to medium and cook the duck breasts for 10 to 12 minutes, rendering out the fat in the skin. After 8 minutes, check to make sure the skin isn't over-browned.

10 Turn the breasts over and cook until medium-rare or until they reach 140°F on an instant-read thermometer, about 1 minute longer. Remove the skillet from the heat, cover with aluminum foil, and let sit for 5 minutes, allowing the juices to redistribute.

11 Transfer the duck breasts to a cutting board and slice on the bias. Scoop the lentils into a mound on a warm plate or platter and top with the duck breast slices. Drizzle the sauce over the lentils and duck breasts and around the plate before serving.

Makes 4 servings

Wizards of wood and masters of hops, the folks at *Firestone Walker* have used their intuition and daring to develop their brewery into one of the most recognized and awarded midsize craft breweries in the country. One of the special things about the brewery is that some of its beers are fermented in toasted American oak barrels, which impart an earthy quality to the beer. In fact, Firestone Walker is the only American brewery to use this particular method. After the new barrels spend about five months fermenting beer, they are emptied and then put into service in the brewery's aging program, along with retired spirits barrels. It is that process that has brought many deeply flavorful and uniquely spiced beers to the glasses of eager fans. Under the direction of brewmaster Matthew Brynildson, Firestone Walker has inspired not only drinkers but fellow breweries to examine ingredients and aging options. And while many of the beers are built to be aged, most drinkers find it difficult to wait long to open them up.

Lemongrass Chicken

UNCOMMON BREWERS

SANTA CRUZ, CALIFORNIA

A wonderful thing about chicken is that it's the perfect blank canvas to absorb and highlight the ingredients it's cooked with. In this dish, the humble bird gets a vibrant boost from fresh herbs and spices that create an inspiring floral bouquet. The beer called for is Uncommon Brewers Siamese Twin, a dubbel infused with lime and spices like coriander. However, a more traditional dubbel works as well if you cannot find Siamese Twin (see note). This recipe requires a few hours of marinating time and is quite tasty served with a grapefruit, avocado, and endive salad. Try pairing with a spicy, hoppy Belgian pale ale.

2 lemongrass stalks, trimmed and minced
¼ cup coarsely chopped fresh cilantro leaves
2 tablespoons minced fresh ginger
1 tablespoon freshly ground black pepper
1 tablespoon light brown sugar
Salt
1 cup Uncommon Siamese Twin Ale, or another dubbel (see note)
4 chicken thighs, preferably skin-on and bone-in

1 Combine the lemongrass, cilantro, ginger, black pepper, brown sugar, salt to taste (about 1 tablespoon), and beer in a plastic ziplock bag. Shake vigorously to combine.

2 Rinse the chicken thighs and pat dry with a paper towel. Add them to the marinade and refrigerate for at least 2 hours, or up to 1 day.

3 Preheat the oven to 375°F. Remove the chicken from the marinade and place skin-side up in a roasting pan or cast-iron grilling pan.

Bake for 15 minutes; turn the chicken over and cook for 20 minutes longer, or until the juices run clear and an instant-read thermometer inserted into one thigh reads 180°F.

4 Switch the oven to broil and broil the chicken for 1 minute. Flip the chicken and broil for 1 minute longer to brown the second side. Remove the chicken from the oven and let rest for at least 4 minutes before serving.

Makes 2–3 servings

Note: If you use another dubbel in the marinade, add 2 tablespoons fresh lime juice and 1 tablespoon coriander to the mixture.

PROFILE ★ **Progress is a delightful thing.** For centuries, Belgian beers have ranked among the finest on the planet. Recipes passed down and perfected over generations delighted and nourished the people. When the American craft beer industry reached its stride, brewers like **Uncommon** came along, studied the established styles, and made some adjustments. The results are traditional ales with untraditional ingredients. The unpasteurized and unfiltered beers from brewer Alec Stefansky are unique to Uncommon, and quite good!

Jerk Pork

Spicy and fragrant, this slow-cooked Caribbean classic reaches perfection when paired with the cooling effect of a refreshingly smooth pale ale, like SBC's 6TH Generation Stock Ale. A favorite of SBC's brewmaster Jaime Jurado, this recipe requires up to a day's worth of marinating.

- 6 tablespoons unsalted butter, at room temperature
- 1 cup firmly packed fresh parsley leaves
- 3 scallions, thinly sliced, white and light green parts only
- 10 garlic cloves
- 3 Scotch bonnet chiles, seeded and roughly chopped
- 1 shallot, roughly chopped
- 2 tablespoons crushed dried oregano
- 2 tablespoons crushed dried sage leaves
- 1 tablespoon dried thyme
- 1 teaspoon ground allspice
- ½ cup pale ale or stock ale
- ⅓ cup apricot preserves
- 1 (2¼-pound) boneless pork loin roast
  Juice of 1 lime
  Kosher salt and freshly ground black pepper

Note: This dish calls for very spicy peppers; feel free to substitute a variety with less heat, such as banana peppers, if you prefer a milder dish.

1 Combine the butter, parsley, scallions, garlic, chiles, shallot, oregano, sage, thyme, allspice, pale ale, and apricot preserves in the bowl of a food processor. Pulse until thoroughly chopped and combined.

2 Rub the entire surface of the roast with the lime juice and then season with salt and pepper to taste. Slather the jerk mixture over the entire surface of the meat. (Alternatively, for a more elegant presentation, cut between the layer of fat and the pork roast, leaving the fat attached to form a flap. Generously slather inside the flap with the jerk mixture.)

3 Tie the pork roast together, cover tightly with plastic wrap, and refrigerate for at least 8 hours or up to 24 hours.

4 Preheat the oven to 250°F. Remove the roast from the refrigerator and discard the plastic wrap. Place the pork in a roasting pan and cook until an instant-read thermometer inserted into the center of the meat reaches 150°F, about 45 minutes. Remove the pork from the oven, allow to rest for 15 to 20 minutes, and then slice or shred with a fork. Serve hot with roasting juices drizzled over the meat.

Makes 8 servings

PROFILE ★ **The Susquehanna Brewing Company** was founded in 2012 by Ed Maier, the great-great-grandson of Charles Stagmaier, who emigrated to America in 1849 and began brewing lager in northeast Pennsylvania in 1851. Maier is joined in the venture by his son, Fred, and a business partner, Mark Nobile. The brewery focuses on German-style beers and benefits from a lot of industry knowledge. Venerable brewmaster Jaime Jurado joined the company, returning to his Pennsylvania brewing roots after a respected stint at Gambrinus in Texas, and Maier and Nobile owned one of the largest wholesale beer distributors before getting into the production end of things. With that kind of knowledge, the odds are with this new brewery.

Baked Ham with #9 Glaze

Fruit and ham are a traditional pairing, and this recipe highlights the compatibility of those two ingredients. The warm apricot notes in Magic Hat's #9 brew combine with spices and orange to make a mouthwatering glaze you won't soon forget. Pair with an ale that makes use of apricot flavors; quite a few are available on the market these days. This is perfect for big holiday dinners with the family (and it's a good excuse to introduce the uninitiated to different beers).

MAGIC HAT BREWING CO.

SOUTH BURLINGTON, VERMONT

1 (5- to 7-pound) bone-in ham
½ cup Magic Hat #9, or similar beer
¼ cup light brown sugar
¼ teaspoon cinnamon
¼ teaspoon ground cloves
Grated zest from 1 orange

1 Preheat the oven to 325°F. Cut a crosshatch pattern in the top layer of fat on the ham, and cook according to the directions on the package label.

2 Make the glaze: stir the beer, sugar, cinnamon, cloves, and orange zest together in a small bowl. Set aside.

3 Remove the ham from the oven about 1 hour before the directions say it will be ready. Spoon the glaze over the ham, return it to the oven, and cook, basting occasionally, until the ham is heated through.

4 Slice the ham and serve warm or at room temperature. Cover and refrigerate any leftovers for up to 5 days, or wrap well and freeze for up to 3 months.

Makes 10–14 servings

> **PROFILE ★**   **Magic Hat Brewing Co.** is home to wacky, inventive, and easy-drinking beers. The brewery made its first sale in early 1994 at the Winter Blues Festival in Burlington, Vermont, and soon fans could find the beers on tap throughout the city. Spurred on by sales from its flagship Not Quite Pale Ale #9, Magic Hat quickly expanded distribution and gained shelf recognition with swirling, colorful, quirky labels and whimsical beer descriptions on bottles and packaging (if you buy bottles, check under the cap for a quirky phrase or message before tossing it). The brewery's headquarters, known as the Artifactory, is a fun place to visit, as it serves many beers only available on site. Its website remains one of the most creative in the beer industry.

Bitch Creek Elk Meatballs

1 (12-ounce) bottle Grand Teton Bitch Creek ESB, or similar brown ale

½ cup panko breadcrumbs

2 tablespoons extra-virgin olive oil

½ green pepper, cored, seeded, and minced

½ sweet onion, minced

2–3 garlic cloves, minced

1 pound ground elk meat

2 eggs

½ tablespoon finely chopped fresh parsley

   Salt and freshly ground pepper

   Vegetable or canola oil, for pan-frying

A Few Beers to Try with This Recipe

- *Big Sky Moose Drool*
- *Brooklyn Brown Ale*
- *Fullsteam Working Man's Lunch*
- *Grand Teton Bitch Creek ESB*
- *Long Trail Harvest*
- *Surly Bender*
- *Tallgrass Ale*
- *Yazoo Dos Perros*

While the meat in this recipe is perhaps not familiar to grandmothers from, say, Brooklyn, one hallmark of a good Italian meatball is that it should taste like meat and let the juicy flavors dominate, with only a modest amount of spices. This simple recipe from the wilds of Idaho uses elk, a readily available meat in those parts. Beef, lamb, pork, veal, or a combination can be used in its place. Enjoy as an entrée with homemade tomato sauce and a pasta of your choosing, though spaghetti is a natural companion. This dish can be paired with a variety of beers, but Grand Teton's brown ale nicely complements the crust that develops on the meatballs.

1 Slowly add the beer to the breadcrumbs in a small mixing bowl, and blend until the mixture has the consistency of wet sand. Set aside.

2 Heat the olive oil in a skillet over medium-low heat. Add the green pepper, onions, and garlic, and cook, stirring occasionally, until golden brown, 5 to 7 minutes. Set aside.

3 Combine the elk meat, eggs, parsley, and salt and pepper to taste in a large mixing bowl. Mix in the breadcrumb mixture with your hands, and then add the vegetable mixture and incorporate thoroughly.

4 With your hands, shape the meat mixture into 1-inch balls, squeezing out any air pockets within the balls while shaping them. Place on a large plate or baking sheet.

5 Heat ¼ inch of vegetable or canola oil in a large skillet over medium heat. Add the meatballs just before the oil begins to smoke. Cook, rotating the meatballs occasionally, until brown on all sides, 8 to 9 minutes. Serve immediately with desired accompaniments.

Makes 6 servings

Though Idaho's Grand Teton Brewing Co. began its life across the border in Wyoming, it now calls the Gem State home, and its distribution covers more than a dozen states. It also has solidified a place in modern beer transport. The brewery tells the story of how founder Charlie Otto was looking for an alternative to bottles when he first opened in 1988, and his father suggested using growlers — metal pails once used to transport beer from taverns and breweries for home consumption. Brewery legend holds that Charlie contacted a manufacturer and had glass growlers created, a design and concept that is now standard for most breweries in the country. Today, helmed by Steve and Ellen Furbacher, the brewery retains its commitment to serving full-bodied beers to those who seek a quality pint.

UPLAND BREWING COMPANY

BLOOMINGTON, INDIANA

Meatless Loaf and Vegetable Mushroom Gravy

GRAVY
- 1 large white onion, diced
- 3 celery stalks, diced
- 1 large carrot, peeled and diced
- 1 cup mushroom stems (from Meatless Loaf mushrooms), roughly diced
- 4 garlic cloves
- 1 tablespoon canola oil
  Salt and freshly ground black pepper
- 2 cups red wine
- 2 quarts vegetable broth
- 1 cup dried mushrooms
- 2 teaspoons black peppercorns
- 1½ teaspoons minced fresh parsley
- 1½ teaspoons minced fresh sage
- 1½ teaspoons minced fresh thyme
- 1 bay leaf
- ½ cup (1 stick) unsalted butter, at room temperature
- ½ cup all-purpose flour

CARAMELIZED ONIONS
- 2 tablespoons canola oil
- 1 large white onion, julienned

This vegetarian twist on the venerable dinner standby is just as flavorful and satisfying as its meaty counterpart. This recipe really allows the vegetables to assert themselves and showcases their unique flavors and textures. It also gets a beer boost from spent grain, which is easy to procure from a local brewery or homebrewer friend. While it's great as an entrée, the loaf can also be sliced, warmed on a griddle, and eaten in a sandwich.

1 **MAKE THE GRAVY:** Preheat the oven to 425°F. Toss the onion, celery, carrot, mushroom stems, garlic, and canola oil in a large bowl and season with salt and pepper to taste. Transfer the vegetables to a baking sheet and bake for 20 minutes, or until the vegetables are darkly roasted.

2 Transfer the vegetables to a stockpot. Deglaze the baking sheet with 1 cup of the red wine, scraping up any bits of fond with a spatula. Transfer the wine and fond into the stockpot and add the remaining 1 cup red wine. Bring the vegetables and wine to a boil over high heat. Reduce the wine by two-thirds, and then add the vegetable broth. Bring the gravy back to a boil, and then reduce to a simmer and add the dried mushrooms, peppercorns, parsley, sage, thyme, and bay leaf. Cook, stirring occasionally, until the vegetables are beginning to fall apart and you are left with about 4 cups of liquid, about 90 minutes.

3 **CARAMELIZE THE ONIONS:** Heat the canola oil in a medium skillet over medium heat. Add the onions, reduce the heat to medium-low, and sauté, stirring occasionally, until browned and caramelized, about 45 minutes. Set aside to cool.

4 **MAKE THE LOAF:** Crumble the tofu into a colander set over a sink or large mixing bowl. Place a mixing bowl that's small enough to fit in the colander on top of the tofu to press out excess moisture.

5 Preheat the oven to 375°F. Mix the button mushrooms, portabella mushrooms, canola oil, and salt and pepper to taste in a mixing bowl. Transfer to a baking sheet and bake for 10 to 12 minutes, or until the mushrooms are dark and soft. Set the mushrooms aside to cool for several minutes and reduce the oven temperature to 350°F.

MEATLESS LOAF

- 1 (14-ounce) package firm tofu
- 1½ cups sliced button mushrooms
- 1 cup diced portabella mushrooms
- 1 tablespoon canola oil
  Salt and freshly ground black pepper
- 2 teaspoons tomato paste
- 1 tablespoon minced garlic
- 1 tablespoon roasted garlic purée, purchased or homemade (see box)
- 1 tablespoon Worcestershire sauce
- 1 teaspoon kosher salt
- 1 egg
- 8 cups panko breadcrumbs
- 1 tablespoon finely chopped fresh parsley
- 1 teaspoon freshly ground black pepper
- ½ cup spent grain (porter), squeezed of any excess moisture
  Nonstick cooking spray

Roasted Garlic Purée

Preheat the oven to 300°F. Carefully cut ½ inch from the tops of 4 whole bulbs of garlic to expose the individual cloves. Coat the bulbs with olive oil and place them in a small baking dish with ½ inch of water.

Cover the pan with aluminum foil and roast the garlic for 1 hour, or until the individual cloves feel soft when pressed. Allow the garlic to cool to room temperature, and then squeeze the soft garlic from the paperlike exterior. Make a purée by smearing the garlic with the flat side of a chef's knife.

6 Combine the tofu, mushroom mixture, caramelized onions, tomato paste, garlic, garlic purée, Worcestershire, salt, egg, breadcrumbs, parsley, and pepper in the bowl of a food processor and pulse slowly until combined. Stir in the grain with a wooden spoon.

7 Spray a 9- by 5-inch loaf pan with cooking spray and transfer the tofu mixture into the pan. Bake for 1 hour, then rotate the pan 180 degrees and cook for 40 minutes longer, or until the mixture is firm and set. Allow the loaf to cool on a wire rack on the counter for 20 minutes.

8 Meanwhile, remove the gravy from the heat, strain, and discard any solids from the liquid. Combine the butter and flour with your hands in a separate mixing bowl to make a thick paste. Whisk the paste into the gravy until it is fully incorporated.

9 Return the gravy to the stovetop and simmer over low heat until it reaches desired consistency, stirring frequently to prevent scorching or lumps. Season with salt and pepper to taste. Turn the meatless loaf out into a kitchen towel held in your other hand and then place it on a cutting board and cut into slices about 1 inch thick. Drizzle the hot gravy over the slices and serve.

Makes 8 servings

On the fringes of the Indiana University campus, *Upland Brewing* occupies a large, squat building with a restaurant in the front and a brewery in the back. Founded in 1998, it's one of the older new-generation breweries in the state and is among the most widely available Hoosier-made beers. The Upland Wheat, a good representation of the style, also makes the occasional appearance in the background of the NBC show *Parks and Recreation*, based in the fictional town of Pawnee, Indiana.

Upland is a bit of a hybrid. It's a commercial brewery that has an excellent restaurant attached, so it's unfair to call it just a brewpub. The brewery also operates a taproom in the capital city of Indianapolis, offering fresh growler fills to thirsty customers.

Colorado Carnitas

Carnitas means "little meats"; the bite-size pieces of pork in this traditional Mexican dish are usually served with soft tortillas. This version of carnitas takes on some Colorado flavoring with the addition of Avery's White Rascal Belgian Wheat. This recipe requires some patience and restraint, as the meat should go untouched for nearly two hours. The end result is worth the wait. Pair with Avery's Ellie's Brown Ale or any brown ale; it will complement the citrus and herbal flavors.

2 pounds boneless pork shoulder or ribs, cut into 2-inch cubes, taking care to keep fat intact
1 (12-ounce) bottle or can Avery White Rascal Belgian Wheat Ale, or similar beer
½ cup orange juice
¼ cup lime juice
2 garlic cloves, crushed
1 teaspoon kosher salt
Water, as needed
Small corn or flour tortillas
Fixings: sliced avocado, cilantro, diced tomatoes, fresh minced jalapeño pepper (optional)

1 Combine the pork, beer, orange juice, lime juice, garlic, and salt in a soup pot. Add enough water so the liquid barely covers the pork. Bring to a boil, and then reduce the heat to medium-low and simmer uncovered until fork-tender, about 2 hours. Do not turn or move the pork.

2 Increase the heat to medium-high and cook the pork while occasionally stirring and turning the pieces

until all of the liquid has evaporated, leaving only the rendered pork fat, 10 to 15 minutes.

3 Continue cooking the pork in the pork fat until brown on all sides, turning the pieces gently so they won't fall apart. Serve the pork in the tortillas, topped with desired accompaniments.

Makes 8–10 servings

PROFILE ★ **Since he founded a brewery** using his family name back in 1993, Adam Avery has overseen the creation and release of some of the country's most respected craft beers. With its *Scarlet Letter*–like logo, **Avery Brewing Company** of Boulder, Colorado, is a brewery that makes the most of flavor. From the floral, room-filling aromas of its India pale ales to the malty, boozy deep flavors of its barley wines and barrel-aged brews, its brews will wake up your taste buds. Avery regularly releases beers that are only available at the brewery, and on those days the crowds arrive early. The taproom features a wall of taps running the gamut of Avery offerings. Pity the visitors who think they will stop in "for just one beer." Available on draft, in cans, and in bottles, an offering from the Avery Brewing Company is worth pouring into your glass.

KNÖDEL

- 8 cups ½-inch cubes pumpernickel bread
- ¾ cup heavy cream
- ⅓ cup whole milk
- 1 tablespoon vegetable oil
- 2 shallots, finely diced
- 4 garlic cloves, smashed
  Salt and freshly ground black pepper
- 4 eggs, lightly beaten
- 3 tablespoon chopped fresh oregano leaves
- 2 tablespoons chopped fresh parsley
- 1 tablespoon unsalted butter, for frying

CRANBERRY SAUCE

- ¾ cup fresh or frozen cranberries
- ¾ cup sugar
- ½ cup Belgian quadrupel, or similar full-bodied dark beer
- 3 (2-inch) strips orange zest, julienned and pith removed
  Juice of 1 orange
- ½ cup veal broth
  Salt

Roasted Pheasant with Pumpernickel Bread Pudding and Cranberry Sauce

Chef Colby Garrelts dreamed up this dish as a more refined alternative to the Thanksgiving turkey. The savory pumpernickel bread pudding is his version of knödel, a German dumpling made from either potatoes or bread, and a wonderful go-to accompaniment for meat and fowl dishes in colder months. This bird pairs remarkably well with a Belgian-style quad, such as Boulevard's The Sixth Glass.

1 **MAKE THE KNÖDEL:** Put the bread in a large mixing bowl. Bring the cream and milk to a simmer over medium heat in a small saucepan and cook for 6 to 10 minutes. Pour the milk mixture over the bread. Set the bread aside to soak up the liquid for 10 minutes.

2 Heat the vegetable oil in a small skillet over medium-high heat. Add the shallots and garlic and sauté until softened, about 2 minutes.

3 Add the shallots and garlic to the bread mixture. Season with salt and pepper to taste. Set aside to cool slightly before stirring in the eggs, oregano, and parsley.

4 Roll the knödel tightly into a log in multiple layers of plastic wrap. Try your best to prevent air pockets from forming. Twist the plastic wrap on both ends tightly and secure

them with kitchen twine. If there are large air pockets under the surface of the plastic wrap, pop them with a small pin.

5 Fill a large roasting pan or stockpot wide and deep enough to submerge the knödel with water and bring to a simmer over high heat. Lower the knödel into the water and reduce the heat to medium. Keep the knödel submerged with a plate or a light weight. Return the water to a simmer and poach the knödel until custardlike, 25 to 30 minutes.

6 When the knödel is almost done poaching, prepare a large ice-water bath. Remove the knödel from the simmering water and submerge it in the ice bath to cool. When the knödel has cooled, remove it from the ice bath and set aside.

PHEASANT

- 4 (4- to 6-ounce) pheasant breasts
- 4 pheasant "oysters" (see note)
- Salt and freshly ground black pepper
- ¼ cup vegetable oil
- 2 tablespoons unsalted butter, cut into small pieces

Note: Pheasant "oysters" are tender rounds of dark meat nested between the small of the bird's back and thigh. A butcher can carve these out for you.

A Few Beers to Try with This Recipe

- *Avery The Reverend*
- *Boulevard The Sixth Glass*
- *Ommegang Three Philosophers*
- *Pretty Things Baby Tree*
- *Sly Fox Ichor*

7 MAKE THE CRANBERRY SAUCE: Bring the cranberries, sugar, beer, orange zest, and orange juice to a boil in a saucepan over medium-high heat. Turn the heat down to medium and simmer until the juices have reduced to a thick syrup, about 25 minutes. Stir in the veal broth, season with salt to taste, and remove from the heat. Cover to keep warm.

8 PREPARE THE PHEASANT: Preheat the oven 375°F. Season the pheasant breasts and oysters with salt and pepper.

9 Heat the vegetable oil in a large ovenproof skillet over high heat. Add the pheasant breasts, skin side down, and the oysters. Brown the meat for about 2 minutes per side. Transfer the skillet to the oven and roast the meat for 6 minutes. Transfer the oysters to a plate and cover to keep warm. Return the skillet to the oven and cook the pheasant breasts for 6 minutes longer. Remove the skillet from the oven, flip the breasts over, add the butter, and let them rest for 5 minutes in the hot pan with the melting butter.

10 To serve, slice the knödel through the plastic wrap into four ½-inch slices; discard the plastic. Heat the butter in a skillet over medium heat. When the butter begins to foam, fry the knödel slices on both sides until golden brown, 2 to 4 minutes per side. Divide the pheasant breasts, oysters, and knödel slices among four dinner plates. Spoon some of the cranberry sauce over the pheasant and serve immediately.

Makes 4 servings

PROFILE ★ **Over a short period of time, Boulevard** grew from a small production brewery to the largest microbrewery in the Midwest, and the second largest in Missouri (behind a brand that claims royalty). The brewery was founded by John McDonald, and the first batches of beer were delivered and poured in 1989. Since then, business has grown steadily, with awards and customers flocking to the brand now known for flavorful ales and lagers. Today, the brewery has a 150-barrel brewhouse inside a 70,000-square-foot complex and has a storage capacity of 600,000 barrels, a sign that Boulevard has room to grow and bring even more pints to happy imbibers.

4 plum tomatoes, blanched,
   peeled, and quartered
Salt and freshly ground
   white pepper
1 garlic clove, thinly sliced
5 tablespoons extra-virgin
   olive oil
1 cup orzo
1 cup kalamata olives, pitted
2 (8-ounce) boneless lamb
   tenderloins
¼ cup chicken stock
¼ cup crumbled feta cheese
4 fresh basil leaves
¼ cup finely chopped dill
¼ cup finely chopped parsley

A Few Beers to Try with This Recipe

- *Bayou Teche LA-31 Bière Pâle*
- *Captain Lawrence Liquid Gold*
- *Coast The Belafonte*
- *Furthermore Fatty Boombalatty*
- *Jolly Pumpkin Luciérnaga, The Firefly*
- *The Lost Abbey Devotion Ale*
- *Uncommon Golden State Ale*
- *White Birch Belgian Style Pale Ale*

Seared Lamb Tenderloin
with Orzo, Feta, Black Olive Purée, and Roasted Tomatoes

Savory and hearty, this dish from the acclaimed beer bar Birch & Barley requires a moderate amount of preparation, but the end result will have guests raving for months. Pair with a Belgian-style IPA.

1 Preheat the oven to 180°F. Scatter the tomatoes on a baking sheet and season with salt and pepper. Sprinkle the garlic slices among the tomatoes and drizzle with 3 tablespoons of the olive oil. Roast for 4 to 6 hours, or until the tomatoes have broken down. Remove from the oven and set aside. Raise the temperature to 400°F.

2 Bring a large pot of salted water to a boil for the pasta. Cook the orzo until al dente, and then drain and set aside.

3 Meanwhile, warm the olives in a small skillet over medium heat until heated through, 2 to 3 minutes. Transfer the olives to a blender, add 1 tablespoon of the olive oil, and blend until puréed.

4 Season the lamb with salt and pepper and heat a large skillet over high heat. Add the lamb and sear on all sides until browned, 2 to 3 minutes per side. Transfer the lamb to a roasting pan and roast for 3 to 4 minutes for medium-rare. Let the meat rest for 8 minutes.

5 Warm the chicken stock in a medium saucepan over low heat. Add the cooked orzo and the remaining 1 tablespoon olive oil; season to taste with salt and pepper and warm over low heat until heated through, about 3 minutes. Stir in the roasted tomatoes, the feta cheese, and the olive purée.

6 Slice the lamb and arrange on a serving platter, garnished with a few torn basil leaves and a sprinkle of dill and parsley. Put the orzo in a serving bowl and garnish with the rest of the basil, dill, and parsley. Serve hot.

Makes 2 servings

Beer nirvana. The *Birch & Barley* restaurant is downstairs and the Churchkey bar is upstairs in this relatively new spot on the D.C. beer scene. It has exploded into a mecca for patrons who treat beer and food as a religion. With temperature-controlled taps and refrigerators (to make sure the beer is always served at the desired temperature), detailed beer menus, and a variety of pours to choose from, it is best to clear your schedule before embarking on a visit, because it's impossible to have just one. Thanks to a masterful staff (including beer director Greg Engert), a kitchen menu that changes daily, and a commitment to the fermented arts, this restaurant has set the bar incredibly high. In 2013, a brewery will join the company, headed by the talented Megan O'Leary Parisi.

Dunkel-Braised Lamb Shanks

As hearty, flavorful, and satisfying as the dunkel beer they're paired with, the lamb shanks in this recipe break down over several hours of cooking, leaving tender meat behind. This plate comes together with side dishes like garlic mashed potatoes (or egg noodles) and fresh green beans. Prost!

4 lamb shanks (20–24 ounces each)
  Salt and freshly ground black pepper
2 tablespoons vegetable oil
6 carrots, peeled and diced
6 celery stalks, diced
2 small onions, diced
3 tablespoons garlic powder
2 tablespoons onion powder
2 tablespoons minced fresh rosemary leaves
15 black peppercorns
8 bay leaves
10 cups Hofbräuhaus Hofbräu Dunkel, or similar dark beer
¾ cup honey
  Veal or beef broth, as needed (about 8 cups)
2 tablespoons cornstarch (optional)
2 tablespoons cold water (optional)

1 Season the lamb shanks with salt and pepper. Place a large braising pan or Dutch oven over medium-high heat and coat the bottom with vegetable oil. Sear the lamb shanks until golden brown on all sides, about 2 minutes per side.

2 Transfer the lamb shanks to a plate and set aside. Add the carrots, celery, and onions to the pan and cook over medium-high heat until caramelized, about 8 minutes. Add the garlic powder, onion powder, rosemary, peppercorns, bay leaves, beer, and honey, and bring to a boil. Boil for 2 minutes and then turn off the heat.

3 Preheat the oven to 350°F. Return the lamb shanks to the braising pan and add enough veal broth to almost cover the lamb shanks. Cover with foil, transfer the pan to the oven, and bake for 1½ hours.

4 Remove the pan from the oven and turn the lamb shanks over. Bake for 1 hour longer, or until the lamb shanks are very tender.

5 Remove the lamb shanks from the oven and place on a serving tray. Strain the pan juices into a sauce pot and pour a small amount over the lamb shanks, reserving the rest to serve as the sauce. Optional: To thicken the sauce, mix the cornstarch with the cold water and whisk into the sauce. Bring to a boil while stirring and remove from the heat when slightly thickened. Serve one shank per person with a generous amount of sauce and side dishes.

Makes 4 servings

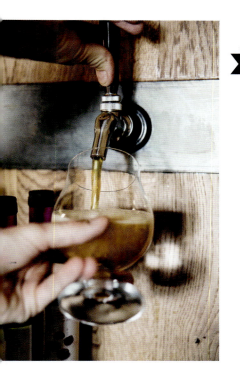

It is not the largest brewery in Munich, but it is likely the best-known globally. Thanks in part to its worldwide availability, its reputation as a must-visit spot for tourists in Germany, and the wonderfully catchy and classic beer-drinking song, Hofbräuhaus is nothing short of sacred.

Nicholas Ellison is keenly aware of that reputation and ensures that the two *Hofbräuhaus* franchises his company operates in the United States are continually striving to match the original. When Ellison and his partners opened their first location in Newport, Kentucky, a suburb of Cincinnati, Ohio, in 2003, they had brewers coming from Munich to make sure their lagers were not just acceptable, but perfect. Today, they have a classically trained German brewer who oversees operations at both locations (the other is in Pittsburgh and opened in 2009). Their state-of-the-art equipment is wired to the Hofbräuhaus headquarters in Munich, where brewmasters there can keep an eye on things. "Germans come in and look at both places, and the comment we hear the most is 'I've never seen a beer garden quite like this in Germany, but if I did I wouldn't be surprised.' We take that as a big compliment," says Ellison.

Maple-Orange Grilled Pork Loin

1 (3-pound) pork loin
Salt and freshly ground
black pepper
3 tablespoons unsalted butter
2 large yellow onions, thinly
sliced
1½ roasted chile peppers,
roughly diced
¾ cup orange juice
⅓ cup pure maple syrup
1 cup dark strong ale
⅓ cup fresh lime juice
2 tablespoons cornstarch
2 tablespoons water
¼ cup finely chopped cilantro

It's the sauce! The combination of citrus, maple, and ale in this sauce will open your eyes to many flavors at once. And the savory and smoky flavor of the pork is perfect with the sauce, creating an overall happy dining experience. Pair this dish with a floral bier de garde, with vibrant hop and yeast flavors that can stand up to the richness of the sauce.

1 Prepare a medium fire in a gas or charcoal grill. Season the pork with salt and pepper and grill, turning several times, to an internal temperature of 160°F, about 1 hour. Allow the pork to rest, tented with foil, for 10 minutes.

2 Meanwhile, melt the butter in a saucepan over medium heat. Add the onions and chile peppers and sauté until the onions are golden brown, about 10 minutes. Add the orange juice and maple syrup, increase the heat to high, and bring to a boil. Reduce the heat to a simmer and continue cooking, stirring occasionally, until the liquid is reduced by half, 7 to 10 minutes. Stir in the beer and lime juice. Whisk the cornstarch and water together in a small bowl to make a slurry. Whisk the slurry into the sauce to thicken it to the consistency of gravy.

3 Slice the roast into ¼- to ½-inch-thick slices. Pour a generous amount of sauce over the pork, and serve the rest of the sauce in a gravy boat. Garnish the pork with the cilantro and serve.

Makes 6 servings

PROFILE ★ **Sometimes, a hobby can become an empire.** Take for example the *Lost Abbey*, where the brother-and-sister team of Vince and Gina Marsaglia began making their own brews when they couldn't find local, flavorful options. Not long after they began brewing, they opened a brewery inside their Pizza Port restaurant. They expanded a few times and eventually took over a location once owned by Stone Brewing Co. That became home to the Lost Abbey and its sister brewery (and American side) Port Brewing. Lost Abbey beers can be hard to classify, and that's the way the Marsaglias and brewmaster Tomme Authur like it. Each bottle is steeped in Belgian tradition, but mixed with American whimsy, ingredient knowledge, and a boldness that translates into complex concoctions sure to delight.

Easy Steak Fajitas

7VENTH SUN BREWING COMPANY

DUNEDIN, FLORIDA

Ever visit a restaurant where sizzling platters of meat and vegetables come through the dining room high above a waiter's head, leaving a mouthwatering trail of spicy scents? Well, now you can stay in and enjoy the same sounds, smells, and flavors. Pair with a refreshing extra pale ale.

1 MAKE THE MARINADE: Combine the onion, garlic, cilantro, pale ale, orange juice, lime juice, canola oil, cumin, and salt and pepper to taste in a blender. Blend until the ingredients are incorporated and the beer foam subsides, about 90 seconds.

2 Place the steak in a shallow container or ziplock bag and add the marinade. Refrigerate, covered, for at least 1 hour or overnight.

3 MAKE THE FAJITAS: Drain the marinade from the steak and discard. Prepare a medium-hot fire in a gas or charcoal grill. Cook the steak on the grill (or in a hot cast iron skillet over medium-high heat) until a dark crust forms, about 4 minutes per side. The steak will shrink a bit and feel slightly firm to the touch.

4 Transfer the steak to a cutting board to rest. Meanwhile, grill or sauté the onion and green, yellow, and red bell peppers. Cook the mixture until the vegetables are tender, about 3 minutes.

5 Slice the steak against the grain and serve with warm tortillas and the sautéed vegetables.

Makes 6 servings

MARINADE
- ½ cup diced red onion
- 2 garlic cloves
- 1 tablespoon chopped fresh cilantro
- 2 cups extra pale ale
- 2 cups orange juice
- Juice of 1 lime
- 3 tablespoons canola oil
- 2 teaspoons ground cumin
- Salt and freshly ground black pepper

FAJITAS
- 2¼ pounds skirt or flank steak
- 1 tablespoon canola oil
- 1 red onion, thinly sliced
- 1 green bell pepper, cored, seeded, and thinly sliced
- 1 red bell pepper, cored, seeded, and thinly sliced
- 1 yellow bell pepper, cored, seeded, and thinly sliced
- 12 flour tortillas

PROFILE ★ **7venth Sun offers a mix** of Belgian-style and sour ales and a variety of hop-forward beers. Owners Devon Kreps and Justin Stange come with industry background: After finishing a food and fermentation science degree at Oregon State University, Kreps began work at Anheuser-Busch. From there, she went to work as the production manager at SweetWater Brewing Company in Atlanta. Stange began volunteering at McGuire's brewpub in Destin, was later hired as a brewer at SweetWater, and also brewed for Cigar City in Tampa. Now they have their own place and have quickly made a quality impression.

Braised Duck Legs with Cabbage and Fingerling Potatoes

4 duck legs
   Salt
1 head green cabbage, cored and cut into ⅛-inch wedges
1 yellow onion, julienned
2 garlic cloves, slivered
¼ cup white wine (optional)
2 cups chicken broth
10 fingerling potatoes

A Few Beers to Try with This Recipe

- *Big Sky Moose Drool Brown Ale*
- *Dogfish Head Indian Brown Ale*
- *Duck-Rabbit Brown Ale*
- *Grand Teton Extra Special Brown*
- *Sierra Nevada Tumblr*
- *Smuttynose Old Brown Dog Ale*
- *Yazoo Dos Perros*

A little bit of work on the front end of this recipe frees you up to leave the rest to the oven. It is a great way to prepare duck; the fat from the legs adds flavor to the vegetables and enriches the broth. This duck pairs well with a brown ale like Half Acre's Over Ale that has mild and earthy notes of chocolate, toffee, and coffee.

1 Preheat the oven to 325°F and season the duck legs with salt. Heat a braising pan over medium heat, and then place the duck legs in the hot pan, skin side down, to render the fat and brown the skin, 8 to 10 minutes. When the skin is golden brown, turn the legs over to sear and lightly brown the other side, about 4 minutes. Remove the duck legs from the pan and set aside.

2 Add the cabbage wedges to the rendered duck fat in the pan and cook over medium heat until the cabbage begins to lightly brown, about 2 minutes. Turn over the cabbage wedges to brown the other side, about 2 minutes longer. Remove the cabbage and set aside on a plate. Add the onions to the pan and sauté until translucent, about 3 minutes. Add the garlic and sauté for about 3 minutes. Season with salt to taste.

3 When the garlic and onions are soft, deglaze the pan with the white wine, if desired. Return the cabbage to the pan, add the chicken broth, and bring the liquid to a simmer. Add the potatoes and duck legs to the pan.

4 Transfer the pan to the oven and bake, uncovered, for 90 minutes, turning the legs every 20 minutes. (Keep an eye on the liquid in the pan, as you do not want to scorch the bottom of the pan; add a small amount of water to the pan if needed.)

5 Remove the pan from the oven and season with salt to taste. Serve immediately.

Makes 4 servings

With a dream of brewing but no experience, the owners of *Half Acre* waded carefully into the business by creating their first beers with the help of an established brewery. They learned, gained experience, and eventually purchased equipment of their own and set up a business in their desired city of Chicago. They have embraced cans as their vessels of choice and produce not only a solid stable of regular beers, but some mighty impressive seasonal and special releases. A visit to Half Acre's Chicago home reveals a trio of attractions. The amply sized brewery is flanked on one side by a retail shop where growlers are filled and sold and on the other side by a warm stone and wood bar that makes even travelers feel like locals.

GORDON BIERSCH BREWING COMPANY

SAN JOSE, CALIFORNIA

Roasted Bell Pepper–Tomato Fettuccine Alfredo

This classic creamy pasta receives added flavor and color from tomatoes and peppers. Try pairing it with an old ale, a hearty brew that can stand up to the sharpness of the Parmigiano and the fresh garlic.

CREAM SAUCE

- 1 stick (½ cup) unsalted butter
- 2 garlic cloves, minced
- 2 cups heavy cream
- 1 cup shredded Parmigiano-Reggiano cheese

PEPPER SAUCE

- 3 tablespoons extra-virgin olive oil
- 4 roasted red bell peppers or 1 (8-ounce) jar roasted red peppers, drained
- 1 (14.5-ounce) can diced tomatoes, drained
  Salt and freshly ground black pepper

TOMATO TOPPING

- 2 tablespoons extra-virgin olive oil
- 1 pound cherry tomatoes, halved
- 10 garlic cloves, chopped
- 4 sun-dried tomatoes, julienned

- 2 pounds fettuccine

1 **MAKE THE CREAM SAUCE:** Melt the butter in a medium saucepan over medium heat. Add the garlic and sauté for 1 minute. Add the cream, and then gradually stir in the Parmigiano-Reggiano. Stir constantly over medium heat until the sauce thickens, about 10 minutes. Cover and keep warm.

2 **MAKE THE PEPPER SAUCE:** Heat the olive oil in a medium skillet over medium heat. Add the roasted peppers and tomatoes and sauté for about 10 minutes. Season with salt and pepper to taste. Transfer the sauce to a blender and purée until smooth.

3 Bring a large pot of salted water to a boil for the pasta.

4 **MAKE THE TOMATO TOPPING:** Heat the olive oil in a large skillet over medium-high heat. Add the cherry tomatoes, garlic, and sun-dried tomatoes and sauté until the cherry tomatoes begin to soften, about 2 minutes.

5 **ASSEMBLE THE DISH:** Cook the fettuccine in the boiling water according to the package instructions, or until al dente. Drain.

6 Spoon the cream sauce into a warm pasta bowl, layer the noodles over the cream sauce, and then top with the pepper sauce and tomato topping. Serve immediately.

Makes 4 servings

Back in 1987, Dan Gordon and Dean Biersch partnered with the idea of opening a brewery restaurant where the food would be hearty, delicious, and made from scratch, and the beer would be modeled on the German tradition. When the first *Gordon Biersch* opened a year later in Palo Alto, it marked the beginning of an impressive brewery run that now includes a growing number of restaurants across the country. In the late '90s, they opened a production brewery in San Jose dedicated to bottling the German-style beers that made them famous. Through that venture, Gordon Biersch has been able to expand into new markets. Gordon continues to be hands-on, and he is well known and respected in the beer community and beyond, appearing on television programs and presenting in-person beer demos.

Chicken-Fried Steak Tips
with ESB gravy

4¾ cups all-purpose flour

2 tablespoons garlic powder

2 tablespoons kosher salt,
plus more for seasoning

2 tablespoons onion powder

1½ tablespoons freshly ground
black pepper, plus more
for seasoning

2½ pounds filet mignon tips,
purchased in "tip" form, or
cut to size from 1 whole
tenderloin

10 eggs

3 cups vegetable oil

½ cup unsalted butter

3 cups whole milk

1 cup Redhook ESB, or any
similar extra-special
bitter

Deep-fried red meat! I love the genius who came up with this idea: it combines what's great about fried chicken and tender steak in one bite. Try pairing this dish, which is accompanied by a creamy and savory gravy, with an extra-special bitter (sometimes called an English pale ale). Optional side dishes might include potato salad, okra, baked beans, or a creamy mac and cheese.

1 Whisk together 4 cups of the flour with the garlic powder, salt, onion powder, and black pepper in a medium bowl until thoroughly mixed.

2 Trim the meat of any tendon (known as silver skin). Dredge the filet mignon tips in the flour mixture and set aside on a plate, in one layer, for 15 minutes.

3 Crack the eggs into a shallow dish and whisk thoroughly for a completely smooth liquid. Lumpy eggs will result in a "spotty" breading.

4 Heat the oil to 350°F in a deep pot over medium-high heat. Dredge the filet mignon tips in the flour mixture again, then toss in the eggs, then dredge again in the flour mixture. Fry the tips in batches until golden brown, 3 to 5 minutes, depending on the size and fat content of the tips. Use a slotted spoon or spider to transfer the tips to a paper towel–lined plate to drain.

5 Melt the butter in a saucepan over medium heat. Add the remaining ¾ cup flour and whisk together over medium heat until golden brown to form a roux. Add the milk and beer and heat to thicken the gravy, stirring often. Increase the heat to medium-high and continue to whisk the sauce for 8 to 10 minutes longer. Season with salt and pepper to taste. Plate the filet mignon tips, smother with gravy, and serve hot.

Makes 4–6 servings

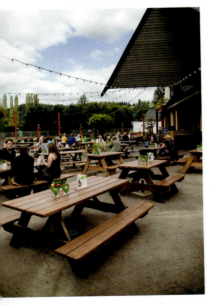

When it outgrew its original location in Seattle, *Redhook* moved slightly northeast to its current location in Woodinville, Washington, to spread out a bit and expand its offerings to a thirsty public. While its flagship ESB has gone through some cosmetic changes over the years, the ale itself has remained a solid, malty, slightly hop-spicy, full-flavored, reliable standby. It has done its part to convert many beer drinkers away from the lighter, yellow, fizzy stuff. The pub in Woodinville is a comfortable spot with an affable and educated staff who are eager to guide visitors through the lineup of beers and offer tastes of brewery-only exclusives. And while its roots are in the West, Redhook has also moved East, operating a second brewery in Portsmouth, New Hampshire.

Saison and Clementine Cornish Game Hens with Roasted Vegetables

4 Cornish game hens
¼ cup extra-virgin olive oil
  Salt and freshly ground black pepper
1 clementine, quartered
6 fresh sage sprigs
1 pound carrots, peeled and chopped
1 pound large Red Bliss potatoes, cubed
2 celery stalks, roughly chopped
½ cup chopped onions
14 garlic cloves
1 cup saison
2⅓ cups low-sodium chicken broth
  Cornstarch, as needed
½ cup chopped scallions or chives
4 fresh rosemary sprigs, for garnish

A Few Beers to Try with This Recipe

- *Bolero Snort Saison de Bull*
- *Bullfrog Busted Lawnmower*
- *Jolly Pumpkin Bam Biere*
- *Swamp Head Saison du Swamp*
- *Upright Four*

Tender, sweet game hens enjoy a welcome enhancement from spicy saison, a sweet clementine, and fresh herbs. With the addition of roasted vegetables that share the same seasonings, this is a dish that brings together many flavors while allowing individual tastes to stand on their own. You'll want to drink a saison with this dish; it will add earthy depth and just a bit of sweetness to the experience.

1 Preheat the oven to 450°F. Rub the hens with 1 tablespoon of the olive oil and lightly season with salt and pepper. Stuff one clementine wedge and one sage sprig into the cavity of each hen.

2 Combine the carrots, potatoes, celery, onions, and garlic in a large, heavy roasting pan. Arrange the hens on top of the vegetables and roast for 25 minutes.

3 Whisk ½ cup of the saison, ⅓ cup of the chicken broth, and 2 tablespoons of the olive oil together in a small bowl. Remove the pan from the oven and pour the beer mixture over the top of the hens. Reduce the oven temperature to 350°F and continue roasting the hens and vegetables, basting with the pan juices every 10 minutes, for 25 minutes longer, or until the hens are golden brown and their juices run clear.

4 Transfer the hens to a platter, pouring any cavity juices into the pan, and tent the hens with aluminum foil to keep warm. Separate the juices from the vegetables and transfer the juices to a bowl.

5 Bring the remaining 2 cups chicken broth to a simmer in a medium saucepan over medium heat. Add the pan juices and the remaining ½ cup saison, and bring to a boil. Continue to boil until the sauce reduces by half, about 5 minutes. Reduce the sauce to a simmer and thicken by whisking in 1 teaspoon of cornstarch at a time, until it reaches the desired thickness. Chop the leaves from the remaining two sage sprigs and stir them into the gravy. Remove the gravy from the heat after it has fully thickened, about 5 minutes.

6 Heat the remaining 1 tablespoon olive oil in a skillet over medium-high heat, and then add the carrots, potatoes, celery, and onions. Sauté the vegetables until slightly browned, 5 to 7 minutes. Toss the vegetables with the scallions in a serving bowl.

7 Remove the clementine and sage from the hens and gently split the birds lengthwise down the middle. Plate the hens and spoon the gravy around them. Garnish with the rosemary sprigs and serve with the vegetable mixture on the side.

Makes 4 servings

PROFILE ★ **So much of the craft beer produced** in our nation's smallest state comes from Sean Larkin. The versatile brewer has been serving up perfected pints from the Trinity Brewhouse in downtown Providence for many years. Then he took on extra responsibilities by helping the classic Narragansett brand return to the market. Now, he's involved in a new project — *Revival Brewing*. Considering the lineup, it doesn't look like he is going to do anything small with this one: a double black IPA, an imperial Oktoberfest, a saison, and an imperial stout. Given his proven track record, these beers from Larkin are ones to seek out and enjoy.

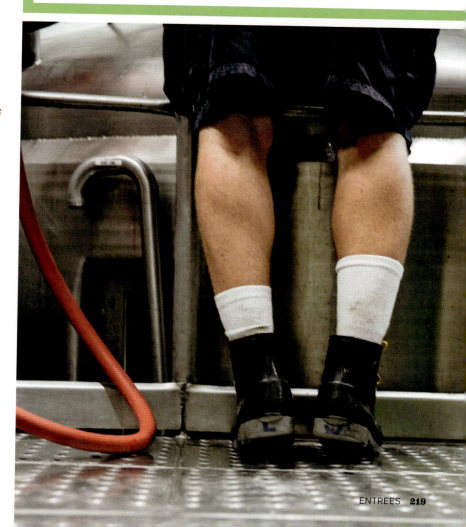

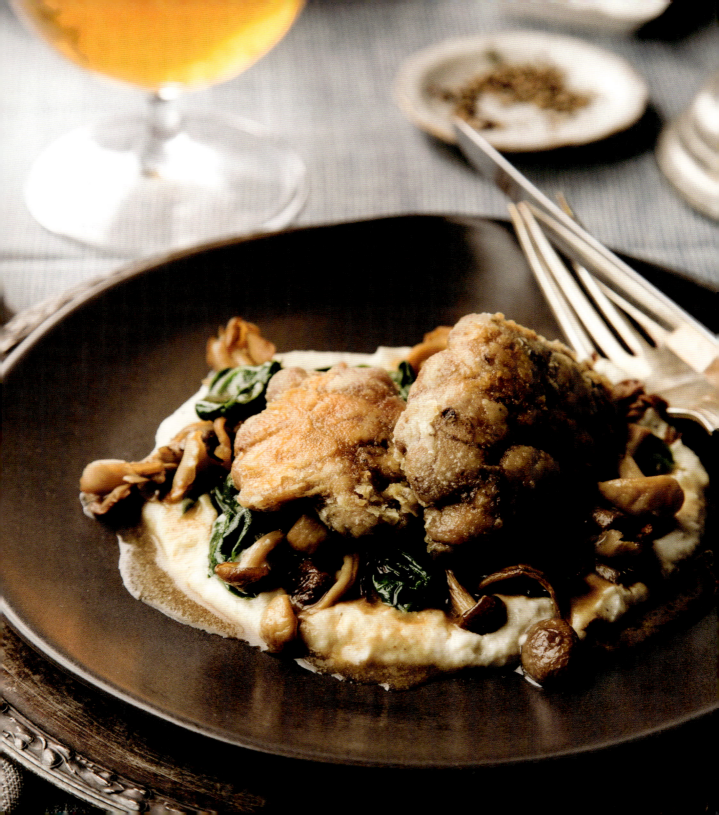

Pan-Roasted Sweetbreads
with Spinach, Cauliflower, Wild Mushrooms, and Sherry-Bacon Vinaigrette

Despite the appealing name, sweetbreads are the thymus glands of a calf and as such often get a bad rap. But for the willing, the brave, and the knowledgeable, sweetbreads are a welcome, silky-textured reward with a crunchy bite. Served alongside a trio of vegetables, this is a meal you won't soon forget. A few days of advance preparation are needed for this recipe, but the end result is a flavorful plate of flavors. Pair with a saison, where the floral sweetness and spice enhance many elements of the dish.

SWEETBREADS

- 1 pound veal sweetbreads
  Salt and freshly ground
  black pepper
- 3 cups grapeseed oil
- 2 teaspooons minced garlic
- 4 thyme sprigs
- 1 bay leaf
- ½ cup all-purpose flour

SAUCE

- 2 tablespoons bacon fat
- 8 shallots, sliced
- ¼ cup light brown sugar
- 1 thyme sprig
- 1 bay leaf
  Pinch of whole black
  peppercorns
- ½ cup sherry vinegar
- 2 cups chicken broth
  Salt and freshly ground
  black pepper

1 PREPARE THE SWEETBREADS: The day before you want to cook, soak the sweetbreads in cold water for 6 to 8 hours, changing the water a few times. Drain and pat dry with paper towels.

2 Preheat the oven to 300°F. Season the sweetbreads with salt and pepper, and set them in an ovenproof dish. Combine the oil, garlic, and thyme, and pour over the sweetbreads. Add the bay leaf and roast for 30 to 45 minutes, or until the sweetbreads are medium-rare.

3 Remove the sweetbreads from the oven. Transfer the sweetbreads from the oil to a plate lined with waxed paper. Place a second sheet of waxed paper and another plate on top of the sweetbreads and weigh down the top plate with heavy cans or other dense objects. Refrigerate overnight to improve the sweetbreads' texture. Pour the oil into a gravy separator and pour off the liquid given up by the sweetbreads. Reserve only the oil and discard the sweetbread liquid, which is a little funky.

4 MAKE THE SAUCE: The next day, preheat the oven to its lowest setting. Warm the bacon fat in a large saucepan over medium heat. Add the shallots and cook, stirring occasionally, until caramelized, 2 to 3 minutes. Add the brown sugar, thyme, bay leaf, peppercorns, and sherry vinegar. Reduce the liquid until almost dry, and then add the chicken broth and cook over medium heat, stirring occasionally,

recipe continues on next page

CAULIFLOWER PURÉE
- 1 cup cauliflower florets
- 2 tablespoons heavy cream
- 1 tablespoon truffle butter
- 1 teaspoon truffle oil
- Salt and freshly ground pepper

MUSHROOMS
- 2 tablespoons grapeseed oil
- 2 cups sliced assorted wild mushrooms
- 1 tablespoon unsalted butter
- 1 tablespoon minced shallots
- ¼ cup saison
- 1 teaspoon fresh lemon juice
- Salt and freshly ground black pepper

SPINACH
- 1 tablespoon grapeseed oil
- 2 cups fresh spinach
- Salt and freshly ground black pepper

until the sauce has reduced by half. Strain the sauce and season with salt and pepper to taste. Keep the sauce warm in the oven.

5 Remove the sweetbreads from the refrigerator and cut into four 4-ounce portions. Set aside.

6 **MAKE THE CAULIFLOWER:** Bring a pot of salted water to a boil and blanch the cauliflower until tender, about 10 minutes. Transfer the cauliflower to a blender and add the cream, truffle butter, and truffle oil. Purée until fully incorporated. Season with salt and pepper to taste. Transfer the purée to a serving bowl and place in the oven to keep warm.

7 **MAKE THE MUSHROOMS:** Heat the oil over high heat in a large skillet. Add the mushrooms and cook, stirring occasionally, until caramelized, 2 to 3 minutes. Add the butter and shallots to the skillet and cook, stirring occasionally, until golden, 2 to 3 minutes. Deglaze the skillet with the beer, add

the lemon juice, and transfer the mushroom mixture to a bowl, and then to the oven to keep warm.

8 **MAKE THE SPINACH:** Heat the oil over high heat in a skillet. Add the spinach and cook until wilted, about 2 minutes. Season with salt and pepper to taste, transfer to a bowl, and then to the oven to keep warm.

9 **FRY THE SWEETBREADS:** Finally, heat the reserved sweetbread oil in a high-sided pan until it reaches 350°F. Place the flour in a small bowl and dredge the sweetbreads in the flour. Pan-fry the sweetbreads until golden brown, 2 to 3 minutes. Transfer the sweetbreads to a paper towel–lined plate to drain, and season with salt and pepper to taste.

10 Divide the sauce among four plates and top with the cauliflower purée, mushrooms, spinach, and sweetbreads. Serve immediately.

Makes 4 servings

Smoke-Braised Pork Belly with Pear Slaw

All good things take time, and while smoking and properly marinating meat can take many hours, this recipe from brewery partner and beervangelist Fred Bueltmann delivers big flavor in a reasonable amount of time. Pair the pork belly with New Holland's Envious, a fruit beer made with pears and aged with oak and raspberries.

¼ cup raisins

1 (12-ounce) bottle New Holland Black Tulip Tripel, or similar beer

1–2 firm medium pears, peeled and thinly sliced into matchsticks

1 medium fennel bulb, trimmed, shaved thin, and sliced

3–4 dried figs, minced

¼ cup minced fresh cilantro leaves

1½ cups plus 2 tablespoons apple cider vinegar, plus more as needed

1 tablespoon stone-ground mustard

1 tablespoon honey

1 teaspoon fresh lemon juice
Salt and freshly ground black pepper

2 pounds whole pork belly, cured or uncured

1 Soak the raisins in 1 cup of the tripel at room temperature for at least 1 hour or until hydrated. Drain the raisins, and then add the pears, fennel, figs, and cilantro to the bowl.

2 Whisk the 2 tablespoons apple cider vinegar, the mustard, the honey, and the lemon juice together in a separate bowl, finishing with salt and pepper to taste. Add to the pear mixture and toss to coat thoroughly. Cover and refrigerate before serving.

3 Preheat the oven or a smoker to 225°F. Place the pork belly in a cast-iron skillet. Add the 1½ cups vinegar and the remaining ½ cup tripel to the skillet (the liquid should cover the pork belly halfway; add more vinegar as necessary) and bring to a simmer.

4 When the liquid simmers, transfer the skillet to a smoker or oven and braise the pork belly for 90 to 120 minutes, or until it reaches an internal temperature of 145 to 150°F. Let the pork belly rest before slicing and serving over the slaw.

Makes 4 servings

PROFILE ★ **Established in 1997, New Holland** began as a scrappy two-man start-up and has since grown into a thriving regional craft brewery, recognized for its creativity and artistry. New Holland currently brews and distills in two locations — a brewpub and a production campus — in the comfortable city of Holland. The pub has a welcoming feel and a constant line at the front door (but you won't wait long). With delicious menu items and pub-only drafts, the brewery is a hub for the thriving beer scene in western Michigan.

Pork Shoulder Braised in Apricot-Beer Sauce

BRINE
- 2¼ quarts water
- ½ cup salt
- ½ cup sugar
- ¼ cup malt powder
- 2¼ quarts ice

PORK
- 2 pounds boneless pork shoulder, cut into 4-inch cubes
- 2 tablespoons extra-virgin olive oil
- 6 cups canola oil, for frying

RUB
- 1½ pounds kosher salt
- 1¼ cups firmly packed dark brown sugar
- ¼ cup freshly ground black pepper
- ¼ cup red pepper flakes

APRICOT-BEER SAUCE
- 1¼ cups Italian apricot jam
- 2 (12-ounce) bottles apricot beer

A Few Beers to Try with This Recipe

- *Ithaca Apricot Wheat*
- *Magic Hat #9*
- *Pyramid Audacious Apricot*
- *Sea Dog Apricot Wheat*

The deep sweetness of the apricot melds into the succulent flavor of pork and creates a delicious marriage of flavors. Flash-frying the pork adds a great crust and subsequent crunch to the still moist meat. At Birreria this dish is served with a side of cucumber and celery salad to offset the richness of the meat. Pair the dish with a refreshing ale such as a witbier; Dogfish Head Namaste would be a good choice.

1 **MAKE THE BRINE:** Bring the water, salt, sugar, and malt powder to a boil in a large pot over high heat. Stir to dissolve the salt and sugar. Remove the pot from the heat and add the ice to cool the brine and bring the liquid measurement to 4½ quarts.

2 **BRINE THE PORK:** Place the pork in a large ziplock bag and pour the brine into the bag. Refrigerate the pork for at least 6 hours or up to 8 hours.

3 **MAKE THE RUB:** Whisk the salt, brown sugar, black pepper, and pepper flakes together in a large bowl.

4 Remove the pork from the brine and pat dry with paper towels. Liberally apply the dry rub to all the pork. Cover and refrigerate for 4 hours.

5 **MAKE THE APRICOT-BEER SAUCE:** Whisk the apricot jam and beer together in a medium bowl until combined. Reserve ½ cup of the sauce in a small bowl and set aside both bowls.

6 **COOK THE PORK:** Preheat the oven to 320°F. Remove the pork from the refrigerator and allow to come to room temperature. Heat the olive oil in a skillet over high heat and sear the pork until browned on all sides, 2 to 5 minutes per side. (The pork will turn almost black because of the brown sugar in the dry rub; do not be alarmed.)

7 Transfer the pork to a deep roasting pan and pour all but the reserved ½ cup apricot-beer sauce over the pork. The pork should be completely submerged. Tightly cover the pork with plastic wrap and then aluminum foil, making sure to completely cover the plastic to keep it from melting or burning. Bake the pork for 3 hours.

8 When the pork is nearly done, heat the canola oil to 350°F in a high-sided pan. Remove the pork from the oven and discard the plastic wrap–foil covering. Transfer all the pork to a plate with a slotted spoon. Carefully add the pork to the hot oil using a slotted spoon and fry for 2 minutes. Work in batches if necessary. Transfer the pork to a bowl and pour the reserved apricot-beer sauce over the top. Serve hot.

Makes 8 servings

In midtown Manhattan, the faithful, curious, and thirsty regularly flock to Eataly, a food market and collection of restaurants with a focus on Italian food. There in a back corner of this Flatiron District gourmand palace, the crowds gather near a host stand, waiting their turn to ride 14 stories up to the rooftop brewery known as ***Birreria***. It is the creation of Sam Calagione of Dogfish Head, Leonardo Di Vincenzo of Del Borgo, and Teo Musso of Baladin, who collaborated on a concept and recipes for the brewpub, which cask-conditions all its housemade beers and serves them from large vessels situated behind the bar. It is by far one of the most scenic breweries in the country, with skyline views of the Empire State Building, Flatiron Building, and other iconic architectural wonders. Taking a break from the views, tuck into the food: rustic Italian fare, such as the Toscana-inspired blood sausage, the pork shoulder, or the roasted maitake mushrooms. In a city that keeps improving its beer scene, Birreria at Eataly quickly established itself as a must-see brewery that deserves regular return visits.

Sake-Braised Beef Cheeks

Beef cheeks are still relatively obscure on menus but are an affordable and flavorful choice for the home cook. Serve the tender meat with sautéed edamame, enoki mushrooms, and tomatoes. The beef cheeks pair well with a rye imperial stout, like the Ex Umbris from Hess Brewing, because the rye and the alcohol cut the fat of the cheek while the sake flavors in the sauce highlight the sweetness of the beer.

2 tablespoons soybean oil

4 (12-ounce) beef cheeks, cleaned and trimmed of visible fat

1 teaspoon salt

1 teaspoon freshly ground black pepper

4 tablespoons unsalted butter

3 medium carrots, peeled and finely diced

2 large celery stalks, finely diced

1 daikon radish, diced

1 medium onion, finely diced

3 garlic cloves, minced

2 tablespoons minced fresh ginger

½ cup tomato paste

2 cups sake

2½ cups water

1 Preheat the oven to 325°F. Heat the soybean oil in a 6-quart Dutch oven over medium-high heat until hot but not smoking. Pat the beef cheeks dry with a paper towel and sprinkle with the salt and pepper. Add the beef cheeks to the pot and cook until browned on all sides, 15 to 20 minutes. Transfer to a plate and set aside.

2 Add the butter, carrots, celery, radish, onion, garlic, ginger, and tomato paste to the pot. Sauté over low heat, stirring occasionally, until the vegetables are soft, 8 to 10 minutes.

3 Stir in the sake and water, scraping up the fond (those little browned bits) from the bottom of the pot with a wooden spoon. Increase the heat to medium-high and bring the liquid to a rapid simmer. Continue simmering until the liquid has reduced by half, 18 to 20 minutes.

4 Return the beef cheeks (along with any juices collected on the plate) to the pot. Cover the pot and cook the beef cheeks for 3 hours, or until tender. Serve hot.

Makes 4 servings

PROFILE ★ **Billed as the city's first nano-brewery,** creating just 1.6 barrels at a time, **Hess Brewing** is the commercial effort of homebrewer-turned-pro Michael Hess. He used to spend about 20 hours a week brewing in 1600-square-foot garage that also served as a tasting room. After two years as a nano, and with a few places around town carrying his beers, Hess decided it was time to grow and made the big jump to a 30-barrel brewhouse in the city's North Park area in late 2012. Being nano was one of the best full-time, lowest-paying jobs, he said, but the demand to grow was too good to resist. Hess said he enjoyed the nano niche because "the homebrewers aren't doing something this big and the big guys aren't doing something this small." So long as it is tasty when served, size doesn't matter.

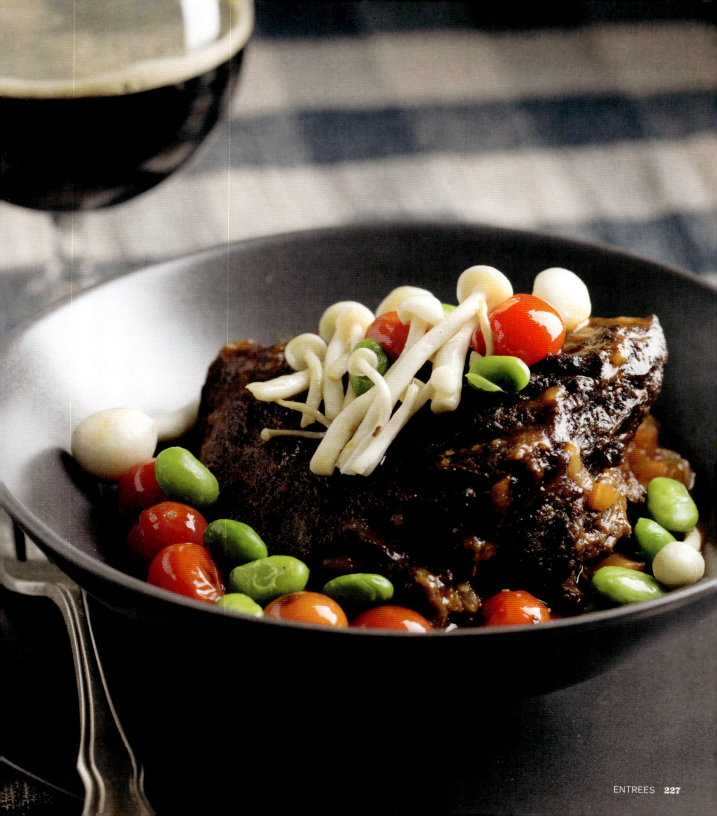

Ginger-Garlic Chicken Stir-Fry

MARINATED CHICKEN

- 1 pound skinless, boneless chicken breasts
- 1 tablespoon plus 1 teaspoon cornstarch
- 2 teaspoons salt
- 1 teaspoon sugar
- ½ teaspoon freshly ground white pepper
- 2 tablespoons vegetable oil
- 2 teaspoons soy sauce

STIR-FRY

- 2 tablespoons vegetable oil
- 2 tablespoons grated fresh ginger
- 1 tablespoon minced garlic
- 1 medium white onion, thinly sliced
- 2 medium carrots, peeled and thinly sliced
- 1 red bell pepper, cored, seeded, and thinly sliced
- 3 scallions, white and light green parts only, thinly sliced on the diagonal
- 1 jalapeño pepper, thinly sliced
- ¼ habañero chile, seeded and thinly sliced (optional)
- 2 tablespoons soy sauce
- ¼ cup pale Belgian-style beer
- 2 tablespoons mirin (Japanese sweet rice wine)
- Jasmine rice, for serving

What fun is subtle? Dinner should be about flavors that pop and are satisfying. This stir-fry is perfect when you crave the fresh flavors of garlic and ginger. As always, quality ingredients are key, so consider using organic chicken and natural soy sauce. Serve jasmine rice and an Asian-inspired spicy cucumber pickle as accompaniments to round out the meal. The complexity and flavors of a saison, such as Surly's Cynicale, enhance this dish and make for a wonderful pairing.

1 **MARINATE THE CHICKEN:** Place the chicken, still in its original packaging, in the freezer for 30 minutes. (Partially frozen meat is easier to slice for stir-frying.) Whisk the cornstarch, salt, sugar, white pepper, oil, and soy sauce together in a small bowl. Remove the chicken from the freezer, slice it into thin strips, ¼ inch thick by 1 inch wide, and place in an airtight container. Pour the marinade on top, shake to coat, and refrigerate for 30 minutes, shaking occasionally.

2 **MAKE THE STIR-FRY:** Heat a wok or large skillet over medium-high heat until a couple drops of water skitter when sprinkled over the surface. Add the oil and swirl the skillet to coat. Add the chicken and the marinade and stir-fry for 2 minutes; some sticking to the pan is normal.

3 Add the ginger and garlic, and cook until fragrant, about 1 minute, stirring to prevent the garlic from burning. Add the onion and cook, stirring occasionally, for 1 minute longer. Add the carrots, bell pepper, two-thirds of the scallions, jalapeño, habañero, and soy sauce, and stir-fry for 30 seconds.

4 Deglaze the pan with the beer and mirin, and cook until the sauce thickens, about 2 minutes. Reduce the temperature to low and put the pan's lid on to let the flavors develop and the vegetables steam, about 3 minutes.

5 Spoon the stir-fry over rice and garnish with the remaining scallions. Serve immediately.

Makes 4 servings

They attended the same junior high school, but *Surly* owner Omar Ansari and brewmaster Todd Haug hadn't seen each other for years. Happily, they reconnected at a brewer's conference, realized they shared brewing philosophies and passions, and decided to get into business for themselves. In the years that led up to the brewery's opening in 2005, Ansari had become a dedicated homebrewer and Haug had risen through the ranks at a few breweries, impressing everyone with his creations. An early adopter of the craft-beer-in-cans movement, Surly has gained a loyal (sometimes rabid) following from those discerning beer people who want the very best. And because good beer needs great food, Todd's wife, Linda, an accomplished chef, has assumed duties as the director of restaurant operations for the forthcoming restaurant and beer garden that will be attached to the brewery.

As for the name? They'll tell you it comes from the anger fueled by the inability to find good beer. Lucky for us, if Surly is close by you don't have to look too hard.

Beer-Braised Pulled Pork

A staple of beer cuisine, pulled pork is a sacred food. Breweries around the country have worked to perfect this flavorful meat, making sure it is falling-off-the-bone tender, with each piece full of the flavors of marinade and spice. Proper application of the dry rub is crucial, and you'll see a difference in taste the longer it's allowed to sit. Shredded and piled high, pulled pork is best enjoyed on a soft toasted roll (topped with coleslaw or red onion slices) but is just as delicious served on top of a salad or alone on a plate. This recipe from Jolly Pumpkin is a harmonious combination of spice and sweet, with an earthy touch from the beer. Because it is so versatile, you can pair this with any number of beers, but a saison (like Jolly Pumpkin Bam Biere) is a particularly good choice.

DRY RUB

- 2½ tablespoons light chili powder
- 2½ tablespoons kosher salt
- 2 tablespoons freshly ground black pepper
- 1 tablespoon granulated garlic
- 1 tablespoon onion powder
- 2 teaspoons ground cumin
- 2 teaspoons dry mustard powder
- 1 teaspoon ground coriander

5–6 pounds bone-in pork butt

BRAISE

- 1 (12-ounce) bottle amber ale, wheat ale, or saison
- 5 garlic cloves, chopped
- 1 small white onion, chopped

SAUCE

- ¼ cup firmly packed light brown sugar
- ¼ cup ketchup
- ¼ cup tomato purée
- 3 tablespoons Worcestershire sauce
- 2 tablespoons whole-grain Dijon mustard
- 1 tablespoon hot sauce

1 MAKE THE RUB: Combine the chili powder, salt, black pepper, granulated garlic, onion powder, cumin, mustard powder, and coriander in a mixing bowl. Rub the mixture over the sides of the pork butt. Wrap the pork butt with plastic wrap and refrigerate for at least 1 hour and up to 8 hours.

2 Preheat the oven to 450°F. Unwrap the pork and place in a roasting pan with sides about 2 inches high. Cook the pork for 45 to 50 minutes, or until browned all over.

3 MAKE THE BRAISE: Remove the pork from the oven and reduce the temperature to 320°F. Pour the beer over the pork butt and add the garlic and onion around the pork. Cover the pan with aluminum foil and poke several holes in the top of the foil. Cook the pork butt for 3 to 3½ hours, or until it reaches an internal temperature of 195°F and is tender enough to pull apart easily.

4 MAKE THE SAUCE: Remove the pork from the pan and pour the pan juices into a saucepan. Add the brown sugar, ketchup, tomato purée, Worcestershire, mustard, and hot sauce, and bring to a simmer over medium heat. Continue to simmer until the sauce has reduced by one-third, about 25 minutes.

5 While the sauce is reducing, pull apart the pork using tongs or forks. Discard any large pieces of fat, transfer the meat to a large bowl, and pour the sauce over the top. Mix until combined and serve.

Makes 8–10 servings

The brewers of Jolly Pumpkin Artisan Ales are sorcerers of sour and wizards of wood. The beers are open-fermented, oak barrel–aged, and then bottle-conditioned before being served. The clear skill of the brewers and the great care that goes into every recipe is apparent. Brewmaster Ron Jeffries has taken Belgian sensibilities and given the ales an American bent. What you get is a solid lineup of beers that cause the eyes to widen with the first sip. From there, it only gets better.

Aside from the main brewery in Dexter, Jolly Pumpkin has a café and brewery in Ann Arbor and a brewery, distillery, and restaurant in Traverse City. Visit all three to get the full experience. You won't be disappointed.

Dungeness Crab Tart,
see page 252

From the Sea

Shellfish to Salmon

Prosciutto-Wrapped Scallops
with Butternut Squash and
Roasted Garlic–Huckleberry Sauce

The meaty scallops and smoky prosciutto combine with a sauce made from whiskey, garlic, and fruit in a perfect symphony of flavors. This dish is especially delightful in late summer when huckleberries reach their peak. Pair with a strong golden ale, like a tripel, with some alcohol heft, assertive yeast, and spice flavors.

1 head garlic
   Extra-virgin olive oil
1 cup fresh or frozen
   huckleberries
½ cup firmly packed light
   brown sugar
½ cup bourbon
1 large butternut squash,
   peeled, seeded, and diced
½ cup mascarpone cheese
5 tablespoons unsalted butter
   Salt and freshly ground
   black pepper
12 large scallops
12 thin slices smoked
   prosciutto
12 fresh rosemary sprigs

A Few Beers to Try with This Recipe

- *Allagash Tripel*
- *Captain Lawrence XTra Gold*
- *Pretty Things Fluffy White Rabbits*
- *Rockmill Tripel*
- *Samuel Adams New World Tripel*
- *Tallgrass Velvet Rooster*

1 Preheat the oven to 300°F. Take the head of garlic and cut off the pointed end to expose the tops of the individual cloves. Coat the head in olive oil, wrap tightly in aluminum foil, and bake for 1 hour.

2 Remove the garlic from the oven and discard the foil. When the garlic is cool enough to handle (about 10 minutes), remove the cloves by gently squeezing the bottom of the head and forcing the cloves out. Combine the garlic cloves, huckleberries, brown sugar, and bourbon in a blender and purée until smooth, about 1 minute.

3 Transfer the sauce mixture to a pot, bring to a boil, and then immediately remove from the heat and strain through a wire-mesh strainer into a bowl. Cover and set aside.

4 Place the butternut squash in a large pot of water and bring to a boil. Cook until tender, 7 to 9 minutes, and then drain. Add the mascarpone and 4 tablespoons of the butter and mash or beat until smooth. Season with salt and pepper to taste.

5 Pat the scallops dry with paper towels and wrap each one in a piece of the prosciutto. Secure the prosciutto by sliding a rosemary sprig through each wrapped scallop.

6 Melt the remaining 1 tablespoon butter in a skillet over high heat. Sear the scallops until the prosciutto is crispy and golden and the scallops have lost their translucence, 2 to 3 minutes per side.

7 Serve the scallops immediately with the butternut squash and a drizzle of the huckleberry sauce.

Makes 4–6 servings

Just south of the center of Ohio, Rockmill sits on a farm that the owners discovered — quite happily — shares water properties similar to those of the Wallonia region of Belgium. With a fondness for beer and tradition, they set out to re-create some of the same styles that Belgian locals have enjoyed for centuries. Rockmill's four beers — finished in cage and cork bottles — are a tribute to history, and using organic ingredients is a compliment to those who work the land.

The brewery takes food seriously and regularly teams up with local restaurants to wow diners with exquisite pairings. It is also one of only a few breweries that has a webpage dedicated to cheese pairings.

HINTERLAND BREWERY AND RESTAURANT

GREEN BAY, WISCONSIN

Seared Diver Scallops
with Roasted Maitake Mushrooms, Cauliflower, and Sweet Potatoes and Coconut–Green Curry Sauce

The natural sweetness of the scallops takes on a new dimension with the fragrant curry sauce and the roasted vegetables. This is a recipe that can be pulled together in less than an hour, making it great for those weeknights when you feel like something special. A tall glass of IPA with just enough hop bite to stand up to the sauce is the perfect accompaniment.

VEGETABLES

- ¾ pound sweet potatoes, diced
- ½ pound cauliflower florets, cut into ¼-inch pieces
- ¾ pound maitake mushrooms, cut into ¼-inch pieces
- 1 tablespoon extra-virgin olive oil
- Salt and freshly ground black pepper

CURRY SAUCE

- 1 tablespoon extra-virgin olive oil
- ⅓ cup chopped carrots
- ⅓ cup chopped celery
- ⅓ cup chopped onion
- 1 tablespoon chopped fresh ginger
- 1 teaspoon chopped garlic
- 1 teaspoon ground coriander seed
- 1 cup coconut milk
- 1 cup shrimp broth
- ½ cup heavy cream
- 2 tablespoons green curry paste
- 1 tablespoon fish sauce
- 1 tablespoon honey
- 1 tablespoon sambal
- 1 cup chopped baby spinach
- ½ cup chopped fresh cilantro
- Salt and freshly ground black pepper

SCALLOPS

- 12 large scallops
- Salt and freshly ground black pepper
- 3 tablespoons clarified butter (see box)
- Chopped fresh cilantro
- Lime zest

1 **ROAST THE VEGETABLES:** Preheat the oven to 375°F. Toss the sweet potato, cauliflower, mushrooms, and olive oil together in a large bowl. Season with salt and pepper to taste and transfer to a baking dish. Roast for 45 minutes, or until tender. Set aside and allow to cool slightly.

2 **MAKE THE CURRY SAUCE:** Warm the olive oil in a large skillet over medium heat. Add the carrots, celery, onion, ginger, garlic, and coriander, and sauté until slightly brown and fragrant, 5 to 10 minutes. Stir in the coconut milk, shrimp broth, cream, curry paste, fish sauce, honey, and sambal, and continue cooking until the liquid is reduced by one-third, 20 to 30 minutes.

3 Let the sauce cool slightly, and then transfer to a blender and blend until smooth. Add the spinach and cilantro and blend until fully incorporated. Season with salt and pepper to taste.

4 **PREPARE THE SCALLOPS:** Pat the scallops dry with paper towels and season with salt and pepper. Warm the clarified butter in a skillet over medium-high heat, add the scallops, and cook until golden brown, 2 to 3 minutes per side. Remove the scallops from the heat, and toss the roasted vegetables into the skillet to reheat. Stir a few tablespoons of the curry sauce into the vegetables to combine all the flavors and heat through.

5 Spoon a puddle of the curry sauce onto each of four plates. Top with the roasted vegetables and three scallops per plate. Garnish with the cilantro and lime zest, and serve immediately.

Makes 4 servings

Clarified Butter

Make the clarified butter by melting 4 tablespoons of unsalted butter in a small saucepan over medium-low heat. When the foam begins to subside, take the pan off the heat and set aside for 5 minutes. Skim off the milk solids; the yellow butterfat left in the pan is clarified butter.

Elevating beer to new heights, Hinterland Brewery is creating flavorful brews and gourmet food, and serving them in a posh location deep in the heart of Packers country. The restaurant flies-in fresh seafood and sources vegetables and meat from local farms and ranches; when it all arrives on your plate, it's a thing of beauty.

And the beer? It's good! In a state where large breweries rule the roost, Hinterland's Bill and Michelle Tressler have come out swinging. Since opening in 1995, they have won over even the most die-hard light lager lovers. Their distinctive pint bottles, unique recipes, and dedication to both tradition and innovation have made Hinterland one of the more respected breweries in the state and region. In addition to their Green Bay headquarters, they also operate a swanky restaurant in Milwaukee. It is the place to be, and to be seen with a beer in hand.

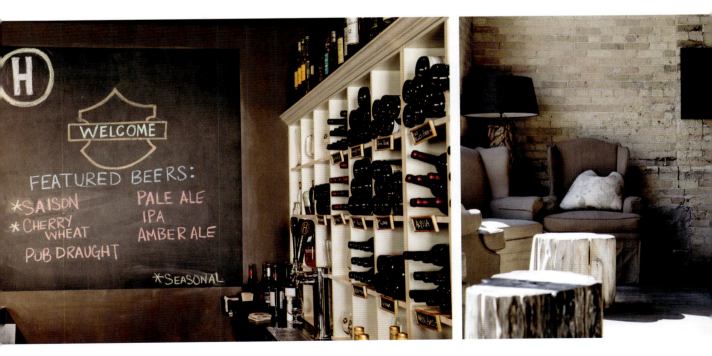

¾ cup extra-virgin olive oil
1 Spanish onion, chopped
1 green bell pepper, cored,
   seeded, and chopped
2 garlic cloves, chopped
1½ pounds boneless chicken,
   diced into 1-inch pieces
½ pound pork, diced into
   1-inch pieces
½ pound crabmeat
½ pound grouper
½ pound lobster meat
½ pound shrimp, peeled
   and deveined
½ cup tomato sauce
6 ounces pimentos
3 tablespoons salt
1 tablespoon saffron
1 teaspoon freshly ground
   black pepper
1 teaspoon ground cumin
3 bay leaves
2 cups dry white wine
2 (12-ounce) bottles Trumer
   Pils, or similar pilsner
   beer
1½ cups Valencia rice
1½ cups water
1 cup sweet peas, fresh or
   frozen
2 pounds steamed clams
   (see box)
1 pound cooked crab claws

Paella Bella

Despite all the ingredients that go into this dish, paella can be relatively simple to prepare. Adding the seafood at the right times ensures that it doesn't become rubbery. The final product is a lively cacophony of flavors and textures. Delicious any time of year, there is a certain enjoyment that comes with serving paella at a sunset dinner in the summer alongside a glass of pilsner. When purchasing the pimentos, clams, and peas, opt for fresh if possible, but canned, frozen, or jarred are acceptable alternatives.

1 Heat the olive oil in a Dutch oven or a large skillet with a lid over medium heat. Add the onion, bell pepper, and garlic, and cook, stirring occasionally, until soft, about 5 minutes.

2 Add the chicken and pork to the dish and sauté over medium heat until golden, about 8 minutes. Add the crabmeat, grouper, lobster, and shrimp, and continue to cook, stirring frequently, until the seafood is lightly golden, about 3 minutes.

3 Add the tomato sauce. Finely chop ¼ cup of the pimentos and add them to the skillet. Add the salt, saffron, black pepper, cumin, bay leaves, and wine. Bring the mixture to a boil and add the beer. Reduce the heat to medium and cook for 10 minutes longer. Remove the seafood with a slotted spoon and set aside in a bowl.

4 Add the rice and water and mix well to combine. Cover and cook over low heat until the rice is done,

approximately 30 minutes, stirring once halfway through. Stir in the peas, reserved seafood, clam meat, and crab claws. Heat through. Chop the remaining pimentos and scatter them over the paella before serving.

Makes 8 servings

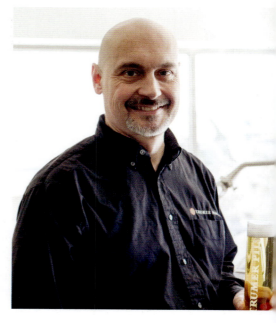

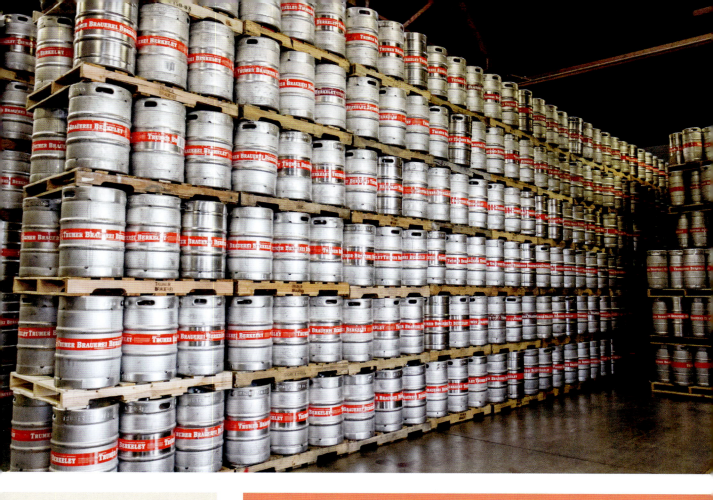

Steamed Clams

Scrub the clams under cool water. Fill a large, wide pot with 2 inches of water, bring the water to a simmer, and put the clams in the water. Simmer until all or most of the clams open. Discard unopened clams and remove the meat from the opened clams.

It is a rarity these days for a brewery — especially one in America — to make just one beer. But the ***Trumer*** brewery does such an outstanding job on its pilsner, there is no need to do anything else. Following the Reinheitsgebot, or German purity law, Trumer's pils is made only with water, malt, hops, and yeast. The result is a revelation in a glass. It is a clear reminder of the way pilsners used to be, before breweries started favoring mass marketing and cutting corners for convenience. This true pilsner is made under the direction of brewer Lars Larson, and the result is a beer with a spicy aroma and kick from the Saaz hops. It is a perfect shade of gold, and endlessly refreshing. Between sips, enjoy the lacing the beer leaves on the side of your glass as it slowly disappears. Each ring brings you closer to the next bottle.

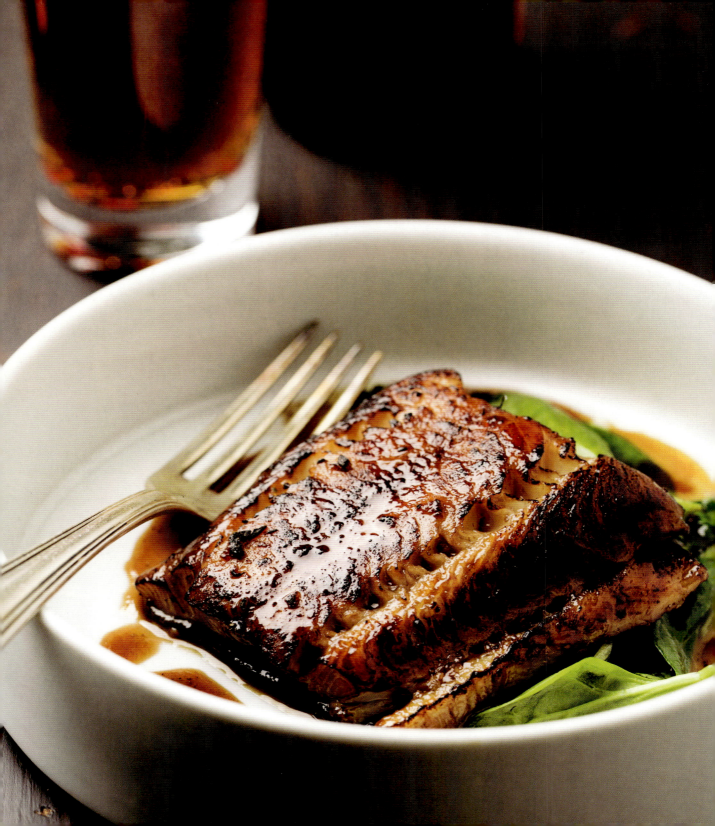

Black Cod Brûlée

This flavorful recipe is also fun to make, thanks to the blowtorch. The marinade gives this full-flavored fish a tangy bite. Pair with a sessionable, malty beer, such as an altbier, so as not to overpower the fish.

1 Bring the beer to a light simmer in a medium saucepan over medium-low heat. Do not boil. Continue to simmer, stirring occasionally, until reduced by one-third, about 1 hour. Remove the saucepan from the heat and let cool completely.

2 Mix the garlic, ginger, cranberry sauce, pomegranate juice, and soy sauce into the reduced beer. Place the cod in a baking dish or roasting pan and cover with the sauce. Cover the dish with plastic wrap and refrigerate for at least 4 hours or up to 24 hours.

3 Preheat the oven to 375°F. Uncover the cod and braise for at least 1 hour, basting every 15 minutes and taking care not to overcook it.

4 Combine the brown sugar and granulated sugar in a small bowl and set aside.

5 Place the cod on a large serving plate and sprinkle each fillet with a fine layer of the sugar mixture. With a kitchen blowtorch, melt the sugar until it forms a crispy topping. Serve immediately.

Makes 8–10 servings

- 2 (12-ounce) bottles Alaskan Amber, or similar beer, or 1¾ cups fruity, non-tannic pinot noir
- 3 garlic cloves, minced
- 3 tablespoons grated ginger
- 2 cups cranberry sauce (preferably homemade)
- 1½ cups pomegranate juice
- ¼ cup dark soy sauce
- 6 pounds whole black cod (sablefish), cut into 8 to 10 fillets
- ½ cup firmly packed dark brown sugar
- 1 cup granulated sugar

PROFILE ★   **A source of pride for locals** and a sought-after brand across much of the country, the *Alaskan Brewing Co.* was founded in 1986 by Geoff and Marcy Larson. Their Alaskan Amber is derived from descriptions of a 100-year-old recipe once served to miners in the nearby city of Douglas, Alaska. Among their seasonal offerings, they make a smoked porter, which is brewed in the fall and is a benchmark of the style. The beer has won a record number of medals — many of them gold — at the Great American Beer Festival.

Alaskan Brewing has been in the forefront of brewery environmental practices, including the installation of a CO_2 reclamation plant to reduce and reuse carbon dioxide produced during fermentation. The brewery also installed a biomass steam boiler, fueled entirely by the brewery's spent grain. The boiler is used to warm the brewhouse and heat the grain dryer. It was also the first American craft brewery to install a mash filter press. As a result, it now uses 6 percent less malt and 1 million fewer gallons of water while still producing upwards of 120,000 barrels of beer per year.

Barbecued Shrimp

This spicy, lip-smacking dish is not what many would consider barbecue, unless you're from Louisiana. First, it's made in the oven, not on a grill, and second, there is none of that sticky sauce to be found. Instead, here, the pride of the Gulf (shrimp) is served with a savory broth. Have some crunchy French bread ready to sop up the broth, and pair this dish with a dark brown ale, such as Abita Turbodog.

1½ cups (3 sticks) unsalted butter
½ cup extra-virgin olive oil
3 tablespoons barbecue spice
3 tablespoons dried onion flakes
3 tablespoons garlic powder
2 bay leaves
1 tablespoon plus 1 teaspoon paprika
1 tablespoon freshly ground black pepper
2 teaspoons dried rosemary leaves
1½ teaspoons cayenne pepper
1 teaspoon ground cloves
¼ cup Worcestershire sauce
  Juice of 1 lemon
1 (12-ounce) bottle dark brown ale, at room temperature
2 teaspoons salt
5 pounds large head-on unpeeled shrimp

1 Preheat the oven to 300°F. Combine the butter and olive oil in a baking pan large enough to accommodate the shrimp (or divide between two pans, if necessary). Place the pan in the oven to melt the butter. This will take about 6 minutes; watch closely so that the butter does not burn.

2 Remove the pan from the oven. Add the barbecue spice, onion flakes, garlic powder, bay leaves, paprika, black pepper, rosemary, cayenne, cloves, Worcestershire, and lemon juice to the pan. Stir to mix. Slowly add the beer and stir until the foam subsides. Add the salt and set the mixture aside to allow the flavors to marry for 10 to 15 minutes.

3 Add the shrimp to the pan and stir to coat with the mixture. Bake, uncovered, basting well every 10 minutes, for about 40 minutes. When there is a slight air space along the back of the shrimp and the shell has pulled away from the meat, remove from the oven and serve.

Makes 4–6 servings

PROFILE ★ **Using water from springs** located 30 miles north of New Orleans, the **Abita Brewing Company** prides itself on sourcing quality ingredients for each of its beers. Founded in 1986, the brewery has become a Louisiana institution, producing more than 126,000 barrels of beer a year and distributing far beyond its bayou borders. Owned and operated by local shareholders, Abita has worked with chefs over the years (and even released a cookbook) to highlight the marriage of good food and beer.

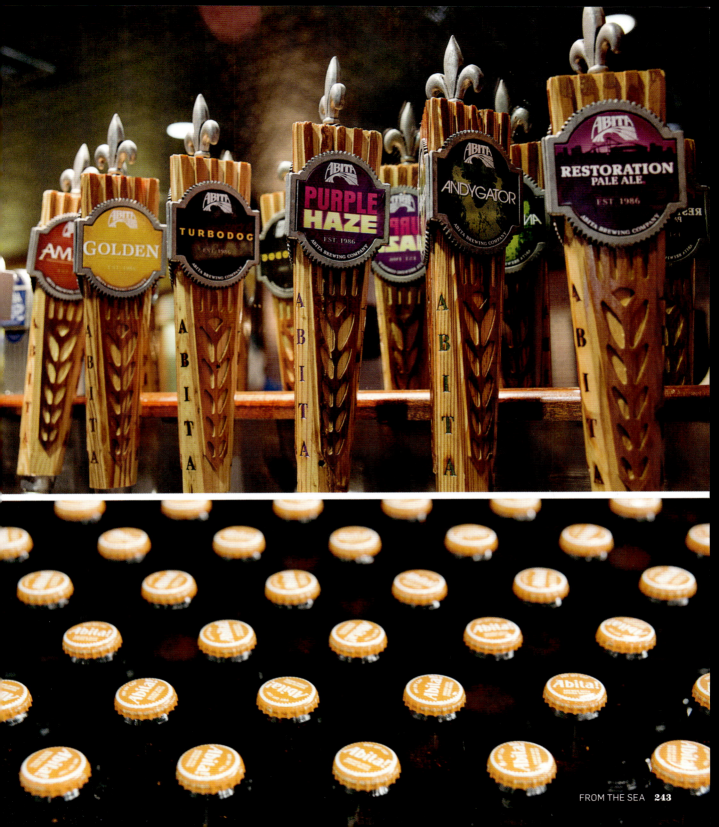

North Carolina Shrimp and Grits with Spicy Pan Sauce

Shrimp and grits are a staple of Carolinas' cuisine, and this spicy and savory take on the classic dish makes it perfect for a hearty lunch or satisfying dinner. Fresh shrimp are best, but it is okay to substitute frozen when necessary. Pair with an India pale ale, like Foothills Hoppyum, which stands up well to the heat and spice.

GRITS

- 3 cups water
- 1 bay leaf
- 1 tablespoon kosher salt
- 1 cup stone-ground grits
- 2 ounces sharp cheddar cheese, shredded (½ cup)

SAUCE

- 2 tablespoons unsalted butter
- ½ cup crumbled Andouille sausage
- 2 tablespoons finely chopped celery stalks
- 2 tablespoons finely chopped yellow onion
- 2 tablespoons cored, seeded, and finely chopped red bell pepper
- ½ garlic clove, minced
- 1 pound fresh shrimp, peeled and deveined
- 1 (14.5-ounce) can fire-roasted tomatoes, drained and puréed
- 2 tablespoons hot sauce

1 MAKE THE GRITS: Bring the water, bay leaf, and salt to a rolling boil in a large pot. Whisk in the grits and simmer over medium-high heat, uncovered, for 15 to 20 minutes. The grits will thicken but remain slightly coarse. Remove the pot from the heat and stir in the cheese until fully incorporated. Cover and set aside.

2 MAKE THE SAUCE: Melt the butter in a skillet set over medium-high heat. Add the sausage, celery, onion, bell pepper, and garlic, and sauté, stirring occasionally, until the sausage is browned and the vegetables are soft, about 10 minutes.

3 Add the shrimp, tomato purée, and hot sauce to the pot. Simmer until the shrimp are pink and cooked through, 3 to 8 minutes, depending on their size.

4 Serve the shrimp hot over bowls of grits.

Makes 2–4 servings

PROFILE ★ **Under the direction of brewmaster** Jamie Bartholomaus, *Foothills*, established in 2004, has quickly become one of the most respected breweries in the country. Thanks in part to flavorful and infinitely drinkable ales, and to special releases like Sexual Chocolate, a chocolate-infused imperial stout, Foothills has grown and thrived. For many serious beer drinkers, no trip to North Carolina is complete without a visit. Moreover, the pub menu features some of the most innovative yet classic cuisine in the city. "Come hungry, leave satisfied" is what many locals say. Finally, in an effort to teach the good word, the brewery holds regular classes for those looking to further their brewing knowledge and acquire some hands-on experience. Start planning your visit now!

Lucky U IPA-Battered Fish

Simple, hearty, and comforting, fried fish is a dish that needs beer. A moderately hoppy pale ale in the batter for these fish fillets provides a slight bitterness that contrasts nicely with the sweetness of the fish. To serve in the traditional style, place the fish in a paper-lined basket and add a splash or two of malt vinegar. A fresh pint — try an American pale ale — to accompany the meal is essential. This recipe calls for cod, but pollock may be substituted.

3 cups all-purpose flour
1 teaspoon freshly ground black pepper
1 teaspoon onion powder
¼ teaspoon ground turmeric
2 eggs, beaten
1 (12-ounce) bottle Breckenridge Lucky U IPA, or similar India pale ale, plus more as needed
 Soy or canola oil, for deep frying
2½ pounds cod, Atlantic pollock, haddock, or hake, cut into 3- to 4-ounce pieces

1 Preheat the oven to 200°F. Line a baking sheet with paper towels and set a wire rack on top.

2 Combine 2 cups of the flour with the pepper, onion powder, and turmeric in a large mixing bowl. Mix in the eggs. Slowly add the beer, stirring constantly until well blended. The mixture should have the consistency of cream. If it is too thick, add more ale. If it is too thin, add more flour.

3 Add 4 inches of oil to a deep pot and heat to 375°F. Put the remaining 1 cup flour in a shallow dish. Dry the fish pieces with a paper towel and dredge them in the flour, shaking off any excess. Dip the floured fish in the batter, taking care to thoroughly coat each piece.

4 Fry the fish, working in batches if needed and turning occasionally, until the batter is crisp and golden brown, about 5 minutes. Transfer the fish to the prepared rack and baking sheet and hold in the warm oven while you fry the remaining fish.

5 Serve hot with your favorite accompaniments.

Makes 6 servings

PROFILE ★ **While it might sound clichéd,** the people who work at *Breckenridge Brewing* say they are living the dream. With a production brewery that's also home to an awesome barbecue joint, two brewpubs, and a separate ale house, Breckenridge is a dominant force in its native Colorado. And with its beers available in half the country, it's easier than ever to have a taste of the Colorado dream at home, wherever that may be.

NEW PLANET BEER

BOULDER, COLORADO

½ cup orange marmalade
¼ cup Dijon mustard
¼ cup honey
¼ teaspoon hot sauce
½ cup gluten-free flour
1½ teaspoons gluten-free baking powder
2 eggs, lightly beaten
⅔ cup gluten-free ale
2 cups medium shredded unsweetened coconut
1 tablespoon sugar
26 large shrimp, peeled and deveined
Coconut or canola oil, for frying

A Few Gluten-Free Beers to Try

- *Bards Tale Gluten Free Beer*
- *Dogfish Head Tweason'ale*
- *Lakefront New Grist Gluten Free Beer*
- *New Planet Gluten Free Beer*

Gluten-Free Battered Coconut Shrimp with Sweet and Spicy Sauce

For those following a gluten-free diet, beer and deep-fried anything used to be among the concessions to be made. But now there are breweries like New Planet and restaurants like Colorado's Gluten-Free Bistro that are aiming to change that. This recipe tastes like the traditional dish but is gluten free.

1 Mix the marmalade, mustard, honey, and hot sauce together in a small bowl. Cover and refrigerate until ready to use.

2 Whisk the flour, baking powder, eggs, and ale together in a medium bowl until the carbonation subsides. Combine the coconut and sugar in a separate bowl.

3 Line a baking sheet or large platter with parchment paper. Dredge the shrimp in the beer batter and then in the coconut-sugar mix. Place the shrimp on the prepared baking sheet and refrigerate for 30 to 45 minutes.

4 Pour enough oil to cover the shrimp into a deep pot and heat to 350°F. Working with five to eight pieces at a time, drop the shrimp into the oil and fry until golden brown, 2 to 3 minutes, or until the shrimp float. Transfer the shrimp to a paper towel–lined plate to drain. Serve immediately with the prepared dipping sauce.

Makes 6–8 servings

When Pedro Gonzalez was diagnosed with celiac disease, he was able to regain a healthy lifestyle after cutting gluten from his diet, but he missed many foods that he had previously enjoyed, like pizza and beer. A few years ago, while on a hike with a brewer friend, they began discussing the possibilities of gluten-free brewing, and the pal offered to try his hand at a few recipes. After some trial and error, they settled on a recipe that would become Tread Lightly Ale, the flagship beer of the brewery the friends founded in 2008, **New Planet Beer**. The ale is a balanced beer brewed with sorghum plus corn extract and orange peel.

Soon after the release of Tread Lightly, Gonzalez released 3R Raspberry Ale, which is similar to Tread Lightly, but with natural raspberry purée added. The brewery also has a pale ale in its lineup, and Gonzalez says he is exploring other styles. "I want to have cream ale, pilsner, IPA, stout, porter, and every kind we can," he said. "I have a passion for giving gluten-free people like me options."

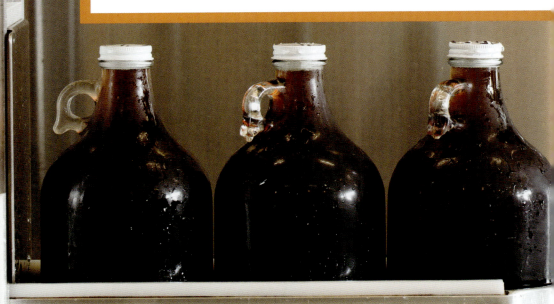

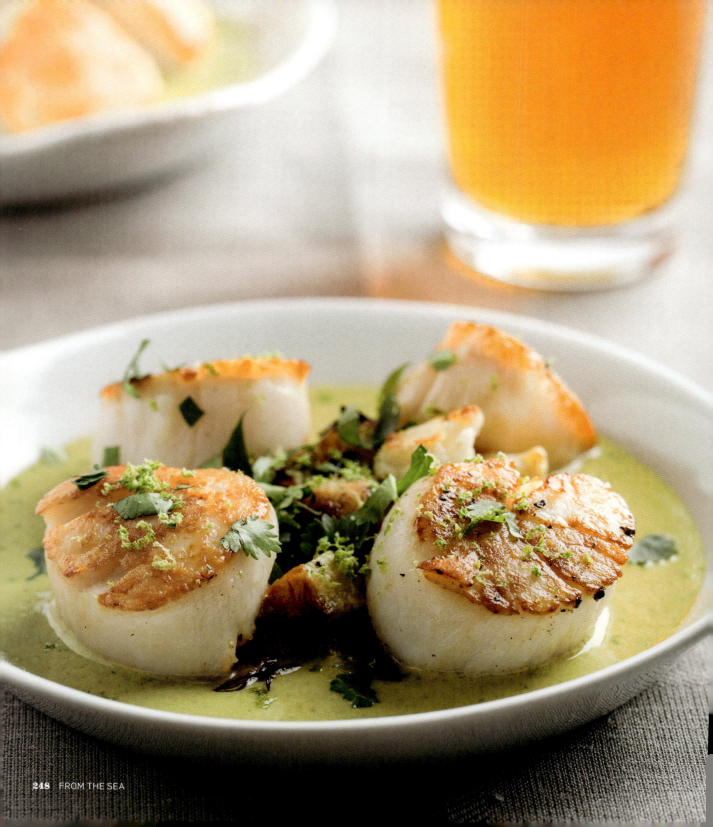

Grilled Diver Scallops and Fall Vegetable Shish Kebabs
with Hazelnut Brown Butter

OSKAR BLUES BREWERY
LONGMONT, COLORADO

For the final cool days before the grill is covered and stashed away for the winter, Oskar Blues offers this recipe that brings autumn flavors and ingredients to the beloved summer outdoor cooking experience. While fennel can have an assertive flavor, it loses some of its licorice-like taste as it cooks; the same is true of parsnips, which sweeten on the grill. The kebabs partner well with a Czech pilsner, a beer that showcases the floral and spicy aroma and finish of Saaz hops.

12 large fresh diver scallops
4 fennel bulbs, trimmed, cored, and diced into 1½-inch cubes
4 large parsnips, peeled and diced into 1½-inch cubes
1 medium butternut squash, peeled, seeded, and diced into 1½-inch cubes
2 tablespoons extra-virgin olive oil
Salt and freshly ground black pepper
1 (12-ounce) can Oskar Blues Mama's Little Yella Pils, or similar beer
8 skewers
1 cup (2 sticks) unsalted butter
1 tablespoon finely chopped toasted hazelnuts

Note: If using wooden skewers, soak them in water for 1 hour before grilling.

1 Remove the scallops from the refrigerator to come up to room temperature. Prepare a medium fire in a gas or charcoal grill. If using charcoal, arrange the coals in a thin layer to evenly control the heat.

2 Combine the fennel, parsnips, and butternut squash in a large bowl and toss with 1 tablespoon of the olive oil. Transfer the vegetables to a cast-iron skillet (or another grill-safe pan), season with salt and pepper, and place the pan on the grill. Cook, with the lid closed, stirring occasionally, until the vegetables are a light golden brown, about 25 minutes.

3 Remove the skillet from the grill and deglaze with ¼ cup of the beer. Remove the vegetables from the skillet and let cool for 5 minutes. Reserve any drippings in the skillet for later.

4 Using two skewers for each shish kebab, alternately thread the scallops, fennel, parsnips, and butternut squash onto the skewers. You should use three scallops on each set of skewers. Using two skewers for each kebab will prevent the ingredients from spinning on the grill.

5 Season the kebabs with salt and pepper and lightly coat with the remaining 1 tablespoon olive oil. Grill the kebabs, turning once, until you've reached the desired level of doneness for the scallops, about 5 minutes per side for medium. Set aside and tent with foil while making the sauce.

6 Return the skillet to the grill; add the butter, hazelnuts, and remaining 1¼ cups beer to the vegetable drippings. Cook, stirring occasionally, until the butter is melted and lightly browned.

recipe continues on next page

A Few Beers to Try with This Recipe
- *Lagunitas Pils*
- *Oskar Blues Mama's Little Yella Pils*
- *Samuel Adams Noble Pils*
- *Saranac Bohemian Pilsner*
- *Summit Pilsener*

7 Transfer the kebabs to a serving plate, pour the brown butter sauce over the scallops, and serve immediately.

Makes 4 servings

An early adopter of cans for craft beers, *Oskar Blues* embraced the aluminum cylinders and gained popularity with outdoor enthusiasts who could suddenly enjoy quality beer in a shatterproof container. Seeing their success, other breweries quickly followed suit.

Oskar Blues has earned a good reputation for its beers, which tend to be higher in alcohol than others on the market. With three locations in Colorado (the brewery in Longmont also features a spirited taproom and a new brewery in North Carolina), the brewery continues to prove that good beer comes in cans.

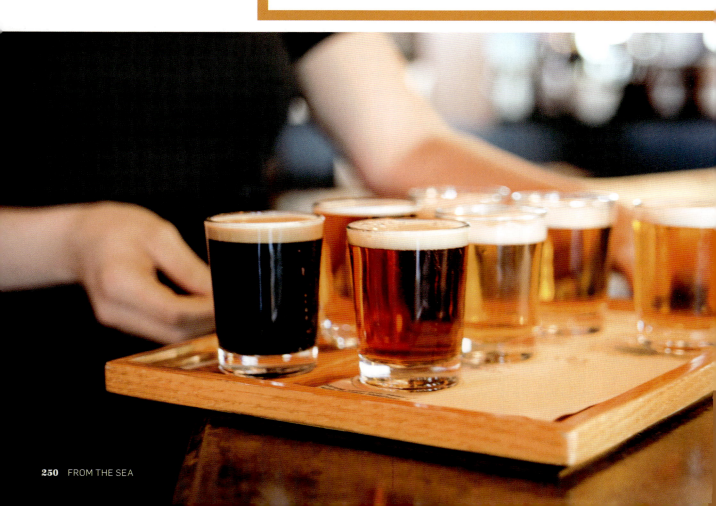

Pomegranate Trout

The mild, nutty taste of trout gets an infusion of tart flavor from the fresh lemon and pomegranate in this recipe. While this dish would be nice with an American wheat like FCB's Major Tom's, also consider drinking an amber or brown ale with a solid malt characteristic.

FORT COLLINS BREWERY

FORT COLLINS, COLORADO

1 pomegranate
4 whole fresh trout, heads
   removed
1 lemon, thinly sliced
1 medium red onion, thinly
   sliced
4 garlic cloves, minced
   Salt and freshly ground
   black pepper
2 tablespoons canola oil
½ cup pomegranate-flavored
   wheat ale
1 tablespoon unsalted butter
2 tablespoons finely chopped
   fresh parsley

1 Cut the pomegranate in half. Thinly slice one half and seed the other half. Reserve the seeds.

2 Stuff the trout cavities with the pomegranate slices, lemon slices, onion, and garlic, dividing the ingredients equally among the fish. Season the skin of the trout with salt and pepper.

3 Heat 1 tablespoon of the oil in a cast-iron skillet over medium-high heat. Sear two of the trout for 3 minutes, and then carefully flip over and sear for 2 minutes longer. Add ¼ cup of the beer to the skillet and cook for 2 minutes longer.

4 Repeat with the remaining 1 tablespoon oil, two trout, and ¼ cup beer in a second skillet.

5 Transfer the trout to a serving platter to rest and combine the beer sauce in one of the skillets. Add the butter and parsley to the sauce and whisk well for 1 minute. Pour the sauce over the trout and serve topped with the reserved pomegranate seeds.

Makes 4 servings

PROFILE ★ **With a solid lineup of ales and lagers, Fort Collins Brewery** is one of many in the happily brewery-crowded northern Colorado city of Fort Collins. However, its reach extends far beyond the Rocky Mountain state, and it has been responsible for spreading the word of good beer to states and areas with a great need. FCB's staples are available in a variety pack known as the brewer's lunchbox, giving first-timers a taste of everything. Any visit to Fort Collins should include a trip to the brewery and its new restaurant, Gravity 1020.

Dungeness Crab Tart with Crab Reduction

CRAB TART

- 4 pounds fresh Dungeness crabs
  Pastry or pie dough for one 9-inch tart
- 2 tablespoons unsalted butter
- 2 shallots, chopped
- 4 fresh basil leaves, chopped
- 2 sprigs fresh parsley, chopped
- 1 fresh tarragon sprig, chopped
- 3 eggs
- 1½ cups heavy cream
- ½ teaspoon salt
- ½ teaspoon freshly ground black pepper

REDUCTION

- 1 tablespoon extra-virgin olive oil
- 1 pound yellow onions, diced
- ½ pound carrots, peeled and diced
- ½ pound celery stalks, diced
- ¼ cup tomato paste
- 1 bay leaf
- 1 fresh thyme sprig
  Water, as needed
- 2 cups heavy cream
  Salt
  Juice of ½ lemon
- ½ cup crème fraîche, for garnish
- ¼ teaspoon tobiko roe, for garnish (optional)

The meaty and salty Dungeness crab is a staple of the Pacific Northwest, and its delicate flavor marries beautifully with fresh vegetables and herbs. This recipe pairs well with a cream ale, as the rich sweet flavors of the crab and the buttery crust tie in nicely with the malt in the brew. The beer also lifts up the fresh herbs to dance with the hops.

1 **MAKE THE TART:** Preheat the oven to 350°F. Steam or boil the crabs for 15 minutes. Pick the meat from the crabs, saving the shells to make the broth. Set aside.

2 Roll out the pastry dough and fit it into a 9-inch pie pan or 9-inch tart pan. Dock the dough with the tines of a fork. Wrap the pan in plastic wrap and refrigerate until ready to use.

3 Melt the butter in a large skillet over medium heat. Add the shallots and sauté until translucent, about 3 minutes. Stir in the reserved crabmeat, basil, parsley, and tarragon, and cook for 3 minutes. Remove the skillet from the heat and set aside.

4 Beat the eggs, cream, salt, and pepper together with a wire whisk.

5 Transfer the crab mixture to the pastry shell and pour the egg mixture over the crab. Bake for 40 to 45 minutes, until the filling is set and the pastry is golden brown.

6 **MAKE THE REDUCTION:** Warm the olive oil in a large stockpot over medium heat. Add the onions, carrots, and celery, and sauté, stirring occasionally, until the vegetables are cooked through, about 6 minutes. Add the tomato paste and cook for 5 minutes longer. Add the crab shells, bay leaf, thyme, and enough water to cover the shells. Simmer, uncovered, for 45 minutes to thicken the reduction.

7 Strain the broth and return it to the stockpot to reduce by half, about 15 minutes. Add the cream and reduce to a saucelike consistency. Season with salt to taste and add the lemon juice.

8 Slice the tart into six pieces and serve warm over a shallow pool of the crab reduction. Top with a dollop of crème fraîche and tobiko roe, if desired.

Makes 6 servings

There are many reasons to visit the *Pelican Pub & Brewery*. There is the beer, of course. And the food, which inspires and delights. And then there is the view — there is nothing between the Pacific Ocean and the brewery except a windswept beach. A table on the outdoor deck yields inspiring views and imparts a deep calm. Combined with the contents on your plate and in your glass, it might be one of the best brewery dining experiences in the country. Looking to top even that? Three times a year the brewery hosts a brewers dinner, a five-course meal that is a culinary journey of beer and food.

Hearth-Baked Salmon with Brewschetta

This is a dish with a lot of great flavors going on! The succulent salmon gets a fresh pop from the herbs and citrus zest, and it is all brought together with Fegley's Brew Works house version of bruschetta. Eat the salmon with fresh vegetables and rice, and drink a Belgian wit, such as Fegley's Brew Work's Steelgaardenwit, that lifts the oiliness of the salmon and enhances and complements the simple and natural flavors.

BREWSCHETTA

- 5½ pounds tomatoes, diced
- 1 cup diced red bell pepper
- ⅓ cup diced red onion
- 2 garlic cloves, minced
- 3 tablespoons chopped fresh basil
- 1 cup balsamic vinegar
- 1 cup Flemish red ale, or similar ale
- ½ cup pomace oil
  Salt and freshly ground black pepper
  Cajun seasoning

CRUSTED SALMON

- Zest of 1 lemon, minced
- Zest of 1 lime, minced
- Zest of 1 orange, minced
- 1 teaspoon minced fresh oregano
- 1 teaspoon minced fresh dillweed
- 1 teaspoon minced fresh basil
- 1 teaspoon granulated garlic
- 1 teaspoon onion powder
- 1 teaspoon minced fresh thyme
- 6 ounces fresh, sustainable North Atlantic salmon
- 1 tablespoon extra-virgin olive oil

1 **MAKE THE BREWSCHETTA:** Combine the tomatoes, bell pepper, onion, garlic, basil, vinegar, ale, oil, and salt, pepper, and Cajun seasoning to taste in a mixing bowl and toss until ingredients are incorporated. Cover and refrigerate for at least 4 hours or overnight.

2 **MAKE THE SALMON:** Toss the lemon zest, lime zest, orange zest, oregano, dill, basil, garlic, onion powder, and thyme together. Spread the blend on a baking sheet for at least 1 hour to allow the mixture to dry out. When the herb mix is nice and dry, you can store it in an airtight container or a ziplock bag for up to 3 days.

3 Preheat the oven to 450°F. Coat the salmon in the olive oil and cover with the herb crust. Bake for 7 to 9 minutes for medium. Remove the salmon from the oven and serve on top of the tomato mixture.

Makes 2 servings

PROFILE ★ **Allentown was the second location** the Fegley family opened in their growing eastern Pennsylvania brewpub chain, and like its sister location in Bethlehem, this one is equipped with expert brewers and accomplished chefs. It is a comfortable, multilevel space in an old furniture store; it now has a lounge in the basement, a great bar and restaurant on the main floor, and a fun party space (and additional restaurant space) above. Add the outdoor patio area, and this Fegley's Brew Works offers a setting for every occasion and mood.

Cumin-Dijon Smothered Baked Halibut

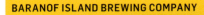
This recipe embodies the spirit of carefree summer days. Due to the simplicity of the preparation, it is as easy to make in your home kitchen as it is to grill it outdoors with friends around a campfire. Serve this flaky and flavorful fish with brown rice, a green salad, and tall glasses of hefeweizen (Baranof makes a good one!) garnished with a sliver of lemon.

1 tablespoon minced onion
¼ teaspoon ground cumin
¼ cup mayonnaise
1½ tablespoons Dijon mustard
   Salt and freshly ground
      black pepper
1 pound fresh halibut steaks
   Cayenne pepper

1 Preheat the oven to 450°F. (If you wish to cook this recipe over a campfire, simply wrap the fish well in foil and place on a rack over some very hot coals.)

2 Whisk the onion, cumin, mayonnaise, and mustard together in a medium bowl until well blended. Season with salt and pepper to taste.

3 Put the halibut in a baking dish and cover the fish all over with the mayonnaise mixture and a pinch of cayenne. Cover with aluminum foil and bake for 20 minutes, or until the halibut is white all the way through and flakes easily with a fork. Serve immediately.

Makes 3–4 servings

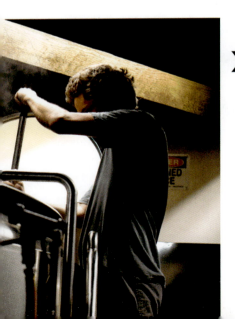

PROFILE ★ **Need directions?** *Baranof Island Brewing Company* is a 1½-mile walk from the roundabout in the middle of Sitka. Find Sawmill Creek Road, keep the ocean at your right, turn left at Smith Street, and keep walking. You'll find it at number 215. The commonsense directions are emblematic of the approach that the brewery takes with its beers. It has become known for no-nonsense, true-to-style brews that use Alaskan glacier water for an authentic local drinking experience. The brewery is so popular that it has expanded quickly and now has an attached tasting room and kitchen where locals and visitors alike can come together and bend elbows over the careful work of a dedicated few.

**Fried Brussels
Sprouts, see page 268**

Side Dishes

Complement Your Main Meal

2 cups heavy cream

3 pounds Yukon Gold
potatoes, peeled and cut
into ¼-inch slices

2 tablespoons unsalted
butter, at room
temperature

¼ pound Pecorino cheese

2 garlic cloves, chopped

16 ounces truffle cheese,
grated

Salt and freshly ground
black pepper

White truffle oil

Truffled Potatoes

Allowing this dish to sit overnight results in a richly flavored *tortino* (a savory pie). Weighting the potatoes is important to help the layers set. The truffle cheese is pricey, but it adds a smooth earthiness that's enhanced by the final drizzle of truffle oil.

1 Pour the cream into a mixing bowl and add the potato slices. Soak for at least 20 minutes, or up to overnight.

2 Preheat the oven to 375°F. Line a 9- by 13-inch baking dish with foil and coat with the butter to create a nonstick surface.

3 Layer half of the potato slices into the prepared pan and sprinkle with the Pecorino and garlic, and then add the truffle cheese in one thick layer and season with salt and pepper to taste. Layer the remaining potatoes over the top and pour any cream left in the bowl over everything. The resulting tortino should be about 1 inch thick. Cover the pan with foil and use another tight-fitting pan or heavy object to weigh down the layers. Bake for 2½ hours.

4 Remove the tortino from the oven, keeping the weight in place, and allow to cool overnight in the refrigerator.

5 When ready to serve, preheat the oven to 350°F. Cut the tortino into 9 or 12 squares, re-cover the baking dish with foil, and reheat for 30 minutes. Serve with a drizzle of white truffle oil.

Makes 8 servings

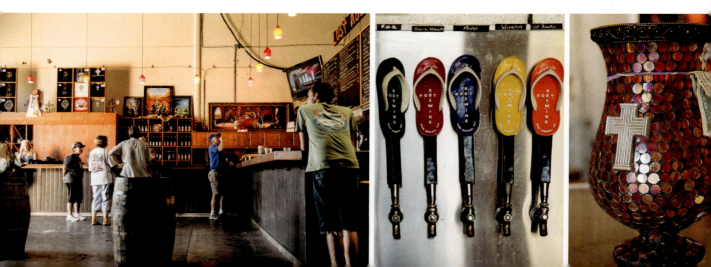

Sometimes a hobby can become an empire. Take, for example, *Port Brewing*, where the brother-and-sister team of Vince and Gina Marsaglia took to making their own brews after they were having trouble finding local, flavorful options. They soon opened a brewery inside their Pizza Port restaurant and were an instant hit. Business was so good that they expanded a few times and eventually took over a location once owned by Stone Brewing Co. That became home to Port Brewing and its sister brewery, the Lost Abbey, which focuses on Belgian styles. With growing distribution, many industry awards, and an impressed customer base, Port Brewing continually produces offerings worth stocking.

BARLEY CREEK BREWING COMPANY

TANNERSVILLE, PENNSYLVANIA

Asparagus Risotto

3½ cups chicken or vegetable broth
4 cups water
1 pound asparagus, trimmed and cut into 1- to 1½-inch pieces
2 tablespoons plus 1 teaspoon unsalted butter
½ cup diced red onion
1 cup Arborio rice
½ cup dry white wine
½ cup grated Parmesan cheese
Salt and freshly ground black pepper

Risotto can be overlooked because people think it is difficult to prepare. It is true that a good risotto requires patience and continuous stirring, but the method is not difficult and the result is a great addition to any meal. Here the asparagus adds a fresh flavor and a bit of crunch to the creamy rice. At the Barley Creek Brewing Company, they serve salmon with the risotto, but it is a nice complement to many meats and fishes, and it is also quite nice on its own as a vegetarian entrée.

1 Bring the broth to a simmer in a small saucepan. Bring the water to a boil in a separate saucepan.

2 Add the asparagus to the boiling water and blanch for 2 minutes. While the asparagus cooks, fill a large bowl with ice water. Drain the asparagus and then plunge into the ice water to stop the cooking. Drain the ice water bath and set the asparagus aside.

3 Melt the 2 tablespoons butter in a wide soup pot over medium heat. Add the onion and sauté until translucent, about 4 minutes. Add the rice; cook and stir until all the rice is coated with butter, about 3 minutes. Add the wine to the rice and continue to cook, stirring frequently, until all the wine is absorbed, about 4 minutes.

4 Reduce the heat to medium-low and ladle ½ cup of the simmering broth over the rice; stir until the liquid is absorbed. Continue adding the broth, ½ cup at a time, and stirring, until all the broth is incorporated into the rice and the rice is tender. The total cooking time will be 15 to 25 minutes.

5 Stir in the reserved asparagus, the 1 teaspoon butter, the Parmesan, and salt and pepper to taste. Serve immediately.

Makes 2 main-course servings or 4 appetizer servings

At the base of Camelback, a ski area in the Poconos, *Barley Creek* has been serving quality beers and food since 1995. Owner Trip Ruvane has created the perfect après-ski bar for the area — comfortable and fun, satisfying yet relaxing. On any given day the parking lot is packed and the bar is humming, even during warmer weather. The bar's Pint-Sized Park has a whiffleball field, horseshoe pits, and its own bar. Perfect for large parties or gatherings, it's another standout feature of Barley Creek.

But it's not just skiers or outdoor types who have made the brewery a success. Its proximity to a large outlet mall means plenty of shopping warriors are resting their weary feet and baggage-heavy arms while sipping a pint of IPA or a black lager. Daily brewery tours help spread the word about craft beer and how it's made, giving customers some happy knowledge before heading on their way, and ensuring they'll come back for more.

Patatas Bravas

This is a vegetarian dish whose name literally means "brave potatoes." With a plethora of spices, this flavorful side dish livens many meals. No courage required. The brewery uses its hop-forward amber ale in this recipe, and it's suggested you pour some into a glass for yourself as well.

1½ pounds small Red Bliss potatoes
1 teaspoon red pepper flakes
1 teaspoon smoked Spanish paprika
½ teaspoon ground cumin
2 tablespoons extra-virgin olive oil
1 medium red bell pepper, cored, seeded, and thinly sliced
2 garlic cloves, chopped
½ cup Crazy Mountain Amber Ale, or similar amber ale
2 teaspoons red wine vinegar
Salt

A Few Beers to Try with This Recipe

- *Bear Republic Red Rocket Ale*
- *Crazy Mountain Amber Ale*
- *Duck-Rabbit Amber Ale*
- *Flying Fish ESB Ale*
- *Fort Collins 1900 Amber*
- *Gritty's Red Claw Ale*
- *Odell Red*
- *Rogue American Amber Ale*
- *Widmer Brothers Drop Top Amber Ale*

1 Bring a large pot of salted water to a boil. Add the whole potatoes and boil until tender, about 10 minutes. Drain the potatoes, then quarter them and transfer to a large bowl.

2 Mix the pepper flakes, paprika, and cumin together in a small bowl and sprinkle the spice mixture over the warm potatoes.

3 Heat the olive oil in a skillet over medium-high heat. Add the potatoes and bell pepper and cook until the potatoes are browned and the bell pepper is soft, about 5 minutes. Stir occasionally to brown the potatoes on all sides. Add the garlic and cook for 1 minute longer. Add the beer and stir until it has almost completely evaporated, about 2 minutes. Stir in the vinegar, taking care to coat all the potatoes. Season with salt to taste and serve immediately.

Makes 4 servings

PROFILE ★ **In a state that's as crowded** with breweries as Colorado, you would think that there wouldn't be much ground left to pioneer. But it wasn't until January 2010 that the Vail Valley welcomed its first production brewery. *Crazy Mountain* is the realized dream of Kevin Selvy and Marisa Aguilar. Their brewery produces a line of solid canned offerings with brightly colored labels and has an attached tasting room that, in addition to serving up pints, also features three friendly employee-owned dogs who are happy to mingle with guests.

Grilled Texas Creamed Corn

SWEETWATER BREWING COMPANY

ATLANTA, GEORGIA

Thick and satisfying, this creamy dish receives a jolt of flavor from the char on the grilled corn. A tasty accompaniment for all kinds of barbecue, this side dish is easy to whip up at the last minute. This recipe, developed by Atlanta's D.B.A. Barbecue for the SweetWater Brewing Company, pairs very well with a porter.

6 ears yellow corn, husked
2 cups heavy cream
1 cup grated Parmigiano-Reggiano
1 cup mayonnaise
2 teaspoons cayenne pepper
Juice of 1 lime

1 Prepare a medium-high fire in a gas or charcoal grill. Grill the corn until lightly charred, about 5 minutes, turning to evenly grill the entire ear.

2 Combine the cream and ½ cup of the Parmigiano-Reggiano in a large saucepan over medium-high heat and reduce until it coats the back of a spoon, about 7 minutes.

3 Cut the corn off the cob and add it to the cream mixture. Stir over medium heat until the corn is warmed through, about 5 minutes. Remove the corn from the heat and let rest for 1 minute.

4 Combine the mayonnaise, the remaining ½ cup Parmigiano-Reggiano, the cayenne, and the lime juice in a serving bowl. Stir the corn into the mayonnaise mixture and serve immediately.

Makes 6–8 servings

PROFILE ★ **Freddy Bensch and Kevin McNerney** were roommates at the University of Colorado at Boulder when they discovered good beer and the possibility of making it a career. After they decided to open their own place, a trip to Atlanta confirmed that the great Southern city was in need of a beer education. So they opened *SweetWater*, bringing the hoppy, aggressive ales they had been homebrewing for years to Georgia. Since their opening in 1997, the partners' hard work has paid off with quality ales and a brewery that continues to grow at an impressive clip. Their annual Brew Your Cask Off event has become one of the more celebrated in the beer community and draws thirsty folks and aspiring brewers from around the country.

Sautéed Spinach

This lively spinach side dish has a lot of personality, thanks to an inspired combination of supporting ingredients. Particularly great with summer fare, this dish cooks up quickly and elevates the otherwise humble leafy green.

2 tablespoons extra-virgin olive oil
3 garlic cloves, chopped
1 large shallot, finely diced
¼ cup Belgian white beer
¼ cup chicken stock
2 tablespoons unsalted butter
10 ounces fresh spinach, washed and stemmed
Kosher salt and freshly ground black pepper

1 Heat the olive oil in a large skillet over medium heat until hot but not smoking. Add the garlic and shallots and sauté for 1 minute. Add the beer and chicken stock and cook until the liquid is reduced by half.

2 Add the butter, spinach, and salt and pepper to taste. Cook, stirring frequently, until the spinach is just barely wilted, about 3 minutes. Transfer to a serving dish and toss well. Serve hot.

Makes 2–4 servings

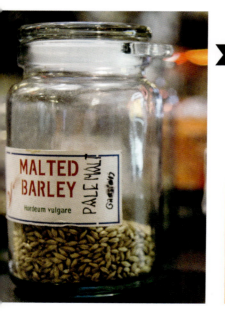

PROFILE ★ **If it isn't fresh,** the brewery doesn't want it. Every day, produce, meat, and other ingredients stream in from local, small organic farms near *5 Seasons*. The supplies are used in the 20 to 30 special dishes that are conceived by the remarkable team of chefs. It's not just the veggies that come in fresh. Just about everything made in the 5 Seasons kitchens (there are two in the local chain) is from scratch. Seafood and meats are also delivered from local sources and farms and butchered on site. Even salad dressings are whipped up on the premises. The South has been a notoriously difficult region for craft beer to gain a foothold in, but by serving up fresh and inspired food 5 Seasons has developed an enthusiastic following. The brewery also keeps things interesting by creating upwards of 100 beers each year — no small feat for a brewery its size. A fun place to spend an evening, the restaurant is modern and inviting, with an expansive outdoor space and large garage door–style windows that offer a distant view of the Atlanta skyline. A brewpub like this is great no matter what the season.

Szechuan Green Beans

Have fun with your vegetables! The spicy/sweet/zesty Szechuan sauce livens up almost any vegetable but works particularly well as a quick (and easy) way to dress up the humble green bean. This dish can be prepared in a flash and also makes a great appetizer. Pair with an amber ale that can stand up to the flavors of the sauce without being muted.

1 Heat the 1 tablespoon canola oil in a large skillet over medium heat. Add the ginger and sauté until fragrant and soft, 2 to 3 minutes. Add the garlic and sauté until it turns light brown, about 1 minute longer.

2 Quickly stir in the brown sugar, pepper flakes, fermented black beans, vinegar, soy sauce, plum sauce, sambal oelek, water, white wine, sesame oil, and Kitchen Bouquet sauce. Bring the mixture to a boil, and then stir in the cornstarch and remove from the heat.

3 Heat the 2 cups canola oil in a deep skillet to 350°F. Add the green beans and flash-fry for 40 seconds. Quickly remove the beans from the oil and toss with the sauce in the skillet. Transfer to a serving plate and garnish with the carrots before serving.

Makes 4 servings

- 2 cups plus 1 tablespoon canola oil
- 1 teaspoon minced fresh ginger
- 1 teaspoon minced garlic
- 1 tablespoon firmly packed light brown sugar
- ½ teaspoon red pepper flakes
- ¼ teaspoon fermented black beans
- ¼ cup rice wine vinegar
- ¼ cup soy sauce
- 2 tablespoons plum sauce
- 1 tablespoon sambal oelek
- 1 tablespoon water
- 1 tablespoon white wine
- ½ teaspoon dark sesame oil
- ½ teaspoon Kitchen Bouquet sauce
- ½ teaspoon cornstarch
- 1 pound green beans, trimmed
- ½ carrot, shredded

PROFILE ★ **The philosophy at Squatters is People, Planet, Profit.**
These three focal areas guide the growing brew chain as its team seeks to bring quality beer and sustainable food to the people in the central Utah area. They are community minded and support a few dozen charities that seek to do good work in the area, from health clinics to community gardens to youth sports. They are just as committed to the planet. Their trucks run on biodiesel made from their kitchen oil, and they are heavily involved in recycling, reducing waste, and using water wisely. And because they are a business they are focused on the bottom line. Their thought is that the more customers they bring in, the more good they can do. They are walking that walk and talking that talk, so if you're in Salt Lake (or its airport) or in Park City, visit one of their locations. See the brewery in action while enjoying quaffable pints and helping its people continue the good work.

Fried Brussels Sprouts with Fish Sauce Vinaigrette

While the potent small sprout can sometimes get a bad rap, this simple recipe uses the strength of several assertive ingredients to create a great end result that's a welcome departure from recipes that rely on bacon and butter for flavor. A note of caution: Brussels sprouts contain a lot of water that makes them pop and explode when they hit oil, so either stand back or use a splatter screen.

VINAIGRETTE

- ½ cup sugar
- 2 garlic cloves, minced
- 1 (1-inch) piece fresh ginger, minced
- ½ cup rice wine vinegar
- ¼ cup fish sauce
- ¼ cup honey
- 2 tablespoons canola oil
  Juice of 3 limes
  Salt

BRUSSELS SPROUTS

- 2 quarts peanut or vegetable oil, for frying
- 2 pounds Brussels sprouts, trimmed and halved lengthwise
- 1 tablespoon *kochukaru* (Korean chile flakes), or red pepper flakes
  Kosher salt

1 **MAKE THE VINAIGRETTE:** Whisk the sugar, garlic, ginger, vinegar, fish sauce, honey, canola oil, and lime juice together in a small mixing bowl. Season with salt to taste and set aside.

2 **MAKE THE SPROUTS:** Heat the oil to 375°F in a cast-iron Dutch oven or a deep fryer. Fry the Brussels sprouts, working in batches, until they are deep brown, about 1 minute. Transfer the sprouts to a large mixing bowl and toss with the chile flakes and a few pinches of salt.

3 Pour the vinaigrette over the sprouts, using just enough to coat them but not drown them. Toss and adjust the salt and chile to taste. Serve hot. If you have leftover vinaigrette, it will keep in an airtight container in the refrigerator for up to 1 week.

Makes 4–6 servings

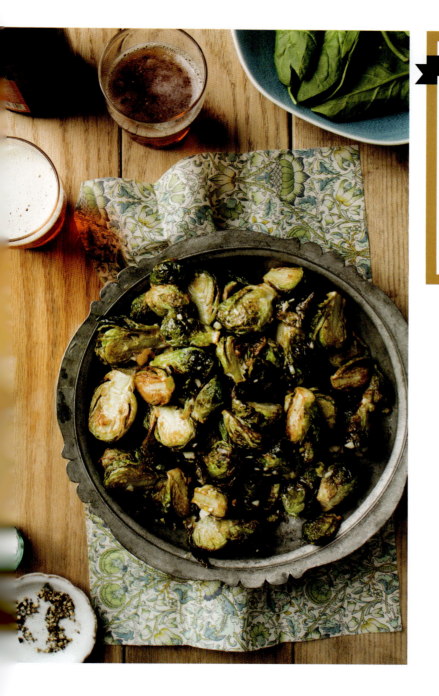

TRIUMPH BREWING COMPANY
PRINCETON, NEW JERSEY

Vidalia Onions Stuffed with Spring Foraged Vegetables

Roasty, rich, herbal, and earthy, this recipe celebrates the very best of spring. The vibrant bite of ramp comes through in a hearty way and mingles with the sweetness of the onion and the spring freshness of the foraged vegetables. This recipe serves two but can easily be scaled up for a crowd.

STUFFED ONIONS

- 2 medium Vidalia onions
- 1 tablespoon plus ½ teaspoon extra-virgin olive oil
- ½ cup nettles
- 2 tablespoons minced fresh ramps
- 1 cup fiddlehead ferns
- ½ cup minced hedgehog mushrooms
- 2 tablespoons dried breadcrumbs

BÉCHAMEL

- ¼ cup extra-virgin olive oil
- ½ cup chopped onions
- ¼ cup white wine
- ¼ cup all-purpose flour
- 2 cups milk
- ¼ cup roasted ramps (see box)
- ¼ teaspoon grated lemon zest
  Salt and freshly ground black pepper

Roasted Ramps

Preheat the oven to 425°F. Wash and trim the root ends from one bunch of ramps and spread them out on a baking sheet. Drizzle ¼ cup of olive oil over the ramps and sprinkle with salt and pepper. Toss to coat the ramps. Roast for 10 to 15 minutes, until the roots are soft and the leaves are beginning to crisp.

1 **PREPARE THE ONIONS:** Preheat the oven to 400°F. Coat the onions with the ½ teaspoon olive oil. Fill a small roasting pan or baking dish with about 1 inch of water, place the onions in the water, and bake for 20 minutes, or until tender. Remove the onions from the oven. When the onions are cool enough to handle, cut off the top of each onion and scoop out most of the inside, leaving an onion bowl ¼ inch thick. Set aside.

2 Bring a saucepan of water to a boil, add the nettles, and cook for 1 minute. Drain and roughly chop.

3 Heat the 1 tablespoon olive oil in a medium skillet over medium heat. Add the ramps and sauté until golden brown, about 1 minute. Add the fiddleheads, mushrooms, and nettles, and cook, stirring occasionally, for about 5 minutes. Cover the skillet and set aside.

4 **MAKE THE BÉCHAMEL SAUCE:** Heat the olive oil in a saucepan over medium heat. Add the chopped onions and cook, stirring occasionally, until golden brown, about 4 minutes. Add the white wine and cook until the liquid is reduced by half, 1 to 2 minutes. Add the flour and cook for 30 seconds, stirring constantly, then whisk in the milk and cook, stirring frequently, until the sauce thickens and the flour is cooked out, about 20 minutes longer.

5 Remove the sauce from the heat and let cool to room temperature. Combine the roasted ramps and sauce in a blender and purée until smooth. Add the lemon zest and season with salt and pepper to taste.

6 **STUFF THE ONIONS:** Preheat the oven to 350°F. Return the béchamel sauce to the saucepan, add the fiddlehead mixture, and bring to a boil to warm everything through. Remove the filling from the heat and stuff each onion with half the filling. Place the onions on a baking sheet and bake for 15 minutes, and then top with the breadcrumbs and bake for 2 to 3 minutes longer, until golden. Remove the onions from the oven and serve.

Makes 2 servings

The now-regional Triumph chain had its start in a cavernous space just across the road from Princeton University. At that spot, scores of undergrads, professors, and guests were introduced to craft beer and the concept of pairing it with fine food. The initial success led to the opening of a second location across the Delaware River in New Hope, Pennsylvania.

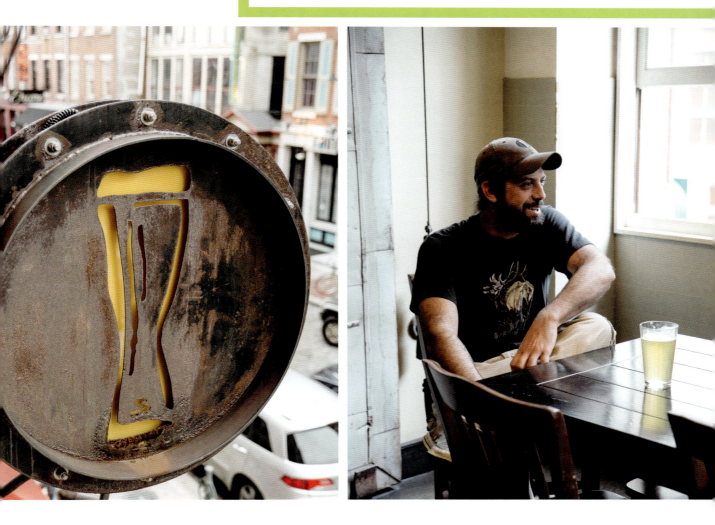

Duck Fat Home Fries

3 large Idaho baking potatoes,
  peeled
2 tablespoons duck fat
  Sea salt
  Freshly ground black
  pepper

This is the ultimate easy and satisfying side dish from Brooklyn's brewmaster Garrett Oliver, and the fries are so versatile that you'll likely end up making them many times a year. Duck fat, once a rare specialty item, is now easily found at any good butcher or at more upscale retailers, such as Whole Foods. You can make this dish in about 20 minutes, and it goes with virtually any meat or fish entrée. The fries are also great with eggs at brunch, especially if you add some chiles. If you can't find duck fat, or it doesn't appeal, you can substitute olive oil for most or all of the fat. These fries are crunchy on the outside and pillowy on the inside, and they're almost foolproof.

1 Bring a large pot of salted water to a boil over high heat. Cut the potatoes cross-wise into 1/2-inch slabs, and then cut the slabs into 1/2-inch cubes. Add the potatoes to the boiling water and return the water to a boil. Adjust the heat to keep the water at a simmer and cook the potatoes until tender, about 4 minutes. Drain well and let the potatoes sit in the strainer for a few minutes.

2 Heat the duck fat in a deep skillet or wok over high heat. Add the potatoes, which should no longer be wet. Be careful to avoid splattering.

Toss the potatoes in the duck fat over high heat, turning constantly, until the potatoes start to turn golden. Reduce the heat to medium and continue cooking, turning constantly, until the potatoes are a deep golden brown, about 10 minutes.

3 Sprinkle the potatoes with sea salt and freshly ground black pepper to taste. Drain on a paper towel–lined plate, and then transfer to a serving dish and serve immediately.

Makes 4 servings

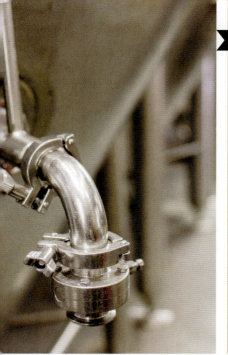

Since opening in 1988, Brooklyn Brewery has fostered the New York City area's brewing renaissance and done quite a bit of good work for the world of craft as well. Cofounders Steve Hindy and Tom Potter saw a need to bring brewing back to New York City and burst onto the scene with a lineup of impressive beers. They have been wildly successful and prompted scores of others to follow in their footsteps. Under the direction of brewmaster Garrett Oliver (one of the most respected, sought-after, and prolific writers in the business), the brewery staff has continually released innovative beers that break boundaries and start trends.

In the earlier years, much of its brewing was done in upstate New York, but in 2011 the brewery in Williamsburg, Brooklyn, underwent an expansion that quintupled capacity. In addition to serving nearly half the country with beer, Brooklyn Brewery probably exports more beer than any other American craft brewery. Brewery employees know what it means to be a good neighbor, so many employees serve on not-for-profit boards, and each year the company supports many charitable and arts organizations and partners with food purveyors across the country to produce beer dinners and tasting events.

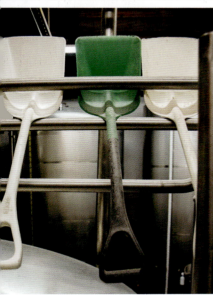

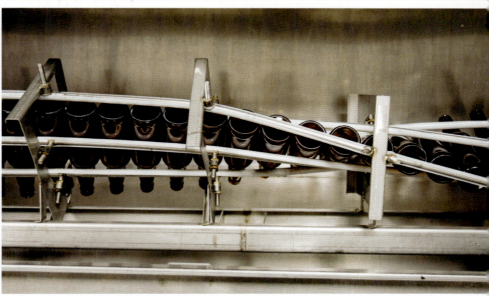

Pale Ale Pineapple Brown
Sugar Cupcakes, see page 292

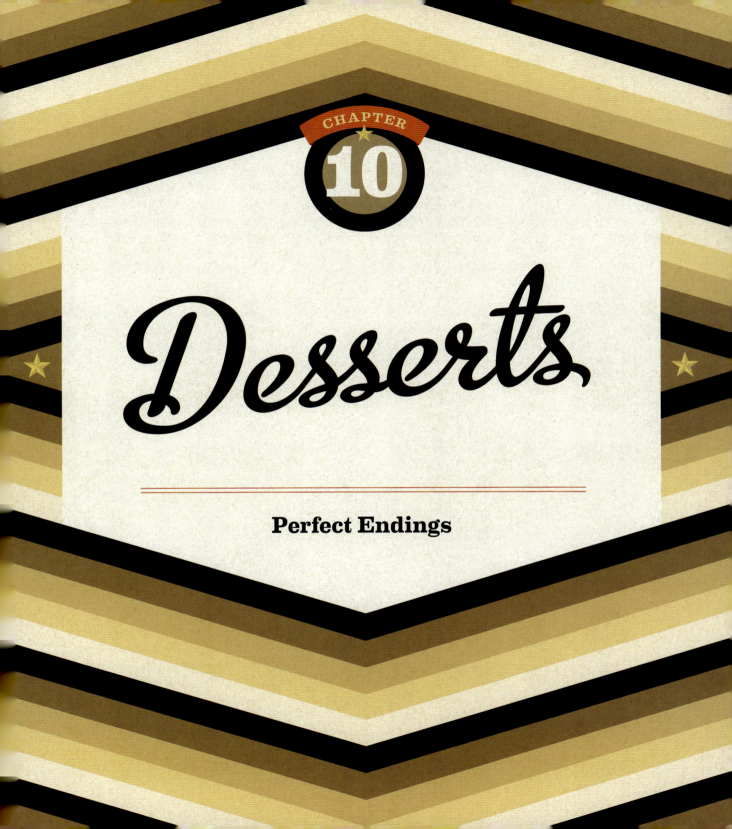

Desserts

Perfect Endings

CRUST

- ½ cup (1 stick) unsalted butter, softened
- ¼ cup sugar
- ½ cup all-purpose flour
- ½ cup finely ground shortbread cookies

FILLING

- 4 (8-ounce) packages cream cheese, softened
- 1½ cups sugar
- ¼ cup all-purpose flour
- 3 eggs
- 1 tablespoon plus 1 teaspoon vanilla extract
- 2 pomegranates
- 1 (16-ounce) container sour cream
- Zest of 1 lemon
- ½ cup Shmaltz He'Brew Origin Pomegranate Ale, or similar beer

TOPPING

- ½ cup pure pomegranate juice
- 1½ cups Shmaltz He'Brew Origin Pomegranate Ale, or similar beer
- ¼ cup firmly packed light brown sugar
- 1 tablespoon cornstarch, flour, or arrowroot

He'Brew Origin Pomegranate Cheesecake

Recent studies have shown that pomegranates have many health benefits. They contain antioxidants and other healthful nutrients. Adding them to a cheesecake won't save you any trips to the gym, but you're sure to enjoy every bite. Some brewers have even joined the pomegranate bandwagon and are experimenting with putting the juicy fruit into beer. This recipe, from the fun folks at Shmaltz, blends fruity goodness with the smooth density of cheesecake. Pair with a pomegranate beer for an extra kick of fruit.

1 MAKE THE CRUST: Preheat the oven to 350°F. Mix the butter and sugar together in a large bowl with an electric mixer on medium-high speed until fluffy, 3 to 4 minutes. Add the flour and ground shortbread cookies to the mixture and blend until fully incorporated, 3 to 4 seconds.

2 Press the mixture evenly into the bottom of a 9-inch springform pan. Bake for 20 to 25 minutes, or until golden brown. Remove the crust from the oven and place on a cooling rack to cool completely.

3 MAKE THE FILLING: Reduce the oven temperature to 325°F. Combine the cream cheese and 1¼ cups of the sugar in an extra-large mixing bowl using an electric mixer until fluffy, 3 to 5 minutes. Beat in the flour on low speed until smooth, about 3 minutes. Mix in the eggs and the 1 tablespoon

vanilla on low speed until just combined, about 3 minutes.

4 Cut off the pointy end and score the flesh of the pomegranates, all the way around the fruit. In a bowl of cool water, separate the fruit into pieces and separate the seeds from the membrane. The seeds will sink and the membrane will float. Fish out the membrane pieces and strain the water to retain the seeds. Don't get too picky about making sure every bit of membrane is removed — it's tasteless and small amounts will not affect the overall recipe.

5 Stir into the batter ½ cup of the sour cream, half the pomegranate seeds, the lemon zest, and ¼ cup of the ale. Pour the filling into the prebaked crust. Place the cheesecake on a baking sheet and bake for 65 minutes, or until the edges are puffed and the center jiggles slightly when gently shaken. Remove from the oven.

6 Mix the remaining 1/4 cup sugar, 1 1/2 cups sour cream, 1/4 cup ale, and the 1 teaspoon vanilla together in a medium bowl until evenly blended. Spread the sour cream mixture over the surface of the baked cheesecake. Return to the oven and bake for 10 minutes longer.

7 Cool the cheesecake on a wire rack for 15 minutes. Loosen the crust from the sides of the pan and cool for 30 minutes longer. Remove the sides of the pan, and cool completely. Cover the cheesecake with plastic wrap and chill for at least 4 hours or overnight before serving.

8 **MAKE THE TOPPING:** Bring the pomegranate juice and ale to a boil in a medium saucepan. Reduce the heat and boil gently, uncovered, until reduced to 1 cup, 10 to 12 minutes.

9 Stir the brown sugar and cornstarch together in a small bowl and add it to the reduced liquid. Continue cooking over medium-low heat until the sauce thickens and becomes bubbly, about 4 minutes.

10 Transfer the sauce to a medium bowl and cover the surface with plastic wrap. Cool to room temperature. Store, covered, in the refrigerator until ready to serve.

11 Remove the cheesecake and pomegranate sauce from the refrigerator 15 minutes before serving. Spoon some sauce over the top of cheesecake and pile the remaining pomegranate seeds in the center. Slice the cheesecake and serve with the remaining sauce.

Makes 1 (9-inch) cheesecake, or about 16 servings

A Few Beers to Try with This Recipe

- *Peak Organic Pomegranate Wheat Ale*
- *Saranac Pomegranate Wheat*
- *Shmalz He'Brew Origin Pomegranate Ale*

PROFILE ★ **Back in 1996,** Jeremy Cowan launched *Shmaltz Brewing Co.* — makers of He'Brew — in San Francisco and bottled, labeled, and delivered the first cases himself. It would have been easy to mistake the brewery as just another gimmick, a way to make a quick buck before becoming nothing more than another piece of craft beer history. In fact, Cowan admits that the whole thing started as a joke with friends. Soon, however, he realized that he could run a legitimate business and was not content to be just another fad or a joke label (although the bottle artwork and tongue-in-cheek phrasing helped propel that mantle), and he backed up the marketing with quality-made lagers and ales. In recent years, the brewery has added Coney Island Craft Lagers as a sister brand. It even opened a carnival attraction in the form of an eighth-barrel brewhouse, designed to be a side show, much like its neighbors, the Bearded Lady and the Human Blockhead, on New York's Coney Island. There the brewery invites contest winners and others to come and brew for a day. Given the small amount of beer produced, it goes quickly. Good thing Shmaltz's other brewery in upstate New York keeps the rest of the country stocked.

Wake 'n' Bake Chocolate-Coconut Dessert Bars

This tiered dessert brings together many sweet flavors that are guaranteed to please. Perfect for parties, these bars will impress your guests with your seemingly professional baking skills. Don't let the name fool you; there is no actual baking involved in this recipe. Serve with oatmeal stout to bring out additional flavors of chocolate and graham cracker.

BOTTOM LAYER

- 1 cup unsweetened coconut flakes
- ⅓ cup plus 2 tablespoons Terrapin Wake 'n' Bake Coffee Oatmeal Imperial Stout, or similar oatmeal stout
- ½ cup (1 stick) unsalted butter, cut into small cubes
- ¼ cup plus 1 tablespoon unsweetened cocoa powder
- ¼ cup sugar
- 1 egg, well beaten
- 2 cups graham cracker crumbs (from about 10 crushed crackers), plus more as needed
- ½ cup walnuts, finely chopped

SECOND LAYER

- 2 cups confectioners' sugar
- ½ cup (1 stick) unsalted butter
- 2 tablespoons custard powder
- 2 tablespoons Terrapin Wake 'n' Bake Coffee Oatmeal Imperial Stout, or similar oatmeal stout

TOPPING

- ½ cup dark chocolate morsels
- 2 tablespoons unsalted butter
- 2 tablespoons Terrapin Wake 'n' Bake Coffee Oatmeal Imperial Stout, or similar oatmeal stout

Note: Place parchment or waxed paper in the pan with its edges draping over the sides prior to building the layers. Simply lift the entire dessert out for cutting.

1 **MAKE THE BOTTOM LAYER:** Mix the coconut and 2 tablespoons of the beer in a small bowl.

2 Stir the butter, cocoa powder, sugar, and the remaining ⅓ cup beer together in a bowl set over hot water until the butter melts. Remove the butter mixture from the bowl of hot water, cool slightly, and stir in the egg until well combined. Add the graham cracker crumbs, the coconut mixture, and the walnuts, and stir thoroughly. (If the mixture is too wet, add additional graham cracker crumbs by the tablespoonful until the mixture holds together in a clump.)

3 Press the mixture into the bottom of an 8-inch square pan. Cover and refrigerate while mixing the next layer.

4 **MAKE THE SECOND LAYER:** Combine the confectioners' sugar, butter, custard powder, and beer in a mixing bowl. Using an electric mixer, beat until light and creamy, 3 to 4 minutes.

5 Remove the baking pan from the refrigerator and evenly spread the second layer on top of the bottom layer. Return the pan to the refrigerator and allow the second layer to set, about 20 minutes.

6 **MAKE THE TOPPING:** Melt the chocolate in a bowl set over hot, not boiling, water. Add the butter and beer, and mix until the ingredients are well combined. Pour the topping over the second layer, spreading equally. Return the baking pan to the refrigerator and chill until the layers set, at least 1 hour and up to overnight.

7 Cut into squares for serving. Any reserved squares may be covered and stored in the refrigerator for up to 4 days.

Makes 16 small squares or 9 larger squares

While some breweries prefer to zig, the ***Terrapin Beer Company*** usually zags. Founded by John Cochran and Brian "Spike" Buckowski, the brewery was ahead of the curve in bringing flavorful beers to the Southeast and has not let up since the moment its first beers hit the shelves. With tongue-in-cheek names, or less than subtle nods to extracurricular activities, Terrapin has the goods to back up the fun it has with titles and labels. Located in Athens, a city as cool as the brewery itself, Terrapin is growing and becoming available in more and more markets. Pick some up, or go in person for the real experience.

Beer Float

2–3 scoops ice cream
1 (12-ounce) bottle beer
2–3 maraschino cherries
Whole mint leaves or finely grated Mexican chocolate, for garnish (optional)

The beauty of this recipe is its simplicity. After all, who doesn't like beer and ice cream? Together they create an adult treat that will please your inner child. This recipe cries out for your creativity. Try rocky road with a pecan nut brown ale. A stout with chocolate, vanilla, or mint chocolate chip ice cream. With an ice cream beer float, you're limited only by your imagination. One word of caution: Always place the ice cream in the glass first. If you attempt to add the ice cream after the beer is poured, you'll get a foamy mess.

When experimenting with beer float combinations, first stick with malt-forward beers before expanding into super hoppy or barrel-aged beers. There are so many beer styles and ice cream flavors, this recipe should keep you busy for a long time.

Place the ice cream in a pint glass. Slowly pour the beer over the ice cream. Add the cherries and the mint or grated chocolate, if using, and serve with a spoon and a straw.

Makes 1 serving

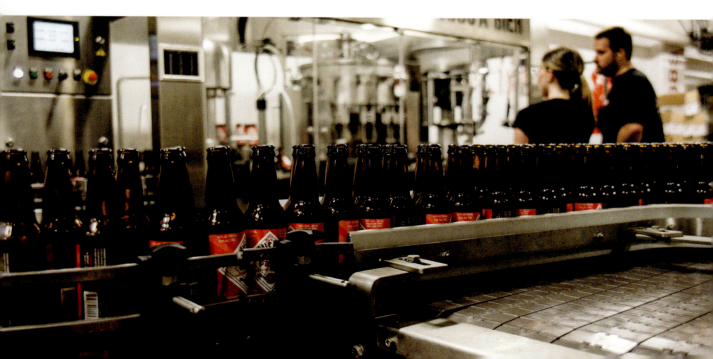

Chocolate-Covered Strawberries with Sprinkles

This is a simple recipe, but one that finishes with a professional look. It's sure to be a crowd pleaser. The sprinkles are optional, but they do give the dessert a nice splash of color.

CROW PEAK BREWING COMPANY

SPEARFISH, SOUTH DAKOTA

1½ cups rainbow sprinkles
1½ cups milk chocolate chips
1 tablespoon vegetable shortening
20 large strawberries (about a pound)

1 Line a large baking sheet with waxed paper and fill a shallow bowl with rainbow sprinkles. Set aside.

2 Stir the chocolate chips and vegetable shortening together in a heatproof bowl set over a pot of simmering water until the mixture is smooth, 3 to 5 minutes. Remove the bowl of chocolate from the pot of water.

3 Hold one strawberry by its top and dip it into the melted chocolate. Let excess chocolate drip off, and then dip into the rainbow sprinkles and place on the prepared baking sheet. Repeat the process with the remaining strawberries.

4 Refrigerate the strawberries until the chocolate coating is firm, about 45 minutes. Serve.

Makes 20 strawberries

Beer to Drink with Strawberries

- *Crow Peak Pile O' Dirt Porter*
- *Rogue Chocolate Stout*
- *Lancaster Strawberry Wheat*
- *Sam Adams Chocolate Bock*
- *Terrapin Moo Hoo*

PROFILE ★ **Crow Peak Brewing Company** is proof that if you build it, people will come. In the relatively dry state of South Dakota, the brewery opened its doors in 2007 with a five-barrel system and, just two years later, expanded to a 30-barrel brewhouse to meet demand. The beer-minded locals flock there and stock their refrigerators with fresh beer. Located just an hour's drive from Mount Rushmore and next door to a seasonal farmers' market that's stocked with cheeses and produce, Crow Peak is a South Dakota destination all by itself.

Chocolate Jefferson Stout Cupcakes

Stouts and chocolate were made for each other. Maybe it's because they share so many of the same flavors thanks to the chocolate malts used to make stouts. This recipe marries the two quite well and is sure to satisfy the chocoholic in your life. Plus it takes just under 30 minutes to bake, so you can quickly soothe chocolate cravings.

CUPCAKES

- 2 cups sugar
- 2 cups all-purpose flour
- ¾ cup unsweetened cocoa powder, plus more for dusting the cupcakes
- 1 teaspoon baking soda
  Fine salt
- 1 (12-ounce) bottle Lazy Magnolia Jefferson Stout, or similar stout
- ½ cup (1 stick) unsalted butter, melted
- 1 tablespoon vanilla extract
- 3 eggs
- ¾ cup sour cream

ICING

- 1 (8-ounce) package cream cheese, at room temperature
- ¾–1 cup heavy cream
- 1 (1-pound) package confectioners' sugar

1 MAKE THE CUPCAKES: Preheat the oven to 350°F. Lightly butter and flour 24 muffin cups.

2 Whisk the sugar, flour, cocoa powder, baking soda, and salt together in a large mixing bowl.

3 Combine the stout, melted butter, and vanilla in a large mixing bowl. Beat in the eggs, one at time. Mix in the sour cream until thoroughly combined and smooth. Gradually mix the dry ingredients into the wet mixture.

4 Divide the batter equally among the muffin cups, filling each three-quarters full. Bake for 12 minutes and then rotate the pans. Bake for 12 to 13 minutes longer, or until risen, nicely domed, and set in the middle, but still soft and tender. Cool the cupcakes for 10 minutes in the tins on a wire rack before turning out onto the rack to cool completely.

5 MAKE THE ICING: Beat the cream cheese with an electric mixer on medium speed until light and fluffy. Gradually beat in ¾ cup of the cream. Slowly mix in the confectioners' sugar on low speed until incorporated and smooth. If the icing is too thick to be spreadable, beat in more cream, 1 tablespoon at a time. Cover the bowl with plastic wrap and refrigerate until ready to use. (The icing can be made several hours ahead and kept covered and chilled.)

6 Top each cupcake with a generous layer of frosting and dust with cocoa powder.

Makes 24 cupcakes

As Mississippi's first craft brewery, Lazy Magnolia has helped turn a relatively dry state into a respected beer destination. Its use of native Southern ingredients in recipes (sweet potatoes and pecans, to name two) adds authenticity and charm to its beers. Founded in 2003 by husband-and-wife team Mark and Leslie Henderson (and now backed by a team of dedicated, enthusiastic employees), the brewery stays true to its Southern heritage and educates out-of-towners in the process. Two words of caution: If y'all plan to visit the brewery in person, follow the directions page on its website. (Using a GPS could find you in the middle of the woods with no beer in sight.) And know that state law currently prohibits the brewery from giving or selling samples on-site. After your tour, head to a local tavern for pints; you won't be sorry.

CARAMEL SAUCE

- ½ cup (1 stick) unsalted butter
- 1 cup firmly packed light brown sugar
- ¼ cup Maui Gold Rum, or similar rum
- 1¾ cups heavy cream

BREAD PUDDING

- 1 cup shredded coconut
- 1 loaf French or sliced white bread, cut into 1-inch cubes
- ¾ cup sugar
- 2 teaspoons ground cinnamon
- 4 eggs
- 2 cups heavy cream
- ½ cup Maui Gold Rum, or similar rum
- 2 teaspoons vanilla extract

COCONUT PORTER BATTER

- 4 quarts vegetable oil
- 1⅓ cups all-purpose flour
- 1 cup Maui CoCoNut PorTeR, or similar porter

A Few Beers to Try with This Recipe

- *Great Crescent Coconut Porter*
- *Maui CoCoNut PorTeR*

CoCoNut PorTeR Bread Pudding

Bread pudding, with its association with Dickensian England, gets a decidedly Hawaiian twist with the addition of coconut. Forget Oliver Twist; porter and rum make this recipe one to enjoy after the kids are off to bed. Take note that this is a preparation that requires the batter to settle for at least four hours (and as long as overnight) and is made in stages, so it can be time-consuming. However, the ultimate sweet reward is worth the work. Pair this with the coconut porter from Maui Brewing or a robust porter sans coconut if a coconut porter is hard to come by.

1 **MAKE THE CARAMEL SAUCE:** Heat the butter and brown sugar in a skillet over low heat to slowly caramelize the sugar, 8 to 10 minutes. Remove the skillet from the heat promptly.

2 Flambé the rum in a separate pan: Warm a small skillet for 30 seconds over medium heat. Turn off the heat and pour the rum into the skillet. Tilt the pan so the rum pools along one side, and then light the rum with a long match or butane stick lighter. Carefully add the heated rum to the caramelized sugar. Do not stir the mixture.

3 Heat the cream slowly in a separate pot over medium-high heat until scalded, about 10 minutes, and then slowly stir into the caramelized sugar and rum. Transfer to a heatproof bowl to cool, reserving 1/4 cup to drizzle over the finished dessert.

4 **MAKE THE BREAD PUDDING:** Preheat the oven to 350°F. Spread the coconut out on a baking sheet and toast for 10 minutes, or until golden. Remove the coconut from the oven and set aside.

5 Grease a 9- by 13-inch baking pan and fill the pan with the cubed bread. Whisk the toasted coconut, sugar, cinnamon, eggs, cream, rum, vanilla, and the caramel sauce together in a large bowl.

6 Pour the mixture over the bread, mixing the ingredients thoroughly with your hands. Cover the pan with plastic wrap and refrigerate for at least 4 hours and up to overnight.

7 Preheat the oven to 350°F. Bake the bread pudding in a water bath (made by placing the pan in a larger pan filled halfway with hot water) for

1 hour, or until a toothpick inserted into the center of the bread pudding comes out clean. If the toothpick doesn't emerge clean, return the pudding to the oven and bake for 10 minutes longer. Cool to room temperature and refrigerate until ready to serve.

8 **MAKE THE COCONUT PORTER BATTER:** Heat the oil to 375°F in a large cast-iron pot or deep fryer. Remove the bread pudding from its pan and cut into square portions. Whisk the flour and porter together in a large bowl until well combined. Dip the bread pudding pieces into the batter. Deep-fry the pieces, working in batches, until light golden brown, 3 to 4 minutes for each piece.

9 Drain the pudding squares on paper towel–lined plates. Serve with the reserved caramel sauce drizzled over the top.

Makes 8–10 servings

HARPOON BREWERY

BOSTON, MASSACHUSETTS

Winter Warmer Pumpkin Pie

1 cup sugar
1 teaspoon ground cinnamon
½ teaspoon ground allspice
½ teaspoon ground cloves
½ teaspoon ground ginger
½ teaspoon ground nutmeg
½ teaspoon salt
2 eggs
1 cup light cream
⅔ cup Harpoon Winter Warmer, or similar medium-bodied ale with 6% ABV or less
1½ cups pumpkin purée
1 tablespoon all-purpose flour, as needed
Pastry for a 9-inch single-crust pie, homemade or purchased
Ice cream, for serving (optional)

Pumpkin pie is the quintessential kitchen smell of the season. The heavenly combination of spices, pumpkin, and buttery crust comes together in a way that can envelop a home like a warm blanket. To bring out the most flavor, I recommend using whole spices and grinding them yourself. Winter Warmer, a hearty alcoholic brew that staves off the outside chill and offers a bit of spice, is the perfect companion and a pleasing way to settle in for that long winter's nap.

1 Preheat the oven to 350°F.

2 Whisk the sugar, cinnamon, allspice, cloves, ginger, nutmeg, and salt together in a medium bowl.

3 Whip the eggs, cream, and ale together in another mixing bowl with a whisk or an electric mixer. Slowly add the cream mixture to the spice mixture, using an electric mixer to fold the ingredients together. Blend in the pumpkin purée until smooth. If the pie filling seems too loose, add the flour and stir in well.

4 Fit the pie crust into a pie plate and pour the filling into the crust. Bake for about 1 hour, until a butter knife inserted into the center of the pie comes out clean.

5 Let the pie cool slightly, then slice and serve warm with a scoop of ice cream, if desired.

Makes 1 pie, serving 6–8 people

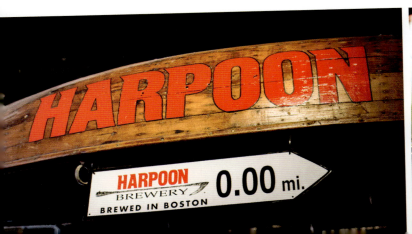

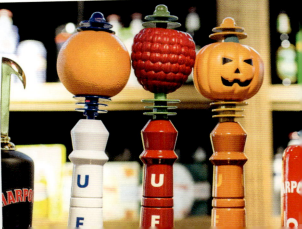

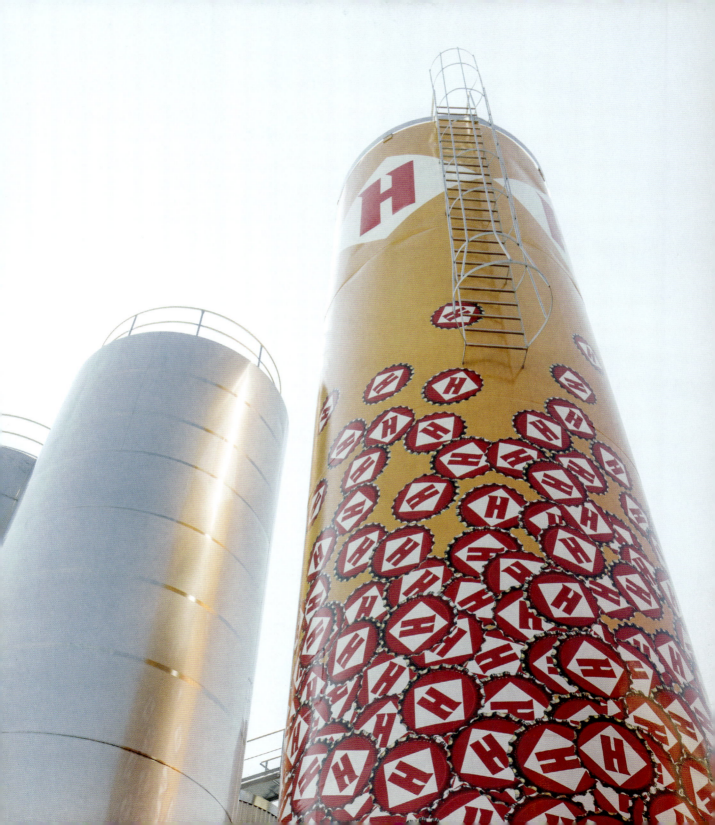

What is currently one of the largest craft breweries in America started off as a school project back in the '80s. *Harpoon Brewery's* co-founder Rich Doyle was in his second year at Harvard Business School when he prepared a report on microbreweries and what it would take to open one in Boston. Doyle repurposed the report into a business plan, partnered with his old friend Dan Kenary, and, in 1986, set out to open what became the first modern microbrewery in Massachusetts. In the beginning, Doyle and Kenary focused on ales, and the beer that first grabbed customers' attention was a mild English ale. In 1993, they introduced an impressive India pale ale as a summer seasonal. The next year, they released the pale ale year-round, and now Harpoon IPA is the brewery's flagship beer. The brewery's first location on the Boston waterfront is a major tourist attraction, as is a second brewery in Windsor, Vermont. With a strong commitment to charity and an inventive brewery staff that churns out new styles as well as fresh takes on old favorites, Harpoon is an American classic.

Fresh Berries with Homemade Maple-Bourbon Whipped Cream

LAWSON'S FINEST LIQUIDS
WARREN, VERMONT

Real maple syrup — not the artificially sugary nonsense that comes cheap in plastic bottles at the supermarket — is a special thing. And in Vermont, where the real stuff is precious and treated like gold, it is serious business. This simple recipe highlights the flavor of the sweet syrup and pairs it with fresh fruit for a light, lip-smacking dessert. Choose berries in season, and mix and match to your heart's content. Pair with a — what else — maple-flavored beer. Lawson's makes a number of maple brews, including an ale, a stout, and a specialty beer, a delightful blend of deep sweetness with notes of vanilla and wood. Other breweries are incorporating real maple into their beers as well. Experiment. Enjoy!

1 pint fresh, seasonal berries
1 tablespoon sugar
2 cups heavy cream
3 tablespoons premium bourbon
1 tablespoon pure maple syrup, preferably from Vermont, plus more for serving
½ teaspoon vanilla extract

1 Slice the berries, if desired, and divide among four serving bowls.

2 Blend the sugar, cream, bourbon, maple syrup, and vanilla together with an electric mixer on medium-high speed until stiff peaks form, about 4 minutes.

3 Scoop the whipped cream onto the fruit, dividing it equally among the bowls. Top with a drizzle of maple syrup, if desired, and serve.

Makes 4 servings, with plenty of whipped cream

PROFILE ★   **There is a certain pleasure** with small-batch beer. Recipes can vary from batch to batch, revealing new subtleties or a dialing in of flavors. Sean *Lawson* is a man who knows his way around beer, and his fine liquids are continually a source of delight for the beer drinkers lucky enough to taste them. He is a wizard of hops to be sure, but he's also skilled with other ingredients, such as maple syrup, herbs, and spices. With Lawson ever experimenting and ever creating, you might not know what to expect next except that it will be exceptional.

Chocolate Ice Cream with Gonzo Imperial Porter

2 cups Flying Dog Gonzo Imperial Porter, or similar porter
½ cup dried malt extract
¼ cup sugar
3 tablespoons unsweetened cocoa powder
2 cups heavy cream
1 cup half-and-half
Kosher or sea salt
4 egg yolks
2 tablespoons whiskey or bourbon

Selecting a flavor from the frozen aisle at your local grocery store is a fine option, but for those days when you feel like stepping things up a bit, why not make your own ice cream? The best part about this recipe (aside from the taste) is that it's decidedly an adult treat thanks to the beer and whiskey. So wait 'til the kids are in bed and enjoy dessert.

1 Bring the porter to a simmer in a medium saucepan over medium heat; simmer until reduced by half, about 20 minutes. Add the malt extract and sugar to the beer and stir continuously to dissolve the sugar. Add the cocoa powder, cream, half-and-half, and salt to taste, and continue to stir to fully incorporate. Once the mixture is smooth and reaches 180°F on a digital thermometer, about 5 minutes, remove from the heat.

2 Beat the egg yolks in a small bowl and whisk in ¼ cup of the hot cream mixture to temper the eggs. Slowly pour the egg mixture into the cream mixture, whisking constantly to prevent the eggs from scrambling.

3 Gradually bring the mixture back up to 165°F, stirring with a wooden spoon. (The mixture should be thick enough to coat the back of the spoon.) Remove the saucepan from the heat and add the whiskey. Pour the mixture into a shallow pan and chill

it in the refrigerator until very cold, at least 2 hours. Alternatively, pour the mixture into a ziplock bag and chill the bag in an ice bath until very cold.

4 Transfer the mixture to an ice cream machine and process according to the manufacturer's instructions. (This recipe will take about an hour longer than most homemade ice creams to freeze in the churn, as the added whiskey lowers the freezing point.)

5 Once the ice cream has reached a semisoft state, transfer it to an airtight container and freeze for no less than 2 hours and no more than 1 week before serving.

Makes about 2 pints

Flying Dog beers are immediately recognizable on shelves, thanks to the erratic label etchings by famed illustrator Ralph Steadman, who was introduced to brewery owner/founder George Stranahan through their mutual friend, Hunter S. Thompson. The Flying Dog name was inspired by art Stranahan saw while in a bar in Pakistan after successfully scaling K2 in 1983. The brewery began its life in Colorado and, along with its full-flavored, unapologetic beers, has been an advocate for free-speech rights. After Steadman finished his first label for the brewery, he added the slogan "Good Beer. No Shit." The label was federally approved, but then a challenge from certain groups saw the removal of the beer from shelves. With the help of the American Civil Liberties Union, the brewery argued that the labels were art and, as such, could not be censored. The slogan was restored and remains to this day.

Pale Ale Pineapple Brown Sugar Cupcakes

Sweet, but a little sour, pineapple is a fruit that brings so many flavors to any recipe it touches. These sweet treats get an added boost from a pale ale that's made with hop varieties that present mango and other tropical fruit flavors. A gentle and floral pale ale also pairs very well with this three-bite dessert. This recipe comes from chef Erin Austin, who owns the Cupcake Brewery in North Carolina. Austin makes delicious baked treats, not beer, but regularly uses the state's generous craft beer offerings to enhance her stellar recipes.

CUPCAKES

- 1 cup (2 sticks) salted butter
- 1¼ cups firmly packed light brown sugar
- 1 cup granulated sugar
- 2 teaspoons vanilla extract
- 4 eggs
- 1 (15-ounce) can crushed pineapple, drained and juice reserved
- 4¼ cups cake flour
- 1 tablespoon plus 1 teaspoon baking powder
- 1 cup whole milk
- 1 (12-ounce) bottle pale ale

ICING

- 1 cup (2 sticks) salted butter
- 1½ cups firmly packed light brown sugar
- 1 tablespoon vanilla extract
- 4 cups confectioners' sugar, plus more as needed
- 2 tablespoons half-and-half, as needed
- Candied pineapple (optional)

Note: The recipe will work best if all ingredients are at room temperature.

1 **MAKE THE CUPCAKES:** Preheat the oven to 350°F and line muffin cups with paper liners.

2 Cream the butter, brown sugar, and granulated sugar together in a large mixing bowl with an electric mixer until light and fluffy, about 5 minutes. Add the vanilla. Beat in the eggs, one at a time, until well blended. Slowly add 1/4 cup of the reserved pineapple juice.

3 Combine the cake flour and baking powder in a medium mixing bowl. Add one-third of the flour mixture to the butter mixture, using the electric mixer on low speed, until just combined. Add the milk, beating until just combined. Add another one-third of the flour mixture to the batter, beating until just combined. Add the pale ale. Add the remaining one-third of the dry mixture, beating until just combined. Fold in the crushed pineapple until evenly distributed.

4 Divide the batter equally among the prepared muffin tins. Bake for 17 minutes, or until just lightly golden. Cool completely on wire racks, about 45 minutes.

5 **MAKE THE ICING:** Melt 1/2 cup of the butter in a medium saucepan over medium heat. Stir in the brown sugar and vanilla until well mixed. Add the remaining 1/2 cup butter and stir until slightly thickened, like a runny caramel, about 17 minutes. Remove the mixture from the heat and let cool to room temperature.

6 Pour the confectioners' sugar into a large mixing bowl. Slowly mix in the brown sugar mixture with an electric mixer until the frosting is light and fluffy. (If the icing is too stiff, slowly add the half-and-half, 1 tablespoon at a time, until it's spreadable. If the icing is too thin, add more confectioners' sugar, 2 tablespoons at a time, until spreadable.)

7 Pipe the icing on the cooled cupcakes and top each one with a small piece of candied pineapple, if using.

Makes 24 cupcakes

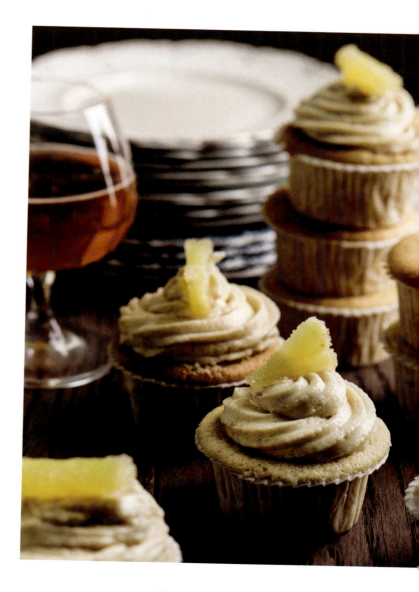

Beer Sorbet

2 cups New Belgium 1554
    Enlightened Black Ale, or
    similar black ale
¾ cup sugar
1 cup water

One of the nice things about a beer sorbet is that you can scoop it within seconds of taking it out of the freezer. The alcohol in the beer will never truly freeze, so the sorbet will have a smoother, less grainy texture. If done correctly you should almost be able to taste the carbonation in the sorbet, and you'll certainly be able to taste the beer. Remember . . . this one isn't for the kids!

1 Pour the beer into a glass to release some of the carbonation and let the foam settle. Place the beer in the refrigerator to chill.

2 Mix the sugar and water together in a medium saucepan over medium heat, stirring occasionally, until the sugar dissolves. Remove the saucepan from the heat as soon as it reaches a soft boil. Place the sugar mixture in the refrigerator to chill, about 2 hours.

3 When the beer and simple syrup are cold, combine the two liquids in a large bowl. Pour the mixture into an ice cream maker and process until thick, about 40 minutes.

4 Transfer the sorbet to a cold storage container and place it in the freezer for at least 2½ hours to set. Serve the sorbet in a chilled bowl or frosted glassware to keep it cold and creamy.

Makes about 3 cups

PROFILE ★ **Inspired to brew** after completing a bicycle trip through Europe, Jeff Lebesch built himself some homebrewing equipment when he returned home to Colorado. Initial response was positive, so he and his then-wife Kim Jordan decided to open their own brewery in 1991. It's been a helluva ride ever since, with their **New Belgium Brewing** becoming one of the largest craft breweries in the United States. Their flagship brew, Fat Tire Amber Ale, is a favorite of many beer drinkers and has helped introduce new customers to the dizzying array of beers New Belgium produces. They rightfully, and proudly, point out that the brewery runs on wind power through credits purchased through wind farms. This and other environmental efforts are highlighted on the brewery tour, where, yes, you can ride a bike around the grounds.

Pots de Crème

BLACK TOOTH BREWING COMPANY

SHERIDAN, WYOMING

French in nature and simple to prepare, this elegant dessert is delicious and offers a satisfying crunch when your spoon breaks apart the caramelized sugar topping. This sweet treat requires eight 6-ounce ramekins, so be prepared. Try pairing this with a creamy milk stout, a fruit beer, or an Irish red ale.

½ cup beet sugar
11 egg yolks
  Pinch of sea salt
2¼ cups heavy cream
¾ cup whole milk
¾ cup sour cream
½ cup raw sugar, for the topping

1 Preheat the oven 300°F.

2 Beat the beet sugar, egg yolks, and salt together in a large bowl with an electric mixer until pale yellow, about 2 minutes. Set aside.

3 Bring the cream to a simmer in a medium saucepan over medium heat. (Do not bring to a hard boil.) Gradually whisk the heated cream into the yolk mixture, adding a few tablespoons at a time so that the eggs don't scramble. Whisk in the milk and sour cream, and then pour the mixture through a fine sieve into a large glass measuring cup.

4 Divide the mixture equally among eight 6-ounce ramekins. Cover each ramekin with foil and place in a large roasting pan. Add enough water to the roasting pan to reach halfway up the sides of the ramekins. Bake for about 1 hour, rotating halfway through, until the custards are set in the center. When the ramekins are cool enough to handle, carefully remove the custards from the pan and refrigerate until cool, at least 2 hours and up to 2 days.

5 When ready to serve, gently pat the top of each custard with a paper towel to remove excess moisture. Sprinkle each custard with a tablespoon of the raw sugar and caramelize either with a kitchen torch or under a broiler for 2 to 3 minutes, turning to achieve an even shell. Cool for 3 minutes and serve.

Makes 8 servings

PROFILE ★ **The modern-industrial decor** that represents the bar at **Black Tooth Brewing** in Wyoming stands in contrast to the surrounding city's Main Street U.S.A. feel. So it is understandable that the beers served up by Travis Zeilstra and his team are something special. The brewery's flavorful, award-winning ales are awakening taste buds in the region east of Yellowstone National Park, and with its plans to grow in the coming years, more people in this mountainous area will have another excellent option for at-home consumption.

1½ cups spent grain
1 cup firmly packed light brown sugar
¾ cup all-purpose flour
½ teaspoon baking soda
½ teaspoon ground cinnamon
½ teaspoon salt
6 tablespoons extra-virgin olive oil
3 tablespoons unsweetened applesauce
1 teaspoon vanilla extract
1½ cups old-fashioned rolled oats
1 cup dried cranberries
1 cup crushed walnuts

A Few Beers to Drink with Cookies:

- *Buffalo Bill's Pumpkin Ale*
- *Elysian Night Owl Pumpkin Ale*
- *New Holland The Poet*
- *Ninkasi Oatis*
- *Portneuf Valley Midnight Satin*
- *Rogue Shakespeare Oatmeal Stout*
- *Samuel Adams Old Fezziwig Ale*

Oatmeal Cranberry Spent-Grain Cookies

Obtaining spent grain is not difficult. Brewers are faced with an abundance of the nutrient-rich mash and are usually happy to help it find a second life. Just call your local brewery and ask. For this recipe, a caramel or a lighter wheat malt will work best. These versatile cookies are also vegan-friendly, high in fiber and healthy oils, and great pairings for a spiced beer, a pumpkin ale, or even an oatmeal stout.

1 Preheat the oven to 350°F and grease a large baking sheet.

2 Mix the spent grain, brown sugar, flour, baking soda, cinnamon, and salt together in a large mixing bowl. Stir in the olive oil, applesauce, and vanilla. Add the oats, cranberries, and walnuts, and mix until thoroughly incorporated.

3 Roll walnut-size balls of the dough in your hand and place 2 inches apart on the prepared baking sheet. Bake for 10 to 14 minutes, or until golden brown. Cool the cookies on the baking sheet for 5 minutes before transferring them to a wire rack to cool completely. Store cookies in an airtight container for up to 3 days.

Makes 2 dozen cookies

PROFILE ★ **Determination and the goal of living out a dream** led to the founding of ***Portneuf Valley Brewing***. Owner Penny Pink had been a home-brewer and went legit by opening a small brewery inside a sports bar in the late '90s. But she soon saw the need to open in a larger space after an enthusiastic response from customers. She moved into the brewery's current location a short distance away, once occupied by the East Idaho Brewing Company, and revived the brewing tradition. Now the brewery is a hub for well-crafted pints, a good meal, live music, and camaraderie. When you visit, ask about their ghost.

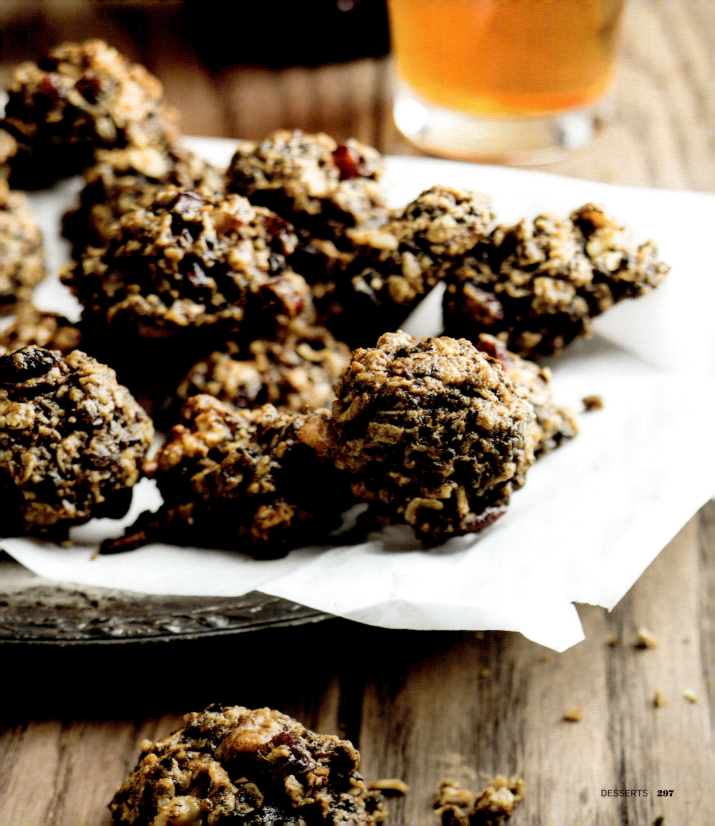

Carrot Cake with Bourbon-Mascarpone Icing

This is not your traditional bake-sale carrot cake. A mascarpone and bourbon icing gives this treat a more adult flavor and refined texture. Pair with an IPA for an added spicy kick.

CAKE

- 2 cups sugar
- 1¼ cups vegetable oil
- 4 eggs
- 2 teaspoons vanilla extract
- 2 cups all-purpose flour
- 2 teaspoons baking powder
- 2 teaspoons baking soda
- 2 teaspoons ground cinnamon
- ½ teaspoon salt
- ¼ teaspoon ground allspice
- ¼ teaspoon ground cloves
- ¼ teaspoon freshly ground nutmeg
- 3 cups grated carrots
- 1 cup chopped walnuts
- ½ cup crushed pineapple

ICING

- 12 ounces mascarpone cheese
- 1 (1-pound) package confectioners' sugar
- 2 tablespoons bourbon
- 1 teaspoon vanilla extract

1 MAKE THE CAKE: Preheat the oven to 350°F and grease and flour a 9- by 13-inch cake pan.

2 Beat the sugar, vegetable oil, eggs, and vanilla together with an electric mixer at medium speed until the mixture is light in color and fully incorporated, about 2 minutes. Mix in the flour, baking powder, baking soda, cinnamon, salt, allspice, cloves, and nutmeg. Fold in the carrots, walnuts, and pineapple until just combined.

3 Pour the batter into the prepared cake pan and bake for 40 to 50 minutes, or until a toothpick inserted into the center of the cake comes out clean. Let the cake cool in the pan for 10 minutes, and then turn out onto a wire rack to cool completely.

4 MAKE THE ICING: Beat the mascarpone, sugar, bourbon, and vanilla together with an electric mixer at medium speed until smooth and creamy, 2 to 3 minutes. Frost the top and sides of the cooled cake.

Makes 1 cake, serving 8–10 people

PROFILE ★ **Steamworks Brewing Co.** opened its doors in 1996 and quickly became a favorite watering hole for locals and visitors alike. While its beers are enough to inspire a visit, it's the menu that routinely elicits oohs and ahhs. With locally raised meats and sustainable seafood, inventive salads and pizzas, and spicy Southwestern-style dishes, there is something for everyone on the menu, and plenty of reasons to visit again and again.

Beer Caramel Sauce

Here is a super simple but delicious caramel sauce that works on ice cream, pancakes, waffles, French toast, and fried chicken. It's a great accompaniment to any food that deserves a sweet and malty boost.

NEW REPUBLIC BREWING

COLLEGE STATION, TEXAS

1 cup loosely packed light brown sugar
1 tablespoon thinly sliced candied ginger
2 cups dunkelweizen

Bring the brown sugar, candied ginger, and beer to a boil in a medium saucepan over medium heat. Reduce the heat and simmer the sauce, stirring frequently, until the caramel is thick, 15 to 20 minutes. Remove and discard the ginger before serving. Stored in an airtight container, the caramel will keep for up to 5 days in the refrigerator.

Makes about 1 cup

PROFILE ★ **Every university town** should have a brewery, and in the loyal town of College Station, students, faculty, and visitors in Aggie-land are lucky to have *New Republic Brewing*. With beers that are English and German by influence, the owners and brewers (mostly alums themselves) are bringing good beer with real flavor to an area that needed it. They also host a regular homebrew club to foster the industry and hobby in the community.

Maria's Favorite Linzertorte

This sweet and flaky treat has been in the von Trapp family for generations and was a favorite of Maria, the matriarch. A perfect way to end a satisfying meal, or a wonderful companion to afternoon tea and coffee, this tart and nutty pastry will impress your guests before it quickly disappears.

1½ cups unsalted butter
1½ cups granulated sugar
1 egg
3 heaping cups all-purpose flour
1½ cups ground walnuts
½ teaspoon ground cinnamon
½ teaspoon freshly ground nutmeg
¼ teaspoon ground cloves
½ cup currant jelly
½ cup raspberry jam
¼ cup sliced almonds
Confectioners' sugar, for dusting

1 Preheat the oven to 350°F. Flour two 8-inch tart or pie pans.

2 Cream the butter and sugar together by hand or with an electric mixer in a large bowl until light and fluffy. Mix in the egg, flour, walnuts, cinnamon, nutmeg, and cloves, and shape the dough into a ball.

3 Divide the dough into quarters. Press a quarter of the dough into the bottom of each pan. Cut one of the remaining quarters in half and press these two pieces up the sides of the two pans. Cut the remaining quarter of dough into 12 pieces and set aside.

4 Mix the currant jelly and the raspberry jam together in a small bowl. Spread half of the mixture into each of the shells. Roll out the remaining dough pieces into rounded strips and crisscross the strips on top of the jam mixture, arranging three pieces each way. Press the side crust down to connect with the strips.

5 Sprinkle the top of the torte with the almonds and bake until the crust is golden brown and the jam mixture is bubbling, 45 to 50 minutes in a conventional oven or 35 to 40 minutes in a convection oven.

6 Cool the tortes to room temperature, remove from the pans, and sprinkle with confectioners' sugar. Slice and serve at room temperature. If you wish to prepare well in advance of serving, this torte freezes very well.

Makes 2 (8-inch) tarts

Thanks to the book and subsequent *Sound of Music* movie, there are not many people who don't know the story of the von Trapp family. Having fled Austria and landed in Philadelphia, the family made their living as performers. Eventually they settled in Stowe, Vermont, purchased a small farmhouse (because the landscape reminded them of home), and continued to sing while also renting out rooms to skiers and running a music camp. Today, Johannes, the youngest of the singing von Trapp children, and his family run the ***Trapp Family Lodge***. The European-style luxury mountain resort sits on 2,500 acres and offers a host of activities or a chance to just get away from it all. With an on-premises brewery and great dining options, it is easy to see why this is a favorite destination for so many people.

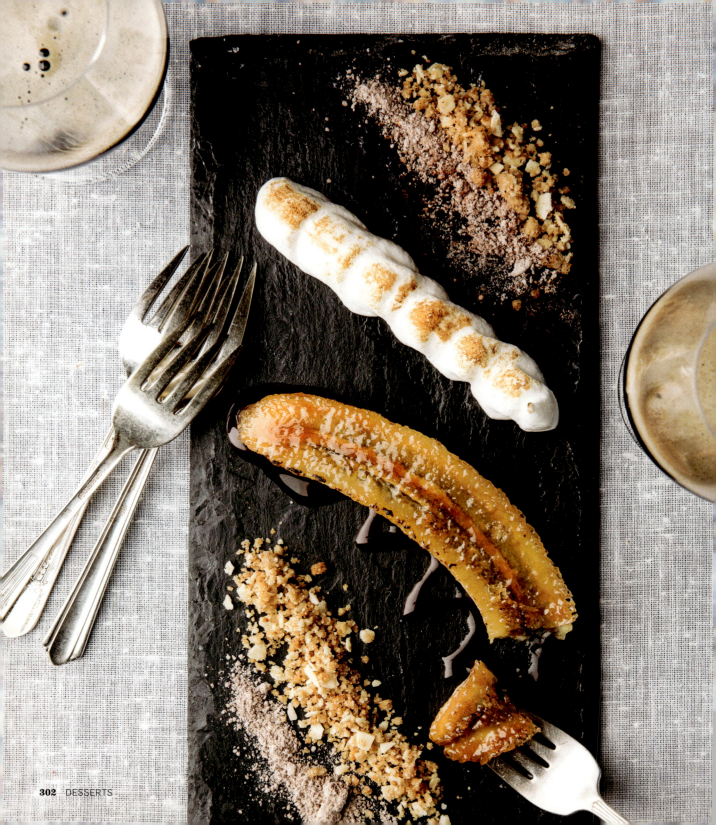

Deconstructed Banana Meringue Pie with Dulce de Leche, Almond Wafer Crumble, and Chocolate Powder

CHAMA RIVER BREWING COMPANY

ALBUQUERQUE, NEW MEXICO

A pie experience with little baking and the use of a kitchen torch? Sign me up! This creative recipe offers all the delicious flavors of the classic pie, but in a more artistic presentation. There is some work involved on the front end, but the end result is worth it. You can even prepare some of the ingredients a few days in advance before bringing it all together prior to serving. This dessert pairs well with a small glass of a bourbon-aged stout, inviting the vanilla notes and darker malts to play with the dessert ingredients.

DULCE DE LECHE
- 1 (14-ounce) can sweetened condensed milk, preferably Eagle Brand
- 1 gallon water
- 1 tablespoon vanilla extract

CHOCOLATE POWDER
- 1 cup tapioca maltodextrin
- 2 ounces 60 percent dark chocolate, melted

ALMOND WAFER CRUMBLE
- 2 cups crushed vanilla wafers
- ½ cup crushed sliced almonds
- 4 tablespoons unsalted butter, melted
- 2 tablespoons sugar
- 1 teaspoon kosher salt
- ¼ teaspoon ground cinnamon

BANANA MERINGUE
- 1 cup sugar
- ¼ cup water
- 4 egg whites
- ½ teaspoon kosher salt

CARAMELIZED BANANAS
- 2 ripe bananas
- ½ cup raw sugar

1 MAKE THE DULCE DE LECHE: Remove the paper label from the can of condensed milk. Place the can in a large pot and cover with the water. Bring the water to a boil and continue boiling for 3 hours, replenishing the water as needed to keep the can submerged.

2 Remove the can from the water and cool to room temperature. Open the can and mix its contents and the vanilla in a small bowl. Set aside.

3 MAKE THE CHOCOLATE POWDER: Combine the tapioca maltodextrin and melted chocolate in the bowl of a food processor and process until it becomes a fine powder, about 30 seconds. Reserve in a dry airtight container.

4 MAKE THE CRUMBLE: Preheat the oven to 350°F and line a baking sheet with parchment paper.

5 Mix the wafers, almonds, melted butter, sugar, salt, and cinnamon together in a mixing bowl until well combined. Transfer the mixture to the prepared baking sheet and bake for 6 to 8 minutes, or until the wafers and almonds are golden. Let cool and reserve in an airtight container.

6 MAKE THE MERINGUE: Combine the sugar and water in a saucepan and cover with a lid. Bring the syrup to a boil, remove the lid, and boil until an instant-read thermometer reads 245°F. Remove the syrup from the heat and allow to cool.

recipe continues on next page

7 With a whisk or an electric mixer, whip the egg whites and salt in a medium bowl until soft peaks form. Slowly add the cooled syrup to the egg whites and whip until firm peaks form. Transfer the egg white mixture to a pastry bag and set aside.

8 **MAKE THE CARAMELIZED BANANAS:** Cut the bananas in half lengthwise and press the cut sides into the raw sugar. Slowly caramelize the sugar using a kitchen blowtorch to brûlée the sugar without burning the bananas.

9 **ASSEMBLE:** Pipe a strip of the meringue onto each of eight serving plates and lightly brûlée the meringue with the kitchen torch. Drizzle the dulce de leche onto the plate parallel to the meringue and top with the brûléed banana. Sprinkle the chocolate powder and almond crumble around the plates. Serve immediately.

Makes 8 servings

PROFILE ★ **Lest you think** that all brewery restaurants are of the burger and nacho variety, Chama River wants you to take a closer look. Here in this upscale eatery, cuisine of the highest order is paired with beers of equal character. The restaurant's sleek, elegant decor is inviting and lends itself to intimate conversations and memorable times. But, being a brewery, there is also some fun afoot with various theme nights (Halloween) and events. Check them out!

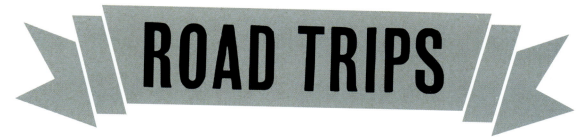

ROAD TRIPS

While one of the satisfying by-products of the American craft beer revolution is that you don't have to go far to experience a unique pint, it is still great fun to travel just to drink beer.

Some of the country's great cities have thriving beer cultures. In the following pages I'll suggest must-visit breweries, dining experiences, and a few local beer-related attractions that provide good local flair.

Everything in moderation, so if you're taking to the streets, please consider using mass transit or having a designated driver.

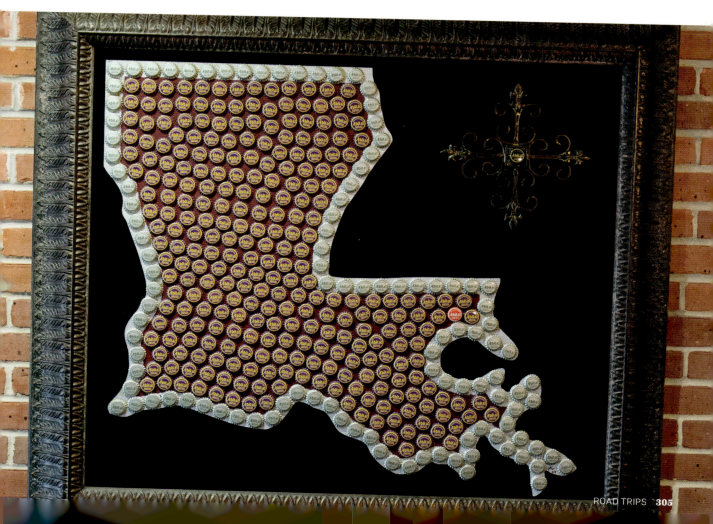

Milwaukee, Wisconsin

One of the country's great brewing cities, Milwaukee has also been at the forefront of the craft-brewing movement. It is too often overlooked because of its proximity to Chicago, but for beer lovers, day-trippers, art and architecture aficionados, and foodies, this city on Lake Michigan deserves a closer look.

Breweries

LAKEFRONT BREWERY
1872 North Commerce Street
Milwaukee, WI 53212
414-372-8800
www.lakefrontbrewery.com

MILWAUKEE BREWING COMPANY
613 South 2nd Street
Milwaukee, WI 53204
414-226-2337
http://mkebrewing.com

ROCK BOTTOM BREWERY
740 North Plankinton Avenue
Milwaukee, WI 53203
414-276-3030
www.rockbottom.com/milwaukee

SPRECHER BREWING CO.
701 West Glendale Avenue
Glendale, WI 53209
414-964-7837
www.sprecherbrewery.com

Restaurants & Beer Bars

CAFE AT THE PLAZA
1007 North Cass Street
Milwaukee, WI 53202
414-272-0515
A familiar countertop feel surrounded by Art Deco architecture, this hidden gem makes everything in-house and from scratch. A breakfast here starts your day off right.

HINTERLAND ERIE STREET GASTROPUB
Hinterland Brewery
222 East Erie Street, Suite 100
Milwaukee, WI 53202
414-727-9300
www.hinterlandbeer.com/Restaurant_Mil.html
An offshoot of Green Bay Brewery, this outstanding restaurant is a gourmand's dream. Try everything on the menu.

SUGAR MAPLE
441 East Lincoln Avenue
Milwaukee, WI 53224
414-481-2393
www.mysugarmaple.com
A wonderful neighborhood spot with impressive craft beer taps, a great menu, and a knowledgeable staff.

Hotel Suggestion

THE BREWHOUSE INN & SUITES
1215 North 10th Street
Milwaukee, WI 53205
414-810-0146
www.brewhousesuites.com
Once home to the famed Pabst brewery, an extensive remodeling and construction project has turned the 1877 building into a modern boutique hotel. Much of the original brewery has been preserved — including the giant copper brew kettle tops — and stained-glass windows feature the legendary King Gambrinus. With 90 suites and rooms of varying sizes, the hotel has more to choose from than standard lodging, and it is steeped in beer history.

Beer-Related Attractions

BEST PLACE
901 West Juneau Avenue
Milwaukee, WI 53233
414-630-1609
www.bestplacemilwaukee.com
Located inside the old Pabst brewery, here the history of the iconic beer comes alive. Visitors are invited to belly up to the bar inside the refurbished beer hall.

HARLEY-DAVIDSON MUSEUM

400 West Canal Street
Milwaukee, WI 53201
877-436-8738
www.harley-davidson.com/en_US/Content/
Pages/HD_Museum/museum.html
Celebrating the iconic motorcycle
brand, this is a must-visit for anyone
passionate about the two-wheeled
machines. With historic bikes and
interactive exhibits, it's great for the
whole family.

MILWAUKEE ART MUSEUM

700 North Art Museum Drive
Milwaukee, WI 53202
414-224-3200
http://mam.org
Designed by architect Santiago
Calatrava, this iconic museum building
has a "wing-like sun screen" that raises
and lowers, creating a unique moving
sculpture. There are rotating exhibits
as well as one on historic beer steins —
a must for any brew historian.

PABST MANSION

2000 West Wisconsin Avenue
Milwaukee, WI 53233
414-931-0808
www.pabstmansion.com
See how the "captain" lived. Tours of
Frederick Pabst's grand home offer
a glimpse into the affluent life of one
of beer's great men. It's decorated
to the nines each Christmas season
with theme rooms and stunning
presentations.

Philadelphia, Pennsylvania

Steeped in brewing history, the City of Brotherly Love is a great place for a proper pint of beer. Philadelphia is easy to navigate and offers world-class dining, museums, attractions, and sports. There is a reason this city is a popular destination, and if you've never been (or just haven't been in a while) it's time to book your visit.

Breweries

EARTH BREAD + BREWERY
7136 Germantown Avenue
Philadelphia, PA 19119
215-242-6666
www.earthbreadbrewery.com

IRON HILL BREWERY & RESTAURANT
8400 Germantown Avenue
Philadelphia, PA 19118
215-948-5600
www.ironhillbrewery.com

NODDING HEAD BREWERY & RESTAURANT
1516 Sansom Street, 2nd Floor
Philadelphia, PA 19102
215-569-9525
www.ripsneakers.com/nodding

TRIUMPH BREWING COMPANY
117 Chestnut Street
Philadelphia, PA 19106
215-625-0855
www.triumphbrewing.com

YARDS BREWING COMPANY
901 North Delaware Avenue
Philadelphia, PA 19123
215-634-2600
www.yardsbrewing.com

Restaurants & Beer Bars

HAWTHORNES CAFE
738 South 11th Street
Philadelphia, PA 19147
215-627-3012
www.hawthornescafe.com
You'll need a map to navigate the more than 1,000 bottles, rotating drafts, and growler fill stations. It's the place to stock your cellar.

KHYBER PASS PUB
56 South 2nd Street
Philadelphia, PA 19106
www.khyberpasspub.com
With a bottle list that requires serious reading and a draft selection that moves so quickly, it's written in chalk behind the bar, it's a favorite among locals and tourists alike.

LOCAL 44
4333 Spruce Street
Philadelphia, PA 19104
215-222-2337
www.local44beerbar.com
A neighborhood joint with a great beer selection and memorable food.

MONK'S CAFÉ
264 South 16th Street
Philadelphia, PA 19102
215-545-7005
www.monkscafe.com
The venerable Philly beer bar; no visit is complete without a stop (or three) here.

READING TERMINAL MARKET
12th and Arch Streets
Philadelphia, PA 19107
215-922-2317
www.readingterminalmarket.org
A historic, indoor farmers' market that offers an opportunity to experience all the great, famous Philly foods.

Boston, Massachusetts

The pilgrims landed at Plymouth Rock because they were running low on beer — among other things — thus laying the foundation for Massachusetts's beer history. Today, the city is alive with history, great breweries, fantastic restaurants, and all-star accommodations. With accessible mass transit, it's easy to make the most of a visit without worrying about a car.

Breweries

THE BOSTON BEER COMPANY
(*Makers of Samuel Adams*)
30 Germania Street
Boston, MA 02130
888-661-2337
www.samueladams.com

BOSTON BEER WORKS — FENWAY
61 Brookline Avenue
Boston, MA 02215
617-536-2337
www.beerworks.net

CAMBRIDGE BREWING CO.
1 Kendall Square, Building 100
Cambridge, MA 02139
617-494-1994
www.cambridgebrewing.com

HARPOON BREWERY
306 Northern Avenue
Boston, MA 02210
617-547-9551
www.harpoonbrewery.com

Restaurants & Beer Bars

CAMBRIDGE COMMON
1667 Massachusetts Avenue
Cambridge, MA 02138
617-547-1228
www.cambridgecommonrestaurant.com
Offers many local beers and generous food portions in an upscale college atmosphere.

DEEP ELLUM
477 Cambridge Street
Allston, MA 02134
617-787-2337
www.deepellum-boston.com
This neighborhood spot has great beer and a wonderful menu to boot.

LORD HOBO
92 Hampshire Street
Cambridge, MA 02139
617-250-8454
http://lordhobo.com
A favorite spot for a nightcap.

THE LOWER DEPTHS TAP ROOM
476 Commonwealth Avenue
Boston, MA 02115
617-266-6662
http://thelowerdepths.com
Comfortably close to Fenway, with knowledgeable staff and a rotating selection. One never leaves this establishment disappointed.

Portland, Oregon

For those seeking the finest craft beers, no journey is complete without a visit (and many thereafter) to Portland. Considered the fertile crescent of beer towns, it boasts a brewery for every taste and style. Some of the country's most established breweries call this city home, and the truly ambitious come and hang shingles of their own. With its laid-back attitude, friendly forward-thinking residents, and a pleasant climate, there are many reasons to visit. Here are just a few.

Breweries

BREAKSIDE BREWERY
820 Northeast Dekum Street
Portland, OR 97211
503-719-6475
www.breakside.com

BURNSIDE BREWING COMPANY
701 East Burnside Street
Portland, OR 97214
503-946-8151
www.burnsidebrewco.com

CASCADE BREWING BARREL HOUSE
939 Southeast Belmont Street
Portland, OR 97214
503-265-8603
www.cascadebrewingbarrelhouse.com

HAIR OF THE DOG BREWING COMPANY
61 Southeast Yamhill Street
Portland, OR 97214
503-232-6585
www.hairofthedog.com

HOPWORKS URBAN BREWERY
2944 Southeast Powell Boulevard
Portland, OR 97202
503-232-4677
http://hopworksbeer.com

UPRIGHT BREWING
240 North Broadway, Suite 2
Portland, OR 97227
503-735-5337
www.uprightbrewing.com

WIDMER BROTHERS BREWING
955 North Russell
Portland, OR 97227
503-281-3333
http://widmerbrothers.com

Restaurants & Beer Bars

APEX
1216 Southeast Division Street
Portland, OR 97202
503-273-9227
http://apexbar.com

GREEN DRAGON BISTRO AND BREWPUB
928 Southeast 9th Avenue
Portland, OR 97214
503-517-0660
www.pdxgreendragon.com
Part of the Rogue Ales family, it is fairly new, but is quickly becoming a favorite spot for many in the city.

HIGGINS RESTAURANT AND BAR
1239 Southwest Broadway
Portland, OR 97205
503-222-9070
www.higginsportland.com
An early adopter of beer and food pairings, it offers some of the best meals in the city.

HORSE BRASS PUB
4534 Southeast Belmont Street
Portland, OR 97215
503-232-2202
www.horsebrass.com
A Portland staple. No visit to the city is complete without a stop here.

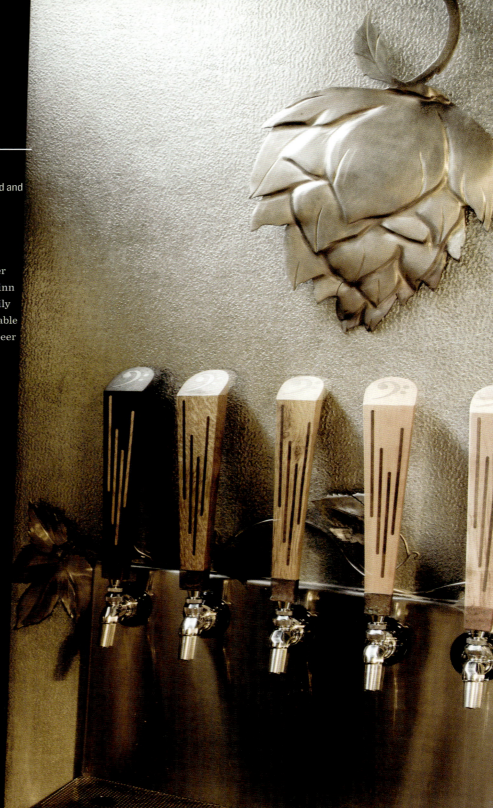

Hotel Suggestion

INN BEERVANA
Near Southeast Hawthorne Boulevard and 39th Avenue
Portland, OR 97214
503-836-7739
http://innbeervana.com
Owned by beer writer Brian Yaeger and his wife Kimberley, this cozy inn is a great spot for couples or a family interested in staying in a comfortable setting in the heart of Portland's beer scene.

San Francisco, California

You could wander the City by the Bay for years and never go thirsty. That's because this delightful city has some proud brewing traditions, a bevy of respected establishments, and an adventurous population who keep things fresh. From the bridge to the wharf, Telegraph Hill to Alcatraz, there are many reasons to leave your heart here.

Breweries

21ST AMENDMENT BREWERY
563 Second Street
San Francisco, CA 94107
415-369-0900
http://21st-amendment.com

ANCHOR BREWING COMPANY
1705 Mariposa Street
San Francisco, CA 94107
415-863-8350
www.anchorbrewing.com

GORDON BIERSCH BREWING COMPANY
Multiple locations; see website for details.
www.gordonbiersch.com

MAGNOLIA GASTROPUB & BREWERY
1398 Haight Street
San Francisco, CA 94117
415-864-7468
www.magnoliapub.com

SOCIAL KITCHEN & BREWERY
1326 9th Avenue
San Francisco, CA 94122
415-681-0330
www.socialkitchenandbrewery.com

TRUMER BRAUEREI
1404 4th Street
Berkeley, CA 94710
510-526-1160
www.trumer-international.com

Restaurants & Beer Bars

CITY BEER STORE
1168 Folsom Street, Suite 101
San Francisco, CA 94103
415-503-1033
www.citybeerstore.com
Come with a heavy wallet and a strong back to carry all your newfound treasures home; this place has an impressive selection.

PUBLIC HOUSE
AT&T Park
24 Willie Mays Plaza
San Francisco, CA 94107
415-644-0240
http://publichousesf.com
Not only is it a great place to warm up before a Giants game, it's a great spot in the off-season. With a commitment to flavorful beers, this is a satisfying and modern spot for a pint.

TORONADO
547 Haight Street
San Francisco, CA 94117
415-863-2276
www.toronado.com
This venerable beer bar is where any good beer journey to the city should begin. And end.

San Diego, California

Southern California — where the sun shines bright, the beaches can't be beat, and the beer in your glass is likely hopped beyond what brewers a century ago thought possible. The beer scene here is fearless and has inspired so many in the industry that it can be considered fertile ground. Mix in the varied architecture, the known attractions, a near-perfect climate, and the constant presence of great food from fish tacos to wood-fired pizza, and it's clear to see why people put down deep roots, or keep coming back for more.

Breweries

ALESMITH BREWING COMPANY
9368 Cabot Drive
San Diego, CA 92126
858-549-9888
http://alesmith.com

BALLAST POINT BREWING COMPANY
10051 Old Grove Road
San Diego, CA 92131
858-695-2739
www.ballastpoint.com
@bpbrewing

GREENFLASH BREWING CO.
6550 Mira Mesa Boulevard
San Diego, CA 92121
858-622-0085
www.greenflashbrew.com

HESS BREWING
3812 Grim Avenue
San Diego, CA 92104
619-786-4377
www.hessbrewing.com
@hessbrewing

KARL STRAUSS BREWING COMPANY
5985 Santa Fe Street
San Diego, CA 92109
858-273-2739
www.karlstrauss.com
@Karl_Strauss

PIZZA PORT BREWING COMPANY
1956 Bacon Street
Ocean Beach, CA 92107
619-224-4700
www.pizzaport.com
@PizzaPortBeer
Multiple locations; see website for details.

PORT BREWING COMPANY / THE LOST ABBEY
155 Mata Way, Suite 104
San Marcos, CA 92069
800-918-6816
www.portbrewing.com
@lostabbey

STONE BREWING CO.
1999 Citracado Parkway
Escondido, CA 92029
760-471-4999
www.stonebrewing.com
@StoneBrewingCo

Restaurants & Beer Bars

HAMILTON'S TAVERN
1521 30th Street
San Diego, CA 92102
619-238-5460
http://hamiltonstavern.com

LOCAL HABIT
3827 5th Avenue
San Diego, CA 92103
619-795-4770
www.mylocalhabit.com

O'BRIEN'S AMERICAN PUB
4646 Convoy Street
San Diego, CA 92111
858-715-1745
http://obrienspub.net

TORONADO
4026 30th Street
San Diego, CA 92104
619-282-0456
www.toronadosd.com

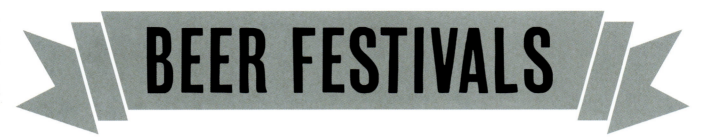

BEER FESTIVALS

Seems like these days you can't swing a hop vine without hitting a beer festival. They are being held in the unlikeliest of places and many offer unlimited samples, food, live music, and the chance to "meet the brewers." The problem is that with so many out there, quite a few are duds. That's not to say you won't have a good time, but too often these festivals pour familiar beers and are frequented by people just looking to tie one on.

Fortunately, there are festivals and events that rise above the rest. Here is a list of a few worth your time and dollars.

BOULDER STRONG ALE FESTIVAL
Avery Brewing Company
Boulder, Colorado
303-440-4324
www.averybrewing.com
Hosted annually by the Avery Brewing Co., this event is a celebration of beers over 8% ABV. Designated driver required.

GREAT ALASKA BEER & BARLEY WINE FESTIVAL
Anchorage, Alaska
http://auroraproductions.net/beer-barley.html
Malt lovers rejoice at this annual affair that celebrates the best of barley wine.

GREAT AMERICAN BEER FESTIVAL
Brewers Association
Denver, Colorado
303-447-0816
www.greatamericanbeerfestival.com
The king of them all. Now in its third decade, the GABF is the premier beer festival, attended by thousands.

Breweries from around the country come to showcase their very best. Held each autumn in Denver, this festival is a mecca for beer lovers.

GREAT TASTE OF THE MIDWEST
Madison Homebrewers and Tasters Guild
Madison, Wisconsin
greattaste@mhtg.org
www.mhtg.org/great-taste-of-the-midwest
More than one hundred breweries and brewpubs come to Madison each summer for this unique festival featuring the best of the Midwest.

MICHIGAN BREWERS GUILD WINTER FESTIVAL
Grand Rapids, Michigan
www.michiganbrewersguild.org
Leave it to the bold folks in Michigan to hold their annual winter gathering outdoors — sun or snow. Attendance by only Michigan breweries means you'll drink local all day long. Go at least once — you won't regret the trip.

NIGHT OF THE BARRELS
BeerAdvocate
Boston, Massachusetts
http://beeradvocate.com/ebf
Part of the *BeerAdvocate* Extreme Beer Festival, this annual event regularly features more than 60 rare barrel-aged beers.

PHILLY BEER WEEK
Philadelphia, Pennsylvania
info@phillybeerweek.org
www.phillybeerweek.org
The original beer-week city is showing no signs of slowing down. Brewers mark this on their calendars early, and you should too. The best beer in the country rolls into the City of Brotherly Love and leaves everyone happy.

SAN FRANCISCO BEER WEEK
The San Francisco Brewers Guild
San Francisco, California
www.sfbeerweek.org
The Bay Area knows how to put on a show. With some of the best breweries

calling this region home, they pull out all the stops. Restaurants get into the act as well and some of the best beer dinners of the year happen during this week.

SAVOR: AN AMERICAN CRAFT BEER AND FOOD EXPERIENCE
Brewers Association
New York, New York
303-447-0816
www.savorcraftbeer.com
An annual event hosted by the Brewers Association, this brings together some of the country's best breweries and pairs their finest offerings with ambitious and expertly prepared dishes. The event regularly sells out within minutes.

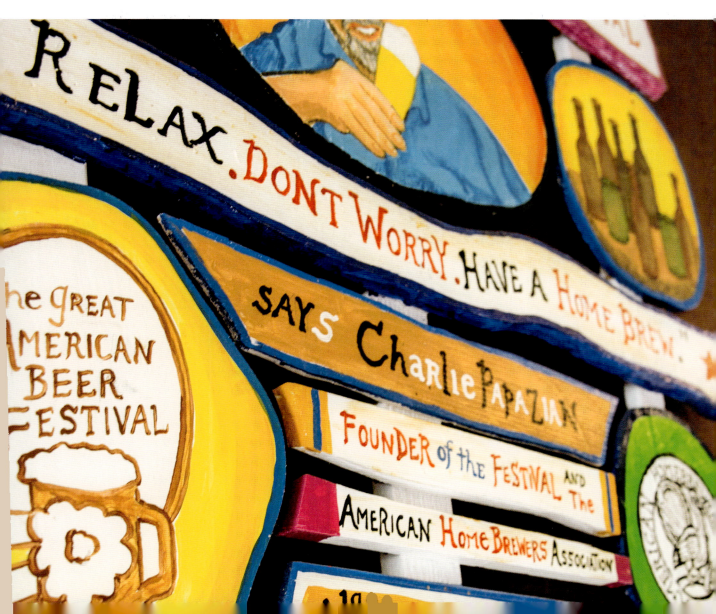

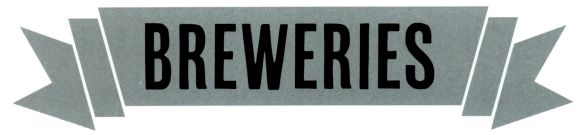

BREWERIES

The following breweries contributed recipes and are listed by state.

Alabama

BELOW THE RADAR BREWHOUSE
220 Holmes Avenue N.E.
Huntsville, AL 35801
256-469-6617
http://btrbrew.wordpress.com
Bill Harden, chef
Fried Green Tomatoes with Sun-Dried Tomato Ale Mustard, 30

Alaska

ALASKAN BREWING COMPANY
5429 Shaune Drive
Juneau, AK 99801
907-780-5866
www.alaskanbeer.com
@AlaskanBrewing
Michael King, chef
Black Cod Brûlée, 241

BARANOF ISLAND BREWING COMPANY
215 Smith Street
Sitka, AK 99835
907-747-2739
www.baranofislandbrewing.com
Rowan Chevalier, chef
Cumin-Dijon Smothered Baked Halibut, 255

California

21ST AMENDMENT BREWERY
563 Second Street
San Francisco, CA 94107
415-369-0900
http://21st-amendment.com
@21stAmendment
Brew Free! Chili, 152

ANDERSON VALLEY BREWING COMPANY
17700 Highway 253
Boonville, CA 95415
800-207-2337
www.avbc.com
@avbc
Fal Allen, chef
Khmer Wild Boar Curry, 150

BEAR REPUBLIC BREWING COMPANY
345 Healdsburg Avenue
Healdsburg, CA 95448
707-433-2337
www.bearrepublic.com
@brbcbrew
Noel Zuazo, chef
Grilled Italian Sando, 118

DRAKE'S BREWING
1933 Davis Street, Building 177
San Leandro, CA 94577
510-568-2739
www.drinkdrakes.com
@DrakesBrewery
Adam Pechal, chef
Hopocalypse Ceviche, 31

FIRESTONE WALKER BREWING COMPANY
1400 Ramada Drive
Paso Robles, CA 93446
805-225-5911
www.firestonebeer.com
@FirestoneWalker
Sean Z. Paxton, chef
Moroccan-Cured Duck Breasts with Pomegranate, Prune, and §ucaba Sauce and Black Beluga Lentils, 92

GORDON BIERSCH BREWING CO.
Multiple locations; see website for details.
www.gordonbiersch.com
Dan Gordon, chef
Roasted Bell Pepper–Tomato Fettuccine Alfredo, 214

HESS BREWING COMPANY
3812 Grim Avenue
San Diego, CA 92104
619-786-4377
www.hessbrewing.com
@HessBrewing
Nate Soroko, chef
Sake-Braised Beef Cheeks, 226

KARL STRAUSS BREWING COMPANY
5985 Santa Fe Street
San Diego, CA 92109
858-273-2739
www.karlstrauss.com
@Karl_Strauss
Gunther Emathinger, chef
Duck Chiles Rellenos, 179

LADYFACE ALE COMPANIE-ALEHOUSE & BRASSERIE
29281 Agoura Road
Agoura Hills, CA 91301
818-477-4566
www.ladyfaceale.com
@ladyfaceale
Adrian Gioia, chef
Bouillabaisse, 160

MAGNOLIA GASTROPUB & BREWERY
1398 Haight Street
San Francisco, CA 94117
415-864-7468
www.magnoliapub.com
@magnoliapub
Ronnie New, chef
Sardines on Toast with Romesco Sauce and Pickled Onions, 52

MOYLAN'S BREWERY AND RESTAURANT
15 Rowland Way
Novato, CA 94945
415-898-4677
www.moylans.com
@MoylansBrewery
Marco Gongora, chef
Irish Lamb Stew, 166

NORTH COAST BREWING COMPANY
444 North Main Street
Fort Bragg, CA 95437
707-964-2739
www.northcoastbrewing.com
Loretta Evans, chef
Braised Beef Short Ribs, 176

PORT BREWING COMPANY / THE LOST ABBEY
155 Mata Way, Suite 104
San Marcos, CA 92069
800-918-6816
www.portbrewing.com
@lostabbey
Vince Marsaglia, chef
Maple-Orange Grilled Pork Loin, 210
Truffled Potatoes, 258

RUTH MCGOWAN'S BREWPUB
131 East First Street
Cloverdale, CA 95425
707-894-9610
www.ruthmcgowansbrewpub.com
@RuthMcGowans
Monica Bramona, chef
Corned Beef Hash, 18

SIERRA NEVADA BREWING CO.
1075 East 20th Street
Chico, CA 95928
530-345-2739
www.sierranevada.com
@SierraNevada
Michael Iles, chef
Pistachio-Crusted Salmon Sandwich with Meyer Lemon Butter, 112

STONE BREWING CO.
1999 Citracado Parkway
Escondido, CA 92029
760-471-4999
www.stonebrewing.com
@StoneBrewingCo
Alex Carballo, chef
Arrogant Bastard Ale Avocado Tacos, 127

SUTTER BUTTES BREWING CO.
421 Center Street
Yuba City, CA 95991
530-790-7999
http://sutterbuttesbrewing.com
@SutterBrewer
James Beall, chef
Chopped Reuben Salad with Sweet Sauerkraut Vinaigrette, 90

California continued on next page

TAPS FISH HOUSE & BREWERY

101 East Imperial Highway

Brea, CA 92821

714-257-0101

The Promenade Shops at Dos Lagos

2745 Lakeshore Drive

Corona, CA 92883

951-277-5800

www.tapsfishhouse.com

Tom Hope, chef

Curly Endive and Spring Dandelion Salad with Belgian White Apricot Vinaigrette and Pork Rillettes, 86

TRUMER BRAUEREI

1404 4th Street

Berkeley, CA 94710

510-526-1160

www.trumer-usa.com

@TrumerPilsUSA

Paella Bella, 238

UNCOMMON BREWERS

303 Potrero Street, Suite #40-H

Santa Cruz, CA 95060

831-621-6270

www.uncommonbrewers.com

Visitors by appointment only.

A.T. Stefansky, chef

Lemongrass Chicken, 195

Colorado

AVERY BREWING COMPANY

5763 Arapahoe Avenue, Unit E

Boulder, CO 80303

303-440-4324

http://averybrewing.com

@AveryBrewingCo

Ted Whitney, chef

Colorado Carnitas, 203

BOULDER BEER COMPANY

2880 Wilderness Place

Boulder, CO 80301

303-444-8448

www.boulderbeer.com

@BoulderBeerCo

Planet Porter Bison Stew, 140

BRECKENRIDGE BREWERY

471 Kalamath Street

Denver, CO 80204

800-328-6723

www.breckbrew.com

Ron Piscatelli, chef

Lucky U IPA-Battered Fish, 245

CRAZY MOUNTAIN BREWING COMPANY

439 Edwards Access Road, B-102

Edwards, CO 81632

970-926-3009

www.crazymountainbrewery.com

@crazymtnbrewery

Patatas Bravas, 264

EUCLID HALL BAR & KITCHEN

1317 14th Street

Historic Larimer Square

Denver, CO 80202

303-595-4255

http://euclidhall.com

@EuclidHall

Jorel Pierce, chef

Rocket Salad with Camembert Croquettes, 82

FORT COLLINS BREWERY

1020 East Lincoln Avenue

Fort Collins, CO 80524

970-472-1499

www.fortcollinsbrewery.com

Pomegranate Trout, 251

NEW BELGIUM BREWING COMPANY

500 Linden Street

Fort Collins, CO 80524

888-622-4044

www.newbelgium.com

@newbelgium

Cameron Stewart, chef

Beer Sorbet, 294

NEW PLANET BEER COMPANY

3980 Broadway, Suite 103

Boulder, CO 80304

303-499-4978

http://newplanetbeer.com

@newplanetbeer

Gluten-Free Battered Coconut Shrimp with Sweet and Spicy Sauce, 246

ODELL BREWING CO.
800 East Lincoln Avenue
Fort Collins, CO 80524
970-498-9070
http://odellbrewing.com
@OdellBrewing
90 Shilling Rib Eye Marinade, 77

OSKAR BLUES BREWERY
1800 Pike Road, Unit B
Longmont, CO 80501
303-776-1914
www.oskarblues.com
@oskarblues
Jason Rogers, chef
Grilled Diver Scallops and Fall
Vegetable Shish Kebabs with Hazelnut
Brown Butter, 249

PAGOSA BREWING COMPANY
118 North Pagosa Boulevard
Pagosa Springs, CO 81147
970-731-2739
www.pagosabrewing.com
Bavarian Cheese Spread, 74

STEAMWORKS BREWING CO.
801 East 2nd Avenue
Durango, CO 81301
877-372-9200
http://steamworksbrewing.com
@Stmworks
Sean Clark, chef
Carrot Cake with Bourbon-Mascarpone
Icing, 298

TRINITY BREWING COMPANY
1466 Garden of the Gods Road
Colorado Springs, CO 80907
719-634-0029
www.trinitybrew.com
@TrinityBrewing
Brian Blasnek, chef
Watermelon Salad with Endive, 84

WYNKOOP BREWING COMPANY
1634 18th Street
Denver, CO 80202
303-297-2700
www.wynkoop.com
@Wynkoop
Bart Proffitt, chef
Vegetarian Green Chili, 134

Connecticut

HALF FULL BREWERY
43 Homestead Avenue
Stamford, CT 06902
203-658-3631
www.halffullbrewery.com
@halffullbrewery
Jennifer Muckerman, chef
Scotch Egg, 10

WILLIMANTIC BREWING COMPANY
967 Main Street
Willimantic, CT 06226
860-423-6777
www.willibrew.com
@willibrew
Will Deason, chef
Sage Veal Medallions, 183

Delaware

DOGFISH HEAD CRAFT BREWERY
6 Cannery Village Center
Milton, DE 19968
888-836-4347
www.dogfish.com
@dogfishbeer
Dennis Marcoux, chef
Pork Belly Corn Dogs with Truffle
Mustard, 28

District of Columbia

BIRCH & BARLEY
1337 14th Street NW
Washington, DC 20005
202-567-2576
http://birchandbarley.com
Kyle Bailey, chef
Seared Lamb Tenderloin with Orzo,
Feta, Black Olive Purée, and Preserved
Tomatoes, 206

Florida

CIGAR CITY BREWING, LLC
3924 West Spruce Street, Suite A
Tampa, FL 33607
813-348-6363
www.cigarcitybrewing.com
@cigarcitybeer
Mrs. Jadot, chef
Carbonnade à la Big Sound
Scotch Ale, 148

Florida continued on next page

7VENTH SUN BREWING COMPANY
1012 Broadway Avenue
Dunedin, FL 34698
727-733-3013
http://7thsunbrewery.com
@7venthSunBeer
Michael Lukacina, chef
Easy Steak Fajitas, 211

Georgia

5 SEASONS BREWING COMPANY
Multiple locations; see website for details.
www.5seasonsbrewing.com
@5seasonswest
David Larkworthy, chef
Sautéed Spinach, 266

SWEETWATER BREWING COMPANY
195 Ottley Drive
Atlanta, GA 30324
404-691-2537
http://sweetwaterbrew.com
@Sweetwaterbrew
Matt Coggin, chef
Grilled Texas Creamed Corn, 265

TERRAPIN BEER COMPANY
265 Newton Bridge Road
Athens, GA 30607
706-549-3377
http://terrapinbeer.com
@TerrapinBeerCo
Dean Graves, chef
Wake 'n' Bake Chocolate-Coconut
Dessert Bars, 278

Hawaii

KONA BREWING CO.
75-5629 Kuakini Highway
Kailua, Kona, HI 96740
808-334-2739
http://konabrewingco.com
Imu Pork, 173

MAUI BREWING CO.
910 Honoapiilani Highway #55
Lahaina, Maui, HI 96761
808-661-6205
www.mauibrewingco.com
@mauibrewingco
CoCoNut PorTeR Bread Pudding, 284

Idaho

GRAND TETON BREWING COMPANY
430 Old Jackson Highway
Victor, ID 83455
888-899-1656
www.grandtetonbrewing.com
@GrandTetonBrew
Julie Levy and Cody Beach, chefs
Bitch Creek Elk Meatballs, 198

PORTNEUF VALLEY BREWING
615 South 1st Avenue
Pocatello, ID 83201
208-232-1644
www.portneufvalleybrewing.com
@PokyBrewpub
Tim Johnson, chef
Oatmeal Cranberry Spent-Grain
Cookies, 296

Illinois

GALENA BREWING COMPANY
227 North Main Street
Galena, IL 61036
815-776-9917
www.galenabrewery.com
@GalenaBrewery
Roasted Bone Marrow, 49

HALF ACRE BEER COMPANY
4257 North Lincoln Avenue
Chicago, IL 60618
773-248-4038
www.halfacrebeer.com
@halfacrebeer
Michael Carroll, chef
Braised Duck Legs with Cabbage and
Fingerling Potatoes, 212

HAYMARKET PUB AND BREWERY
737 West Randolph Street
Chicago, IL 60661
312-638-0700
www.haymarketbrewing.com
@HaymarketPub
*Christopher McCoy and Pete
Crowley, chefs*
The Riot Sandwich, 100

PIECE BREWERY & PIZZERIA
1927 West North Avenue
Chicago, IL 60622
773-772-4422
www.piecechicago.com
@piecechicago
Piece Green Salad, 93

TWO BROTHERS BREWING COMPANY

30W315 Calumet Avenue

Warrenville, IL 60555

630-393-2337

www.twobrosbrew.com

@TwoBrothersBeer

Tommy Michael, chef

Croque Monsieur with Blackberry Onions, 130

Indiana

BLACK SWAN BREWPUB

2076 East Hadley Road

Plainfield, IN 46168

317-838-7444

www.blackswanbrewpub.com

@BlackSwanBP

Nick Carter, chef

Butternut Squash Soup, 162

NEW ALBANIAN BREWING COMPANY

Bank Street Brewhouse

415 Bank Street

New Albany, IN 47150

812-725-9585

Pizzeria and Public House

3312 Plaza Drive

New Albany, IN 47150

812-944-2577

www.newalbanian.com

@nabcnews

Matt Weirich, chef

Chicken Wings with Bacon Barbecue Sauce, 42

SUN KING BREWING CO.

135 North College Avenue

Indianapolis, IN 46202

317-602-3702

http://sunkingbrewing.com

@sunkingbrewing

Dustin Boyer, chef

Cherry Wee Mac Syrup, 68

UPLAND BREWING COMPANY

350 West 11th Street

Bloomington, IN 47404

812-336-2337

http://uplandbeer.com

@UplandBrewCo

Seth Elgar, chef

Meatless Loaf and Vegetable Mushroom Gravy, 200

Kansas

GELLA'S DINER & LB. BREWING CO.

117 East 11th Street

Hays, KS 67601

785-621-2739

www.lbbrewing.com

Manuel Hernandez, chef

Grebble with Sunflower Seed Pesto, 62

TALLGRASS BREWING COMPANY

8845 Quail Lane

Manhattan, KS 66502

785-537-1131

www.tallgrassbeer.com

@tallgrassbeer

Kurstin Harris, chef

Halcyon Chicken Breakfast Enchilada, 16

Kentucky

HOFBRÄUHAUS NEWPORT

200 East 3rd Street

Newport, KY 41071

859-491-7200

www.hofbrauhausnewport.com

@HofbrauhausNWPT

Vincent Quinzio, chef

Dunkel-Braised Lamb Shanks, 208

Louisiana

ABITA BREWING COMPANY

166 Barbee Road

Abita Springs, LA 70420

800-737-2311

http://abita.com

@theabitabeer

Barbecued Shrimp, 242

BAYOU TECHE BREWING

1106 Bushville Highway

Arnaudville, LA 70512

337-303-8000

http://bayoutechebrewing.com

Karlos Knott, chef

Chicken and Sausage Jambalaya, 142

Maine

GRITTY MCDUFF'S
396 Fore Street
Portland, Maine 04101
207-772-2739
Multiple locations; see website for details.
www.grittys.com
@grittys
Dave French, chef
Blackened Shrimp and Corn Chowder, 157

Maryland

THE BREWER'S ART
1106 North Charles Street
Baltimore, MD 21201
410-547-6925
www.thebrewersart.com
Dave Newman, chef
Pan-Roasted Sweetbreads with Spinach, Cauliflower, Wild Mushrooms, and Sherry-Bacon Vinaigrette, 221

FLYING DOG BREWERY
4607 Wedgewood Boulevard
Frederick, MD 21703
301-694-7899
http://flyingdogales.com
@flyingdog
Larry Pomerantz, chef
Chocolate Ice Cream with Gonzo Imperial Porter, 290

HEAVY SEAS BEER
4615 Hollins Ferry Road
Halethorpe, MD 21227
410-247-7822
www.hsbeer.com
@heavyseasbeer
Kelly Zimmerman, chef
Loose Cannon Wings, 32

Massachusetts

SAMUEL ADAMS
Boston Beer Company
30 Germania Street
Boston, MA 02130
617-368-5000
www.samueladams.com
Ken Oringer, chef
Roasted Venison Saddle with Samuel Adams Chocolate Bock Mole, 174

HARPOON BREWERY
306 Northern Avenue
Boston, MA 02210
617-547-9551
www.harpoonbrewery.com
@harpoon_brewery
Jaime and Mary Schier, chefs
Winter Warmer Pumpkin Pie, 286

Michigan

BELL'S BREWERY, INC.
335 East Kalamazoo Avenue
Kalamazoo, MI 49007
269-382-2332
www.bellsbeer.com
@BellsBrewery
David Munro, chef
Double Cream Stout Mustard, 70
Spicy Two-Hearted Mustard, 71

DARK HORSE BREWING CO.
511 South Kalamazoo Avenue
Marshall, MI 49068
269-781-9940
www.darkhorsebrewery.com
Kyle Marshall, chef
Amber Ale Cheese Bread, 64

FOUNDERS BREWING CO.
235 Grandville Avenue Southwest
Grand Rapids, MI 49503
616-776-2182
http://foundersbrewing.com
@foundersbrewing
Justin Golinski, chef
Devil Dancer Chicken Sandwich, 122

JOLLY PUMPKIN ARTISAN ALES
Cafe and Brewery
311 South Main Street
Ann Arbor, MI 48104
734-913-2730
Restaurant, Brewery, Distillery
13512 Peninsula Drive, Old Mission Peninsula
Traverse City, MI 49686

231-223-4333
www.jollypumpkin.com
@jollypumpkin
Paul Olson, chef
Beer-Braised Pulled Pork, 230

NEW HOLLAND BREWING COMPANY

66 East 8th Street
Holland, MI 49423
616-355-6422
www.newhollandbrew.com
@newhollandbrew
*Fred Bueltmann, partner and
beervangelist*
Smoke-Braised Pork Belly with Pear
Slaw, 223

SHORT'S BREWING COMPANY

121 North Bridge Street
Bellaire, MI 49615
231-498-2300
www.shortsbrewing.com
@Shortsbrewing
Jon Wojtowicz, chef
Northern Michigan Salad with Fruit
Beer Vinaigrette, 80

Minnesota

SURLY BREWING CO.

4811 Dusharme Drive
Brooklyn Center, MN 55429
763-535-3330
www.surlybrewing.com
@surlybrewing
Linda Haug, chef
Ginger-Garlic Chicken Stir-Fry, 228

Mississippi

LAZY MAGNOLIA BREWING COMPANY

7030 Roscoe Turner Road
Kiln, MS 39556
228-467-2727
www.lazymagnolia.com
@lazymagnolia
Chocolate Jefferson Stout
Cupcakes, 282

Missouri

BOULEVARD BREWING COMPANY

2501 Southwest Boulevard
Kansas City, MO 64108
816-474-7095
www.boulevard.com
@boulevard_beer
Colby Garrelts, chef
Roasted Pheasant with Pumpernickel
Bread Pudding and Cranberry
Sauce, 204

O'FALLON BREWERY

26 West Industrial Drive
O'Fallon, MO 63366
636-474-2337
www.ofallonbrewery.com
Gary Brokaw, chef
Cheddar Ale Soup, 145

SCHLAFLY BEER

Schlafly Bottleworks
7260 Southwest Avenue
Maplewood, MO 63143
314-241-2337
Schlafly Tap Room
2100 Locust Street

St. Louis, MO 63103
314-241-2337
www.schlafly.com
@schlafly
Andy White, chef
Imperial Meat Pie, 184

URBAN CHESTNUT BREWING COMPANY

3229 Washington Avenue
St. Louis, MO 63103
314-222-0143
http://urbanchestnut.com
@urbanchestnut
Florian Kuplent, chef
Bavarian Sausage Salad, 85

Nebraska

NEBRASKA BREWING CO.

Shadow Lake Towne Center
7474 Towne Center Parkway, Suite 101
Papillion, NE 68046
402-934-7100
www.nebraskabrewingco.com
@nebrewingco
Adam Graybill, chef
Pork Tenderloin Sandwich, 108

Nebraska continued on next page

UPSTREAM BREWING COMPANY

Legacy
17070 Wright Plaza
171st and West Center Road
Omaha, NE 68130
402-778-0100
Old Market
514 South 11th Street
Omaha, NE 68102
402-344-0200
www.upstreambrewing.com
@UpstreamBrewing
Gary Hoffman, chef
Artichoke Dip, 48

Nevada

BUCKBEAN BREWING COMPANY

(formerly of Reno, Nevada)
Daniel Kahn, chef
Cocoa-Crusted Pork Loin, 172

New Hampshire

SMUTTYNOSE BREWING CO.

225 Heritage Avenue
Portsmouth, NH 03801
603-436-4026
www.smuttynose.com
Todd Sweet, chef
Hanger Steak with Gorgonzola
Sauce, 190

WOODSTOCK INN STATION & BREWERY

135 Main Street
North Woodstock, NH 03262
800-321-3985
www.woodstockinnnh.com
@woodstockbrew
Scott Rice, chef
Spent-Grain Beer Bread, 44

New Jersey

BARCADE

163 Newark Avenue
Jersey City, NY 07302
201-332-4555
www.barcadejerseycity.com
@barcadejersey
Alan V. Bacchiochi, chef
Barcade's Pickled Hop Shoots, 56

BOLERO SNORT BREWERY

65 Railroad Avenue
Ridgefield Park, NJ 07660
201-464-0639
www.bolerosnort.com
@bolerosnort
Robert and Melanie Olson, chefs
Roasted Chipotle Salsa Burger, 102

TRIUMPH BREWING COMPANY

Multiple locations; see website for details.
www.triumphbrewing.com
Nick Devine, chef
Vidalia Onions Stuffed with Spring
Foraged Vegetables, 270

New Mexico

BLUE CORN CAFÉ AND BREWERY

Café
133 West Water Street
Santa Fe, NM 87501
505-984-1800
www.bluecorncafe.com
Brewery
4056 Cerrillos Road
Santa Fe, NM 87507
505-438-1800
@bluecorncafe
David Sundberg, chef
Potato Chip Chicken Sandwich, 120

CHAMA RIVER BREWING CO.

4939 Pan American Freeway
Albuquerque, NM 87109
505-342-1800
www.chamariverbrewery.com
@ChamaRiverBrew
Stephen Shook, chef
Deconstructed Banana Meringue Pie
with Dulce de Leche, Almond Wafer
Crumble, and Chocolate Powder, 303

LA CUMBRE BREWING COMPANY

3313 Girard Boulevard Northeast
Albuquerque, NM 87107
505-872-0225
http://lacumbrebrewing.com
Jeff Erway, chef
New Mexican Posole, 158

New York

BIRRERIA
200 5th Avenue
New York, NY 10010
212-937-8910
www.eataly.com/birreria
@EatalyBirreria
Alex Pilas, chef
Pork Shoulder Braised in Apricot-Beer
Sauce, 224

BREWERY OMMEGANG
656 County Highway 33
Cooperstown, NY 13326
800-544-1809
www.ommegang.com
@BreweryOmmegang
Teddy Folkman, chef
Steak and Blue Cheese Tartare, 55

BROOKLYN BREWERY
#1 Brewers Row
79 North 11th Street
Brooklyn, NY 11249
718-486-7422
http://brooklynbrewery.com
@brooklynbrewery
Garrett Oliver, chef
Duck Fat Home Fries, 272

JIMMY'S NO. 43
43 East 7th Street
New York, NY 10003
212-982-3006
http://jimmysno43.com
@jimmysno43
Jimmy Carbone, chef
Hot Tea Sandwich, 107

SHMALTZ BREWING COMPANY
6 Fairchild Square
Clifton Park, NY 12065
www.shmaltzbrewing.com
He'Brew Origin Pomegranate
Cheesecake, 276

SOUTHERN TIER BREWING COMPANY
2072 Stoneman Circle
Lakewood, NY 14750
716-763-5479
www.stbcbeer.com
@stbcbeer
Laura Anderson, chef
Super Ultra Free-Range Pancakes, 6

North Carolina

BULL CITY BURGER AND BREWERY
107 East Parrish Street, Suite 105
Durham, NC 27701
919-680-2333
http://bullcityburgerandbrewery.com
@BullCityBurger
Seth Gross and CeCe Lopez, chefs;
John Rogers, baker
Soft Rye Pretzels, 50

FOOTHILLS BREWING
638 West Fourth Street
Winston-Salem, NC 27101
336-777-3348
www.foothillsbrewing.com
Shane Moore, chef
North Carolina Shrimp and Grits with
Spicy Pan Sauce, 244

FRONT STREET BREWERY
9 North Front Street
Wilmington, NC 28401
910-251-1935
www.frontstreetbrewery.com
@fsbrewery
Kevin Kozak, chef
Shrimp and Grits, 8

FULLSTEAM BREWERY
726 Rigsbee Avenue
Durham, NC 27701
888-756-9274
www.fullsteam.ag
@fullsteam
Sean Lilly Wilson and Ali Rudel,
chefs
Pork and Porter Hand Pie, 58

Ohio

GREAT LAKES BREWING COMPANY
2516 Market Avenue
Cleveland, OH 44113
216-771-4404
www.greatlakesbrewing.com
@GLBC_Cleveland
Richard Basich, chef
Wild Mushroom and Edmund
Fitzgerald Porter Stuffing, 260

Ohio continued on next page

JACKIE O'S PUB & BREWERY
24 West Union Street
Athens, OH 45701
740-592-9686
www.jackieos.com
@jackieosbrewery
John Lange, chef
Breakfast Pigs in a Blanket, 7

ROCKMILL BREWERY
Rockmill Farm
5705 Lithopolis Road Northwest
Lancaster, OH 43130
740-654-0112
www.rockmillbrewery.com
@rockmillbrewery
John Dornback, chef
Prosciutto-Wrapped Scallops with
Butternut Squash and Roasted Garlic–
Huckleberry Sauce, 234

Oregon

CALDERA BREWING COMPANY
31 Water Street
Ashland, OR 97520
541-482-4677
www.calderabrewing.com
Jim Mills, chef
Caldera IPA, Strawberry, and
Grapefruit Dressing, 72

DESCHUTES BREWERY
Brewery
901 Southwest Simpson Avenue
Bend, OR 97702
541-385-8606
Deschutes Brewery Bend Public

House
1044 NW Bond Street
Bend, OR 97701
541-382-9242
Deschutes Brewery Portland Public
House
210 Northwest 11th Avenue
Portland, OR 97209
503-296-4906
www.deschutesbrewery.com
@DeschutesBeer
Jeff Usinowicz, chef
Venison Stew, 155

FULL SAIL BREWING CO.
506 Columbia Street
Hood River, OR 97031
541-386-2247
www.fullsailbrewing.com
@FullSailBrewing
Jamie Emmerson, chef
Gouda Fondue, 22

NINKASI BREWING COMPANY
272 Van Buren Street
Eugene, OR 97402
541-344-2739
www.ninkasibrewing.com
@NinkasiBrewing
Jamie Floyd, chef
Roasted Root Vegetable Hash, 15

OAKSHIRE BREWING
Public House
255 Madison Street
Eugene, OR 97402
541-688-4555
www.oakbrew.com
@oakshire

Matt Van Wyk, chef
Bourbon Sweet Potato Tarts with
Imperial Stout Sauce, 26

PELICAN PUB & BREWERY
33180 Cape Kiwanda Drive
Pacific City, OR 97135
503-965-7007
www.yourlittlebeachtown.com/pelican
Ged Aydelott, chef
Dungeness Crab Tart with Crab
Reduction, 252

ROGUE ALES
Brewer's on the Bay
2320 OSU Drive
Newport, OR 97365
541-867-3664
Multiple locations; see website for
details.
www.rogue.com
@RogueAles
Alex Gund, chef
Barley-Crusted Tuna Sandwich with
Remoulade, 110

STANDING STONE BREWING COMPANY
101 Oak Street
Ashland, OR 97520
541-482-2448
www.standingstonebrewing.com
@ssbc
Javier Cruz Paso, chef
Mole Poblano, 75

UPRIGHT BREWING

240 North Broadway, Suite 2
Portland, OR 97227
503-735-5337
www.uprightbrewing.com
Alex Ganum, chef
Cauliflower Lavender Soup, 164

WIDMER BROTHERS BREWING

955 North Russell
Portland, OR 97227
503-281-3333
http://widmerbrothers.com
@Widmer_Brothers
Adam Stevens, chef
Grilled Lamb Burgers with Local
Chèvre and Mint-Cilantro Aioli, 104

Pennsylvania

ALLENTOWN BREW WORKS

Fegley Enterprises, Inc.
812 West Hamilton Street
Allentown, PA 18101
610-433-7777
www.thebrewworks.com/allentown-
brewworks
@thebrewworks
Michael Honeywell, chef
Hearth-Baked Salmon with
Brewschetta, 254

BARLEY CREEK BREWING COMPANY

Sullivan Trail and Camelback Road
Tannersville, PA 18372
570-629-9399
www.barleycreek.com
Bobby Fluegel, chef
Asparagus Risotto, 262

BETHLEHEM BREW WORKS

Fegley Enterprises, Inc.
569 Main Street
Bethlehem, PA 18018
610-882-1300
www.thebrewworks.com/bethlehem-brew-
works
@thebrewworks
Jill Oman, chef
Asian Grilled Salmon Salad with Thai
Dressing, 92

EARTH BREAD + BREWERY

7136 Germantown Avenue
Philadelphia, PA 19119
215-242-6666
www.earthbreadbrewery.com
Alexandra Fries, chef
Wheat Berry Salad, 88

SLY FOX BREWING COMPANY

Phoenixville Brewhouse & Eatery
520 Kimberton Road
Phoenixville, PA 19460
610-935-4540
Pottstown Brewery & Tastin' Room
331 Circle of Progress Drive
Pottstown, PA 19464
484-300-4644
www.slyfoxbeer.com
@slyfoxbeer
Craig Coffman, chef
Saison Vos Mussels, 33

SUSQUEHANNA BREWING CO.

635 South Main Street
Pittston, PA 18640
888-725-4902
www.sbcbeer.com
@sbcbeer
Jaime Jurado, chef
Jerk Pork, 196

TROEGS BREWING COMPANY

200 East Hersheypark Drive
Hershey, PA 17033
717-534-1297
www.troegs.com
@troegsbeer
*Christian DeLutis and Matt Hailey,
chefs*
Smoked Bologna Mousse on Chicken
Skin Crostini, 36

VICTORY BREWING COMPANY

420 Acorn Lane
Downingtown, PA 19335
610-873-0881
www.victorybeer.com
@VictoryBeer
Eric MacPherson, chef
Festbier Cheddar Bisque, 146

WEYERBACHER BREWING COMPANY

905-G Line Street
Easton, PA 18042
610-559-5561
http://weyerbacher.com
@Weyerbacher
Mark Myers, chef
Belgian Endive with Gruyère and
Prosciutto, 46

Rhode Island

NARRAGANSETT BREWING CO.
60 Ship Street
Providence, RI 02903
401-437-8970
www.narragansettbeer.com
@Gansettbeer
Rhode Island Clam Chowder, 154

REVIVAL BREWING CO.
95 Chestnut Street
Providence, RI 02903
info@revivalbrewing.com
http://revivalbrewing.com
@revivalbrewing
Sean Larkin, chef
Saison and Clementine Cornish Game
Hens with Roasted Vegetables, 218

South Dakota

CROW PEAK BREWING CO.
125 West Highway 14
Spearfish, SD 57783
605-717-0006
www.crowpeakbrewing.com
@crowpeakbrewing
Chocolate-Covered Strawberries with
Sprinkles, 281

Tennessee

YAZOO BREWING COMPANY
910 Division Street
Nashville, TN 37203
615-891-4649
www.yazoobrew.com
@yazoobrew
Linus Hall, chef
Nashville Hot Chicken Sandwich, 98

Texas

**BLACK STAR CO-OP PUB AND
BREWERY**
7020 Easy Wind Drive, Suite 100
Austin, TX 78752
512-452-2337
www.blackstar.coop
@blackstarcoop
Johnny Livesay, chef
Fried Brussels Sprouts with Fish Sauce
Vinaigrette, 268

BLUE STAR BREWING COMPANY
1414 South Alamo Street
San Antonio, TX 78210
866-813-5506
www.bluestarbrewing.com
Pork Green Chili, 139

FREETAIL BREWING CO.
4035 North Loop 1604 West, Suite 105
San Antonio, TX 78257
210-395-4974
www.freetailbrewing.com
@freetailbrewing
Gary Butler, chef
Cheese Pizza, 188

K. SPOETZL BREWERY
603 East Brewery Street
Shiner, TX 77984
361-594-3383
www.shiner.com
Brook Watts, chef
Shiner Beer Barbecue Sauce, 73

NEW REPUBLIC BREWING
11405 North Dowling Road, Unit C
College Station, TX 77845
713-489-4667
www.newrepublicbrewing.com
@NewRepublicBeer
Andrew Vaserfirer, chef
Beer Caramel Sauce, 299

RAHR & SONS BREWING COMPANY
701 Galveston Avenue
Fort Worth, TX 76104
817-810-9266
www.rahrbrewing.com
@RahrBrewing
Bill Pierce, chef
Ugly Pug Sweet Potato Pancakes, 14

SAINT ARNOLD BREWING COMPANY
2000 Lyons Avenue
Houston, TX 77020
800-801-6402
www.saintarnold.com
@saintarnold
Michael Scott Castell, chef
Lady Cream Pea Salad with Gingered
Beets, 94

Utah

EPIC BREWING COMPANY

825 South State Street
Salt Lake City, UT 84111
801-906-0123
www.epicbrewing.com
@epicbrewing
David Cole, chef
Curried Pumpkin Chicken Soup, 136

MOAB BREWERY

686 South Main
Moab, UT 84532
435-259-6333
www.themoabbrewery.com
Black Bean Soup, 138

SQUATTERS PUB BREWERY

147 West Broadway (300 South)
Salt Lake City, UT 84101
801-363-2739
Multiple locations; see website for details.
www.squatters.com
@SquattersPubs
Vicente Cardenas, chef
Szechuan Green Beans, 267

Vermont

LAWSON'S FINEST LIQUIDS

Warren, VT 05674
802-272-8436
www.lawsonsfinest.com
Sean Lawson, chef
Fresh Berries with Homemade Maple-
Bourbon Whipped Cream, 289

LONG TRAIL BREWING COMPANY

5520 Route 4
Bridgewater Corners, VT 05035
802-672-5011
www.longtrail.com
@Longtrailbrwing
Matt Pond, chef
Portabella Sub, 123

MAGIC HAT BREWING COMPANY

5 Bartlett Bay Road
South Burlington, VT 05403
802-658-2739
www.magichat.net
@magichat
Marialisa Calta, chef
Baked Ham with #9 Glaze, 197

OTTER CREEK BREWING

793 Exchange Street
Middlebury, VT 05753
802-388-0727
www.ottercreekbrewing.com
Jane Costello, chef
Hummus, 35

TRAPP FAMILY LODGE, DELIBAKERY, AND BREWERY

700 Trapp Hill Road
Stowe, Vermont 05672
800-826-7000
www.trappfamily.com
@trappfamily
Maria Von Trapp, chef
Maria's Favorite Linzertorte, 300

THE VERMONT PUB & BREWERY

144 College Street
Burlington, VT 05401
802-865-0500
www.vermontbrewery.com
Chicken Satay with Peanut Sauce, 60

WOLAVER'S FINE ORGANIC ALES

793 Exchange Street
Middlebury, VT 05753
www.wolavers.com
Jane Costello, chef
Marie's Turkey Sandwich, 124

Virginia

DEVILS BACKBONE BREWING COMPANY

200 Mosbys Run
Roseland, VA 22967
434-361-1001
www.dbbrewingcompany.com
@dbbrewingco
Brian Colbert, chef
Crawfish Bordelaise, 76

MAD FOX BREWING COMPANY, LLC

444 West Broad Street, Suite I
Falls Church, VA 22046
703-942-6840
http://madfoxbrewing.com
@MadFoxBrewing
Andrew Dixon, chef
Frickles, 61

Washington

CHUCKANUT BREWERY & KITCHEN
601 West Holly Street
Bellingham, WA 98225
360-752-3377
www.chuckanutbreweryandkitchen.com
@ChuckanutBeer
Joel Shumate, chef
Rolling Chicken with Beurre Blanc, 170

ELYSIAN BREWING COMPANY
Elysian Fields Brewpub
542 1st Avenue South
Seattle, WA 98104
206-382-4498
Capitol Hill Brewpub
1221 East Pike Street
Seattle, WA 98122
206-860-1920
Tangletown Brewpub
2106 North 55th Street
Seattle, WA 98103
206-547-5929
www.elysianbrewing.com
@elysianbrewing
Eric Greenwalt, chef
Black Bean Sliders, 114

PIKE BREWING COMPANY
1415 1st Avenue
Seattle, WA 98101
206-622-6044
www.pikebrewing.com
@pikebrewing
Gary Marx, chef
Kilt Lifter Mac & Cheese, 186

REDHOOK BREWERY
Portsmouth Brewery & Cataqua
Public House
1 Redhook Way
Pease International Tradeport
Portsmouth, NH 03801
603-430-8600
Woodinville Brewery & Forecasters
Public House
14300 Northeast 145th Street
Woodinville, WA 98072
425-483-3232
http://redhook.com
@Redhook_Brewery
Drew Holliday, chef
Chicken-Fried Steak Tips with ESB
Gravy, 216

Wisconsin

**HINTERLAND BREWERY AND
RESTAURANT**
Hinterland Brewery
313 Dousman Street
Green Bay, WI 54303
888-604-2337
Hinterland Erie Street Gastropub
222 East Erie Street, Suite 100
Milwaukee, WI 53202
414-727-9300
www.hinterlandbeer.com
@hinterlandbeer
Kelly Qualley, chef
Seared Diver Scallops with Roasted
Maitake Mushrooms, Cauliflower, and
Sweet Potatoes and Coconut–Green
Curry Sauce, 236

LAKEFRONT BREWERY, INC.
1872 North Commerce Street
Milwaukee, WI 53212
414-372-8800
www.lakefrontbrewery.com
@lakefront
May Klisch, chef
Gluten-Free Fruit and Nut Crisps, 39

SPRECHER BREWING CO.
701 West Glendale Avenue
Glendale, WI 53209
414-964-7837
www.sprecherbrewery.com
@sprecherbrewery
Craig Burge, chef
Slow-Cooked Doppelbock BBQ
Meatballs, 24

Wyoming

BLACK TOOTH BREWING COMPANY
312 Broadway
Sheridan, WY 82801
307-675-2337
www.blacktoothbrewingcompany.com
@blacktoothbrew
Travis Zeilstra, chef
Pots de Crème, 295

ACKNOWLEDGMENTS

Working on a book like this requires a lot of time in the kitchen, in front of the computer, and talking to a lot of great people. I am extremely grateful to the American craft beer community, which has offered a limitless supply of support, help, and delicious ales and lagers. The recipes come from passionate and talented brewers, chefs, and others who embrace the joy of beer and food. From their kitchens to yours, enjoy.

Behind any book is a support network that provides guidance, encouragement, and that occasional jolt of reality that is sorely needed. The staff of Storey Publishing is among the finest in the industry and I'm honored to work with them. Cheers to Pam Art and Dan Reynolds, Mars Vilaubi, Alethea Morrison, Sarah Armour, Adrienne Franceschi, Margaret Lennon, Tina Parent, Suzanne Farr, Maribeth Casey, and in particular Margaret Sutherland, who fostered this project from a simple introductory e-mail to what you hold in your hands. Throughout she was the kind of engaged and thoughtful editor that writers are rarely blessed with.

My admiration and thanks to Lara Ferroni, a talented photographer and all-around good person whose work brings these recipes to life. Thanks also to Garrett Oliver, a man who is passionate about beer, food, and life, for writing the foreword and for his endless hospitality.

A lot of friends offered suggestions, meal memories, and pairing ideas, and this is a richer book because of their generosity. The following people have their fingerprints on the pages that follow: Nate Schweber, Nick Kaye, Tony Forder, Julia Herz, Jason and Eileen Edwards, Tom Troncone, Brian Yaeger, Glen Nile, Nancy Maddaloni, Chris Shepard, Jeannine Sherman, Margaret Casey, Carrie Woods, Randy Sprecher, Lucy Saunders, Russ Klisch, Sandra Evans, Jimmy Carbone, Rick Armon, Brett Joyce, Howie Weber, Randy Clemens, Ashley Johnston, Paul Kermizian, Bill Manley, Jaime Jurado, Charles and Rose Ann Finkle, Dan D'Illippoto, Fred Bueltmann, Sean Lilly Wilson, Win Bassett, Sean Z. Paxton, Mark Spivey, Matthew Brynildson, John Kleinchester, Natasha Bahrs, Craige Moore, Jeff Cioletti, Ted Lane, Kyle Weaver, Joe and Rebecca Biland, Frederick and Jaime Lawson, Stan Hieronymus, Jeff Alworth, Lisa Morrison, Gerard Walen, Dale Miskimins, Pat Battle and everyone at WNBC, Barbara Sullivan, and so many others who provided support, advice, suggestions, and encouragement.

Fellow scribes Randy Mosher and Lew Bryson provided much appreciated advice and contacts. I'm honored to work among their ranks.

Thanks to Raymond A. Schroth, my parents, my siblings (Tom, Bill, Dan, Amanda, and Todd), and my extended family. Thanks also to Theodore J. Romankow.

Testing and tasting recipes is not as easy as you might think. I am blessed with friends and family who enjoy experimenting and who opened their kitchens to make sure you're getting the best dish, possible. Thanks to my expert testers: Richard Alfonzo, Robert and Melanie Olson, Joseph and Rebecca Biland, the Marc Cregan family, Brandon Furhman and Julie Golden, Charlie and Stacey Gow, Teresa Darcy, John and Carolyn Holl, Adel Holl, Jill Darcy Moore, Amanda Theide, Kristen Weber Holding, Peter Kennedy, Charlotte Cusumano, Colby Janisch, Gregory Boland, Rob Hurley, Christopher LaSpata, Drew Jennings, Jonathan Moxey, and John Kleinchester.

Finally, there is not enough appreciation and thanks in the world for my wife, April, who was so loving and patient during the writing of the book. She held her tongue when my prediction that this would "have minimal impact on our daily lives" fell woefully short. She makes me a better writer through her editing skills, and she is a calming force and the love of my life. So much of what I do is because of her.

JOHN HOLL
Jersey City, New Jersey
April 2013

INDEX

Page numbers in *italic* indicate photos.

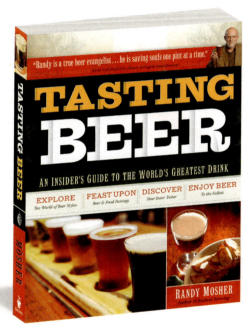
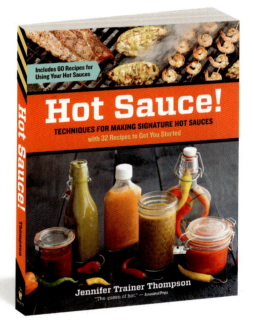

The American
CRAFT BEER COOKBOOK

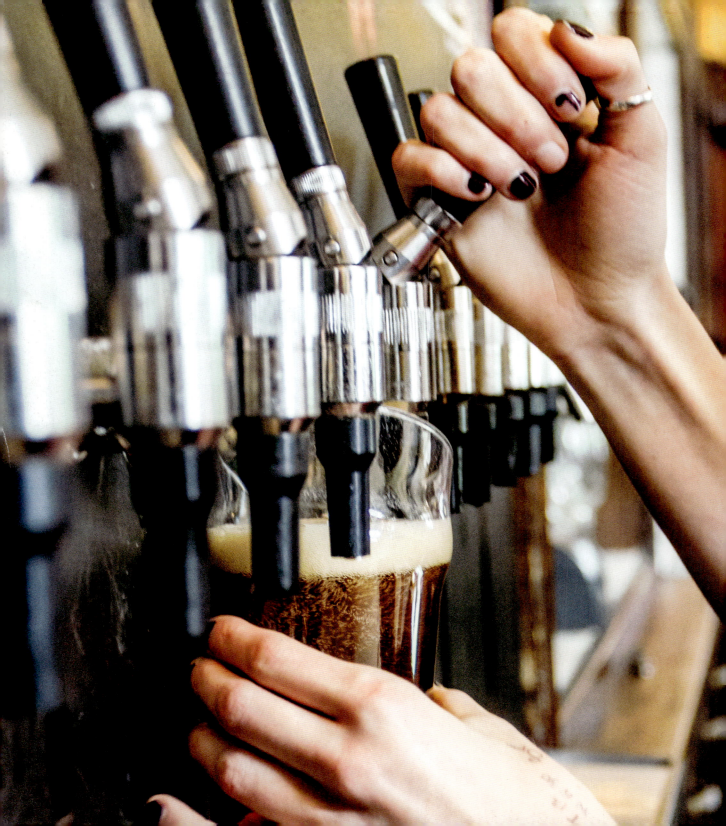